PRAISE FOR

Mastering Patient Flow:

Using Lean Thinking to Improve your Practice Operations,

3rd Edition

"For more than fifteen years, health care professionals and researchers have been advocating for patient-centered care. We have yet to achieve what is still an aspiration. Here in this comprehensive volume, Elizabeth Woodcock demonstrates how physician practices can deliver on the promise at the ground level."

LAWTON ROBERT BURNS, PhD, MBA
Professor of Health Care Systems
THE WHARTON SCHOOL, UNIVERSITY OF PENNSYLVANIA, PHILADELPHIA

"...this book takes complex office systems and breaks them down into real world, useable day-to-day operations in a very easy-to-read format. If you are a first time manager or just need to freshen your approach, this is the book that can help you 'positively affect change' in your office."

LORI BURROWS
HASTINGS ORTHOPEDIC CLINIC PC, HASTINGS, MICH.

"...This is a comprehensive resource detailing how to run an efficient medical office, including real-world examples and updated technology. This book will be valuable to novices and veterans alike."

STEPHEN HILL
Practice Administrator
FAMILY MEDICINE OF ALBEMARLE, CHARLOTTESVILLE, VA.

More praise . . .

MASTERING PATIENT FLOW

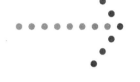

*Using Lean Thinking to
Improve your Practice Operations*

3RD EDITION

Elizabeth W. Woodcock, MBA, FACMPE, CPC

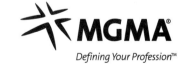

Defining Your Profession™

Medical Group Management Association
104 Inverness Terrace East
Englewood, CO 80112-5306
877.275.6462
Web site: mgma.com

Production Credits
Editorial Director: Marilee Aust
Project Editor: Ruth Gaulke
Page Design, Composition, and Production: Boulder Bookworks
Copy Editor: Robert Redling
Proofreader: Ruth Gaulke
Cover Design: Amy Kenreich – Graphic Design Inc.

LIBRARY OF CONGRESS CATALOGING-IN-PUBLICATION DATA

Woodcock, Elizabeth W.
   Mastering patient flow : using lean thinking to improve your practice operations / by Elizabeth Woodcock. -- 3rd ed.
        p. ; cm.
   Includes bibliographical references and index.
   Summary: "Mastering Patient Flow, 3rd edition will help medical practices manage patient flow to improve operations to create and sustain patient value. Use this book to get up to speed on the fundamentals of managing medical practice operations or as a reference to revisit many familiar concepts from a new perspective."--Provided by publisher.
   ISBN-13: 978-1-56829-283-0
   ISBN-10: 1-56829-283-X
   1. Medicine--Practice. 2. Medical appointments and schedules. 3. Medicine--Practice--Finance. I. Medical Group Management Association. II. Title.
   [DNLM: 1. Practice Management, Medical--organization & administration. 2. Appointments and Schedules. 3. Efficiency, Organizational. W 80 W886m 2007]
   R728.W66 2007
   610.68--dc22

                                                                                                2007021881

Item #6636

ISBN-13: 978-1-56829-283-0

Printed in the United States of America
10 9 8 7 6 5 4 3

Contents

ACKNOWLEDGMENTS

I would like to thank my husband and children, and both of our families, for their continued support of the passion I channel into my professional endeavors.

I owe a debt of gratitude to my colleague, Deborah Walker Keegan, PhD, FACMPE, founder and president of Medical Practice Dimensions, whom I admire and respect as a sage contributor to our industry, as well as a dear friend.

My appreciation for their time and assistance toward this endeavor goes out to Peter Anderson, MD, Riverside Hilton Family Practice, Newport News, Va., Roger Coleman, general manager, Coleman Associates, Santa Fe, N.M., Randy Cook, MHA, senior medical practice Consultant, State Volunteer Mutual Insurance Company, Brentwood, Tenn., Michael Gilligan, FACHE, president and CEO, Mayfield Clinic, Cincinnati, Jeffrey K. Griffin, principal and senior medical planning consultant, Medical Design International, Norcross, Ga., Richard C. Haines, Jr., AIA, president, Medical Design International, Norcross, Ga., Richard Honaker, MD, president, Family Medicine Associates of Texas, Plano, Benjie Johnson, director of professional billing, University of Michigan Faculty Group Practice, Ann Arbor, Sara Larch, MHA, FACMPE, chief operating officer, University Physicians, Baltimore, Md., Annemarie C. Lucas, MHSA, director of operations, Ambulatory Psychiatry, University of Michigan Faculty Group Practice, Ann Arbor, Brian McDonald, MD, chief, Virginia Mason Medical Center, Rosemarie Nelson, MHA, principal, MGMA Health Care Consulting Group, MarieAnn North, director, Navigant Consulting, Charlotte, N.C., Frederic Platt, MD, clinical professor of medicine, University of Colorado Health Sciences Center, Denver, and regional consultant Institute for Healthcare Communication, Kathy Rice, CMPE, administrator, The Plastic Surgery Group and Hayes Hand Center P.C., Chattanooga, Tenn., Philippe Sammour, CPA, MBA, MSA, project manager, University of Michigan Faculty Group Practice, Ann Arbor, Somer Shields, CMPE, administrator, Women's Health Associates, Portland, Ore., Tom Stearns, FACMPE, vice president, Medical Practices Services, Brentwood, Tenn., Todd Tamalunas, CMPE, assistant vice president, Physician Practices, Freeport (Ill.) Health Network, Peter Townes, Jr., president, Ambulatory Innovations Inc., Indianapolis, Pamela Weisse, MSN, FNP, webmaster, logistics manager, and coach, Coleman Associates, Santa Fe, N.M., and Thomas Yaeger, MD, chief, family medicine, Guthrie (Pa.) Clinic.

Preface

As health care costs rise, the U.S. reimbursement system has placed financial responsibility squarely in the hands of patients. Armed with more responsibility to pay, patients are assessing their options about where to receive care and from whom. Because quality and safety are expected, physician practices now compete on access, efficiency, and service. Patients can now access health care through the Internet, the telephone, at grocery stores, retailers, and pharmacies. Entrepreneurs are rapidly expanding the delivery of optional services, and more recently, a small but growing array of insurance-covered services to Americans who travel to providers stationed in Malaysia, Thailand, India, and other places across the globe.

What patients want – access, efficiency and service – are the same characteristics of any sound business operation. Creating a patient-centered practice was a benefit in yesteryear; today, it's essential.

Mastering Patient Flow: Third Edition uses the lean-thinking movement to transfer new and better ideas to improve the operations of a medical practice.

Make *Mastering Patient Flow: Third Edition* your guide to creating and sustaining a patient-centered operation. Not every idea will work for you, nor will every suggestion work every day; the key is to have the skills, knowledge, and tools to try in your practice.

MGMA is pleased to be a partner in delivering the skills, knowledge and tools that lead to mastering patient flow for medical practices.

ABOUT THE AUTHOR

Speaker, trainer, and author **Elizabeth W. Woodcock, MBA, FACMPE, CPC**, has visited countless medical practices in search of how to master patient flow. Believing that efficiency and earnings can be achieved, she presents practical advice sure to create the environment in which every medical practice can improve the patient flow process.

Educated at Duke University (BA) and the Wharton School of Business (MBA), Elizabeth has traveled the country as an industry researcher, operations consultant, and expert presenter. Founder and principal of Woodcock & Associates and an independent consultant with the Medical Group Management Association Health Care Consulting Group, Elizabeth has focused on medical practice operations throughout her career. Formerly, she served as the director of knowledge management for Physicians Practice Inc., group practice services administrator at the University of Virginia Health Services Foundation, and a senior associate at the Health Care Advisory Board.

Elizabeth is a Fellow in the American College of Medical Practice Executives (ACMPE). In addition to co-authoring *Operating Policies and Procedures Manual for Medical Groups* (1st, 2nd, and 3rd Editions) and *The Physician Billing Process*, Elizabeth is a frequent contributor to national health care publications. She currently resides in Atlanta, Ga., with her husband and two children.

ABOUT THE EDITOR

Robert Redling, MS, is a freelance writer and editor. Formerly senior writer and web content editor at the Medical Group Management Association, and practice management editor at Physicians Practice Inc., he is a graduate of San Diego State University and the University of Kansas, Lawrence, where he earned his master's of science in journalism. Robert has been a speechwriter for the American Academy of Family Physicians, a legislative correspondent for United Press International, and a reporter for the Wyoming Daily Eagle, Cheyenne. He currently lives in Tacoma, Wash.

Introduction

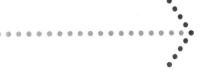

Who should read this book?

This book is a manual to help medical practices manage their patient flow to improve their operations to create and sustain value to the patient. The ideas, descriptions and resources in this updated, third edition will be of value whether you are new to practice management, are changing duties, or face new challenges.

If you are relatively new to practice management, use this book to quickly get up to speed on the fundamentals of managing the operations of a medical practice. If you are more experienced, use this book as a quick reference and refresher course to revisit many familiar concepts from a new perspective.

This book is neither meant to be exclusively for a large practice nor for a small practice, nor is it specific to any specialty. It is an all-purpose primer on improving patient flow in a medical practice to create and sustain value to the patient. Readers at all levels of experience and in all types and sizes of medical practices will find handy tools to monitor current operations and discover areas to improve. Even if you've read the first and second editions, you'll find many new ideas in this revised and updated edition.

Whether you are a nurse, physician, or administrator, this book is valuable to you.

Why should you read this book?

Maybe you picked up this book because you want to learn more about patient flow. Or, you were curious about how lean thinking applies to medical practice operations. Or, you want to improve your practice's bottom line. Maybe you want to enhance patient satisfaction. Maybe you want to boost staff and physician performance, morale and productivity. All these are valid reasons to analyze and improve your patient flow. So, what's standing in your way? Often, it is the bottlenecks in patient flow. As you strive to grow your practice and serve your patients better, don't find yourself struggling to retain patients and referring physicians because of a disgruntled receptionist, a telephone system that always rings busy, or lengthy wait times.

In this book, I walk through every aspect of your practice as it impacts the patient. By evaluating a medical practice quantitatively and qualitatively, you can discover and remove logjams that disrupt the flow of patients through the practice. Smoother patient flow will help your practice generate more cash at lower cost (i.e., lower overhead), achieve better patient satisfaction, retain physicians and employees, and become more competitive in its market and more resilient over the long term. In other words, better patient flow will empower your practice to become stronger.

Loyalty used to keep patients coming back to your physicians, but today's patients are far less tolerant of an inefficient office, no matter how good the quality of care you provide. The same goes for insurance companies and referring physicians when they repeatedly hear patients complain about your practice. Patients, referring physicians, insurance companies, and your other customers relate your quality of service to your quality of care. If your service is sub-optimal, you will lose those patients. Let's make sure that you don't lose those patients — learn to master the patient flow process!

Why this book is different

Many practice management books are structured around the various aspects of running a practice from the point of view of the manager or the physician. This book attacks many of the same issues but from the perspective of that most important person in your medical practice: the patient. In lean thinking, this is exactly how our operations should be built: around our patient. The book's chapters parallel the contact points between patients and your practice with the end result, I hope, being a new perspective on how patients flow through the practice and, where the logjams are that may impede that "flow" and cost you money.

This book differs from many others because it acknowledges that there is no one right way for a medical practice to function. Yet, there are steps that all practices can take to improve efficiency and patient flow while providing exceptional customer service. This, indeed, is the ideal patient encounter.

Rather than tackle every activity of a medical practice, this book focuses on the functions surrounding (and, too often, slowing down) the flow of patients – from telephones to scheduling to provision of care to the conclusion of the encounter. To supplement the patient flow process, I have included sections on the physician's time, costs, and technology, all of which are critical to creating an efficient and cost-effective patient flow process. In addition to updates throughout the book, new to this third edition are chapters on patient access, the management of prescriptions and test results, and the patient-centered practice of the future.

The issue of receivables management is addressed as it relates to the patient flow process, to include patient registration and charge entry. Due to the complexity of the issues, this book does not provide comprehensive coverage of billing and collections, nor the related subject of compliance. Although these subjects are not addressed in-depth, make no mistake, they are critical. Why? Because each member of your staff, including your physicians, is a member of "the business office" and the "compliance team." Thus, when appropriate, I have incorporated tips on the billing process, particularly as it relates to registration, charge capture, and charge entry. (For more information on billing, please see *The Physician*

Billing Process: Potholes on the Road to Getting Paid, an MGMA publication, which I co-authored with Deborah Walker-Keegan, PhD, FACMPE, and Sara Larch, MHA, FACMPE.)

How to use this book

Since this book is organized around the natural flow of patients through your practice, I hope you will follow this path from beginning to end. However, if you wish to focus on only one function, then jump ahead to that section.

Each section is organized around a critical function in the operations process. After introducing you to the concept of lean thinking and how it rightly challenges the way we've operated practices historically, I'll focus on the most important asset in your practice – your physician's time. Then, you'll go on a journey with me to explore ways to improve your patient flow. Finally, you'll conclude with a worksheet to develop an action plan for your practice.

The chapters are outlined as follows:

Chapter 1. The Lean-Thinking Revolution: Our journey begins with a discussion of lean thinking, and the how its principals of reducing waste to increase value also apply to the medical practice industry. Through examples of "muda" (waste), we'll understand why lean thinking holds a bounty of opportunity to challenge our historical ways of thinking to improve our operations, and in the process improve the value for our patients.

Chapter 2. The Physician's Time: I take a look at your practice's most valuable asset – the *time* of your physician or any other billable provider. This provides a meaningful introduction to the patient flow process and the recognition of the necessity of maximizing this asset.

Chapter 3. Telephones: I couldn't discuss patient flow without highlighting telephones, as this is often your patients' first impression of your office operations. This process is explored through the steps of managing patients' demand, as well as through a comprehensive overview of telephone systems and features, and the various telephony applications.

Chapter 4. Scheduling: The patient flow process is created from scheduling. Following an overview of scheduling methodologies, I take an in-depth look at advanced access scheduling, controlling no-shows, and managing patients bumped from the schedule.

Chapter 5. Patient Access: To maintain an efficient operation, the supply of providers and services must be in balance with the demand of patients. Find out how to determine whether or not you're in balance, the consequences of imbalances in supply and demand, and ways to rebalance your practice.

Chapter 6. Reception Services: How to avoid hiccups in the processes that welcome your patient to the practice are explored in this chapter, plus you'll get an in-depth look at how to streamline your pre-visit processes for maximum efficiency.

Chapter 7. Waiting: Although waiting and even occasional delays are inevitable in the medical practice's flow process, I take a close look at waiting, how to reduce it and improve the quality of it.

Chapter 8. The Patient Encounter: The patient flow process revolves around the actual provision of care – the patient encounter. In this chapter, physician efficiency is explored in depth as I follow patients from the reception area into the clinical area until they move to practice services (check-out).

Chapter 9. Prescriptions: An important process in patient flow – the management of prescriptions – is highlighted in this chapter. Practices have implemented a bevy of ways to manage this core process: some work, some don't. Not only do I review historical methods managing the work produced by handling prescription refills, renewals, and drug samples, but I also will examine proven solutions that will increase the value this process provides to your patients.

Chapter 10. Managing Test Results: Critical to risk management, as well as patient satisfaction, is a coordinated process of ordering, receiving, and notifying patients of test results. I examine the steps from ordering to reporting and technologies and tips (new and old) that make them more efficient to you, your referring physicians, and your patients.

Chapter 11. Practice Services: The practice services process, often called the "check-out", varies among specialties but the core objectives remain to provide value to patients at the same time as you capture their charges and collect the revenue they owe. I explore the entire gamut of these critical processes from entering charges to making referrals.

Chapter 12. Technology: New technology offers significant benefits to the patient flow process. The chapter walks you through technologies that can improve patient flow and shows you how to evaluate them.

Chapter 13. Fundamental Financials: Practice operations cannot be managed without an understanding of the core financial concepts embedded in the operations of a medical practice. This chapter takes a concise but informative look at how the numbers establish a solid base from which you can leap from the ideas gathered in this book to implementing operational changes in your practice.

Chapter 14. The Patient-Centered Practice of the Future™: A new day is dawning for medical practices. Patient access, a changing workforce, and a historically poor use of space are only a few reasons why a new model of operations is in order. Explore the patient-centered practice of the future™ to determine if you're ready to innovate.

Chapter 15. Summing Up: I conclude with a summary of the most important concepts discussed in our journey through the perfect patient encounter.

Appendix A: Benchmarks for Staff Performance Expectations: A summary of all of the staff benchmarks presented in the book is included in this table.

Appendix B: Action Plan: Use this comprehensive checklist compiled from the ideas presented in the book, and outlined by chapter, to build an action plan for your practice.

Integrated into each chapter are case studies, best practices, deeper analysis of concepts, terms you need to know, and advice from your peers.

To make it easier for you to revisit this book later on and quickly find what you need, more detailed information about the processes of patient flow appears in separate boxes.

These boxes are:

"Getting started"
Specific questions to ask or materials/resources to assemble before changing key office functions.

"Staff benchmarks"
Productivity by function to evaluate your staffing strategy.

"Steps to get you there"
Actions you need to take in changing a key office function.

"Things to consider"
Issues or logistics to consider as you attempt to make changes.

"Case study"

*How another practice solved a key process problem
and improved patient flow in the practice.*

"You know..."

*Hints that something is or is not working
in your practice.*

"Words of wisdom"

*Just that. Handy tips and insights from the author, industry
experts, health care leaders, and practice managers.*

"Key concepts"

*Explanations that give perspective on key concepts mentioned
in the text.*

"Best practices"

*Industry innovators have tried and proven
these ideas to be successful.*

"Analysis"

Formulas to measure impact and processes.

After you read this book

Before you embark on operational changes, look at your practice
and consider the variables that can affect your ability to change critical processes affecting patient flow. Your facility's physical layout
will have a huge impact on operations as will your management
information systems including accounting and practice management systems, and especially whether or not you have an electronic
health record. Perhaps the most important factor is one that you
cannot see and you cannot buy: your practice's culture.

The "that's the way we've always done it" factor is the most common and most dangerous of all variables in patient flow. As you make changes in your practice, be on the look out for those words. When you hear them, look upon it as an opportunity. This is the one variable which requires no walls to be constructed or software modules to be purchased, only that attitudes change. The assessment tools in this book will give you some of the ammunition you need to overcome this most difficult variable. Using proven change management techniques, and staying focused on what's best for the patient, will allow you to forge a new – and better – path for your practice.

This book will be a useful resource but, rest assured, some of your attempted changes will fail. In fact, if you don't experience some failures, then you might not be trying hard enough to make change.

The path to success is paved with opportunities and challenges: failing at some initiatives is a natural process and should not be looked down upon. There is no right way to operate a practice. Creating the ideal patient flow in your practice is difficult, but I believe that it should be your goal.

There are so many ideas in this book that it may seem overwhelming. For best results, create an action plan to master patient flow in your office. Divide your practice into teams each representing a chapter in this book. Issue a challenge for each team to make at least three improvements, and offer a small prize to the team with the ideas that make the most significant impact.

Even if you only pick up a few ideas to help your practice improve the patient flow process, then this book will have done its job!

CHAPTER 1

The Lean-Thinking Revolution

Key Chapter Lessons

➤ Discover the principles of lean thinking

➤ Learn to apply lean thinking to the operation of a medical practice

➤ Challenge historical ways of thinking

➤ Understand the key concepts of lean thinking

➤ Identify value-stream mapping

➤ Recognize the merits of small improvements to address strategic challenges

To physicians, "lean thinking" may sound like yet another attempt to impose industrial production-line management on medical practices. But the philosophy of lean thinking, also known as lean management, is decades-old – and you may already be practicing some of its techniques. The reason to learn more about lean thinking is that it holds the potential to help improve patient flow in all types of medical practices, and ultimately, improve patient care. A lean-thinking approach can assure that your patients remain at the center of all the processes in your practice.

Once upon a time, there was no question about the physician's ability to keep the focus on the patient. But numerous intrusions have crept into that relationship. These include demands by insurance companies and regulators, plus the more aggressive "take-charge" attitudes on the part of patients. Unless you put careful thought into how you do what you do, your practice and its providers will be caught up in putting out the many little fires that occur each day – locating forms, filing paperwork, and other administrative details. As your practice creates or modifies processes and redeploys person-nel and other resources to get these little jobs done, it begins to shift its focus. Before long your practice, like many others, will end up with more of its processes aimed at serving the practice's needs rather than the patients' needs.

What is lean thinking?

Based on the work of quality guru W. Edwards Deming, the lean production movement got its name from the 1990 book *The Machine That Changed the World: The Story of Lean Production*[1] authored by three researchers at the Massachusetts Institute of Technology. The authors studied the efforts of Toyota to rise to the top of the automobile industry in the 1960s. Their thesis was that market changes, increased competition, and a desire to improve profitability helped auto manufacturer Toyota successfully re-engi-neer not only its core processes, but also its culture. To make the journey from mass production to lean production, Toyota stripped away – and continues to find and eliminate – waste from the manu-facturing process. Instead of relying on inspections of cars after pro-duction to determine their quality, Toyota integrates quality into the production process. This transformation in thinking helped Toyota become the market leader in its industry in terms of sales and mar-ket share. Ultimately, more buyers of automobiles perceive they get better value from purchasing a Toyota than other brands.

How could a medical practice possibly look to an automobile manu-facturer's experience to redesign its operations? How can doing so increase the value that the practice provides to its patients? Consider the teachings of the lean-production movement as they relate to patient flow, and you'll see that the simple-but-powerful teachings of this approach have much to offer for medical practices seeking to survive in this era of reducing reimbursements and rising costs.

Two of the original lean production researchers – James P. Womack and Daniel T. Jones – summarized the lean-thinking approach in their 1996 book, *Lean Thinking*.[2] The five-step process, which took their teachings about lean production from solely a manufacturing environment to any industry espoused:

- Specify value from the standpoint of the customer;
- Identify all the steps in the process (value stream);
- Make the value-creating steps flow toward the customer;
- Let the customer pull value from the next activity; and
- Pursue perfection across the organization.

Replace the word "customer" with "patient" in the five-step process and you'll see how lean thinking can lead the way to reaching many of the same goals your practice sets for patient service and clinical excellence. Of course, there's a bit more to making this process work in a medical practice.

The lean-thinking system aims to provide the best quality at the lowest cost and in the shortest time through eliminating waste. In essence, lean thinking means doing more for your patients with less. We can assume that most physicians are operating with less of everything these days, except paperwork that is. In this era of declining reimbursement and rising costs, translating these teachings into medical practice operations offers more value to our patients – and to our medical practices.

How to spot and eliminate waste

Lean thinking can optimize value for patients by getting them the care they need. Doing this efficiently requires a sharp eye for waste, which can come in many forms – taking too much time to schedule appointments, adding unnecessary steps to a registration process, or doing tasks out of sequence, such as not verifying a patient's insurance coverage until after the service has been provided.

The first critical step in lean thinking is learning how to spot waste, or "muda" as lean thinkers refer to it. This muda may be occurring in a few processes or throughout an entire system. We certainly don't want to think that there is a great deal of waste in our medical practices – except for all of that time spent on filling out paperwork that is. But the fact is, waste exists in all of our practices and often occurs in subtle ways.

Waste is not strictly leaving too many lights on or seeing the nurse use a few too many sterile swabs when cleaning a wound (although that is waste, too). The waste that lean thinking sets its sights on is the amount of time and other resources that are spent on actions that do not optimize the patient's care. This waste can come from using a slow-speed scanner that adds three minutes to the act of processing a patient through registration, losing a positive test result in the shuffle of paperwork, or allowing last-minute cancellations and no-shows to reduce the daily capacity of the practice.

Why can't we always identify waste when it occurs in our own practices? It's an easy answer – we're in the system! We keep waste alive in small ways that we never think about.

The process of referring a patient to a specialist exposes several examples of how we sometimes overlook the waste embedded in the medical system. Patients are asked to describe their symptoms several times as they work through the net of schedulers and registration personnel. They are asked to fill out lengthy demographic information forms at each stop. Then, they may have to wait for weeks to obtain an appointment at the referred specialist. Although the patient will eventually get the care needed from the most appropriate source, it's hard to see how the delays and repetitions in this transfer process add value for the patient.

The referral process also diminishes value for providers. Have you or a physician in your practice ever had to help a friend, relative, or patient get past a long wait or some other hurdle to obtain an appointment or a test sooner than the rest of the crowd?

Perhaps a patient has asked for help scheduling an appointment with an ophthalmologist. Normally, it might take up to three months to be seen at that particular ophthalmology practice. The patient would have to make several telephone calls to describe the symptoms to multiple personnel so the ophthalmology practice could determine where the patient fits into its lengthy appointment queue and complex scheduling criteria.

Acting as an insider to the medical system, the referring physician from your practice could make that long wait go away with just one phone call. In just 60 seconds, that patient could be scheduled in that ophthalmologist's practice perhaps the next day. Likely no one involved would see this as gaming the system. Perhaps, the patient faced several unrelated medical or family issues and it would be very helpful to have the ophthalmology appointment out of the way sooner rather than later. Yet, the fact that anyone had to spend time in stepping up to the plate is the result of waste in the system. How? Remember that we defined waste as doing things that do not add value. Consider that the ophthalmologist always has a three-month wait for new patient appointments. Does that three-month wait add value to the patients or to the practice's referring physicians? Not likely. Does requiring referring physicians to spend time on the phone to sneak their patients to the head of the line add any value to their practice? Or does having a three-month wait indicate that the ophthalmology practice may have inept internal processes of its own that cause waste? Consider that the patient has had to explain his or her symptoms multiple times, and can expect to spend 15 minutes filling out multiple pages of a medical history and other demographic forms at the ophthalmology practice. If having a wait of three months for an appointment somehow added value (helped the patient), then your patient would have gladly waited and you would have been adamant in recommending that the patient wait. If the three-month waiting period is stable over time (i.e., it's consistently three months), but does not add to the patient's care, then why does the three-month wait exist in the first place?

Lean thinking doesn't mean seeing every patient who calls your practice the following day. It means getting the patient to the right provider, in a value-added way; in other words, optimizing the patient's care.

The value stream

Now that we understand what waste is and are learning how to identify it, the challenge becomes eliminating that waste. We do this by designing our work flow processes around the patient's needs, not the needs of our practice.

What would happen if someone visiting your practice, perhaps a consultant, asked your business office manager why new patient charges were entered only by worker A and only every other day. Would the billing manager respond by saying, "that's the way we've always done it." That answer doesn't really get to the "why." Is the employee doing so because some manager who left two years ago wanted it done that way? What about other tasks and functions in your office? Why does your scheduler send calls regarding patient appointments to voice mail only to take care of them later on? Does making patients wait by the phone for a call-back to get test results add value to their care? Why do you have nurses take patients' vital signs and medical histories instead of the medical assistants who escort patients to exam rooms? Does having a bachelor's-level medical professional operate the blood pressure cuff add any value for the patient?

Can you really say you are committed to improving patient flow in your practice if you are not looking carefully at the entire flow of work, including how that flow has been designed?

In this book, we look at the processes leading up to, during, and following the patient encounter in the office. In the medical practice, the goal is to create an ideal encounter for the patient, and our goal is to look at the value stream and the flow surrounding it. How we try to bring value to these processes also relates to what happens when one of our patients visits a hospital, surgery center, diagnostics, or even a pharmacy.

Attacking the familiar

Here's an example of lean thinking in action. Ask yourself candidly, why do you have a front desk reception area? All practices have them so they must be necessary. Or are they? When I ask this question at medical practices, the response is usually that the front desk is needed to greet patients and perform important administrative functions. For the first reason – greeting patients – I doubt that even half of patients are truly greeted by staff when they enter the door of the medical practice. A sign-in list on a clipboard sitting by a closed sliding glass window seems to fulfill that function in many practices. As for the administrative function of the front desk, many if not all of those functions can be performed ahead of the patient's visit by pre-registering patients. Pre-registration can allow you to verify coverage and benefits before the appointment. In doing so, value is added for patients because you can keep them informed. It also can help resolve insurance coverage problems well in advance of the office encounter and identify copayment requirements to patients in advance so as to reduce billing and collection expense.

You may still argue that you need the front desk to assure that medical history forms are accurately completed. But did you ever consider asking patients to fill out those forms ahead of time, either by mail or by directing them to your practice's Web site? Or, capturing the information via a kiosk that you have conveniently placed in your lobby?

You may still try to hold your ground on having a fully staffed front desk by arguing that this is your opportunity to collect the copayment and any other payments. You don't want to do anything that would keep your practice from achieving its goals of a 100 percent time-of-service collection rate. But did you consider that the recent trend of high-deductible plans, health savings accounts, and other steps to shift more financial responsibility to patients means that collections are now being driven by charges incurred. In response, more practices are moving the patient collection function to the end of the encounter so they don't have to bill patients for those charges and wait 30 to 60 days to collect.

In sum, when we really consider the whole front desk process, haven't we designed it around us, and not the patients? Wouldn't patients rather be greeted by a person without a wall or a counter between them? Wouldn't patients prefer to have already had a chance to perform the registration processes with clear knowledge about their coverage, or lack thereof? Wouldn't they like to step immediately into the process by being quickly escorted to an exam room where the remaining administrative functions can be quickly performed and the intake process commenced? Wouldn't patients find value in not having to give much of the same information about their history and chief complaint multiple times to several people before being seen by the physician? In the end, couldn't we save thousands of dollars by not having to invest in the space and furnishings dedicated to a front office and a waiting area? And, what if we no longer had to manage the turnover of a front desk or the infighting that occurs between the front desk staff and the clinical team? Lean thinking gives us a chance to reevaluate our value stream – and in the end, the answer is almost always better for us, too.

Improve value by challenging the norm

In addition to questioning common process steps, lean thinking requires us to challenge all processes in the organization. Instead of looking at individual processes in isolation, such as registration, scheduling, intake, and so forth, lean thinking asks us to consider the entire flow. Now is an opportune time to do so. Consider that as the years have gone by, the level of complexity and sophistication of our operations has increased. In response, we have increased our degree of functionality. Staff positions now include referral clerks, surgery schedulers, phone nurses, master schedulers, and on and on. While the tasks that these individuals are assigned may be more efficiently performed in isolation (that is, the designated surgery scheduler can schedule a surgery in 20 minutes, while someone cross-trained on many functions may need 24 minutes to schedule the same surgery), we may have damaged the larger flow of processes. Worse, our attempts to be more efficient may have reduced the value (to our patient). Let's take surgery scheduling as an example.

In a general surgery practice, there is a designated surgery scheduler. When the surgeons decide to schedule a surgery, the patient is told that he or she must meet the scheduler. The surgeon's nurse completes a series of forms to identify the surgeon's requests (e.g., the type of surgery, timing, and so forth). If the scheduler happens to be available, the patient is brought to the scheduler's office by the nurse, along with the set of completed papers. (If the scheduler is not available, the patient is told to expect a call, and the surgery will be scheduled over the phone). In the scheduler's office, the surgery is scheduled. The process of the scheduling itself is very efficient; the scheduler takes the information from the paperwork and schedules all aspects of the surgery.

Lean thinking asks us to consider not just the efficiency of the scheduling process, but rather the entire flow. From the patient's perspective, the process wasn't ideal. While still reeling from the news, the emotional patient must be moved into another office (or even worse, receive a phone call "sometime" in the near future), only to have the details of the surgery repeated during the scheduling process. Our contention that the surgery scheduling is optimally efficient is shaken when we consider the nurse's time to write down the details of the surgery and escort the patient to the next step, as well as the office required by the surgery scheduler.

Could the nurse schedule the surgery? Sure, the nurse could be cross-trained to perform the function, thereby decreasing the time to document, to transfer the information to the scheduler, and to escort the patient to another office. The value to the patient is higher in the new process as well (remember, the patient considers that the surgery will be scheduled correctly and timely regardless of the process, but now the patient can remain comfortably with the nurse who knows and understands the patient's clinical and emotional condition).

Perhaps there's too much value wrapped up into your surgery scheduling process to deconstruct, but you should still see the point. There are numerous ways that we've become efficient at functions, while not improving the flow of the whole – or the ultimate value that we're providing to patients.

Start assessing your value stream

Lean thinking works best when everyone is thinking about increasing value and reducing waste, not just following orders. To get started on assessing your practice's value stream, gather individuals who work on the process in question, or assemble a smaller team to evaluate several areas for improvement.

Womack and Jones define the value stream as the "set of all the specific actions required to bring a specific product [patient care, in the case of a medical practice] through the three critical management tasks of any business: the problem-solving task from concept through detailed design and engineering to production launch, the information management task from order-taking through detailed scheduling to delivery, and the physical transformation task from the raw materials to placing the finished product in the hands of the customer [patient, in the case of a medical practice]." In sum, the entire process – people, technology, transfer of information, time, as well as every step in the process, should be analyzed and challenged.

Map workflow

Start the redesign effort by holding an intensive work session. This session may last several hours depending on the complexity of the process you are examining. Instead of spreading the session out over several weeks, work intensely – perhaps, spend an entire day or two on it.

This team is charged with evaluating and improving a process. The team starts by mapping the current process flow through every step and, importantly, how each step actually works, not how it should work. By mapping the workflow, and the timing of each step, the individuals (employees and customers) involved, and the total duration of the process, the team can begin to question the process (see Exhibit 1.1). They'll be ready to design a new one – keeping in mind that the process should produce value for the patient.

The value stream map of the appointment scheduling process represented in Exhibit 1.1 demonstrates an opportunity for improvement. The internal process time consumes up to 85 minutes, and the patient waits up to 21 days. Perceived value does not correspond to the wait times. Visualizing the process and associated time spent allows the improvement team to focus on redesigning the process to add value.

In this case, the process team determined that more than 95 percent of patients were "approved" for scheduling when the physician received the new patient folder. Instead of manually reviewing each situation, the physicians developed written protocols that would guide the scheduling process. Based on the protocols, patients would be given an appointment at the time of the request, thus reducing the rework ("muda") associated with rescheduling.

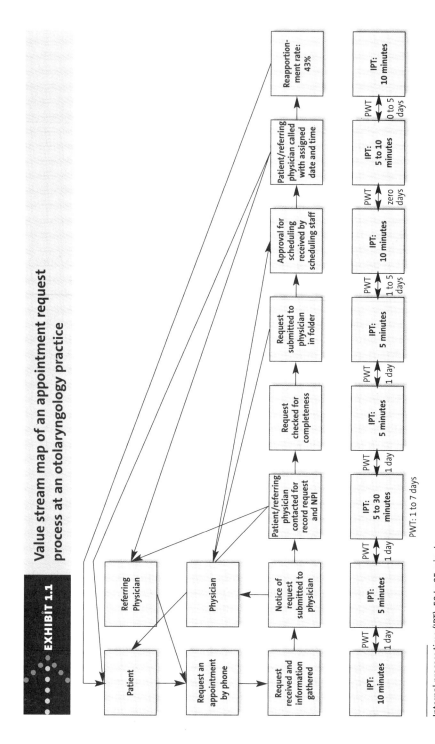

EXHIBIT 1.1

Value stream map of an appointment request process at an otolaryngology practice

Internal process time (IPT): 50 to 85 minutes
Patient wait time (PWT): 6 to 21 days

Upon scheduling, a request for records and chief complaint was initiated with clear expectations that these needed to be received 48 hours prior to the appointment date. (Secure electronic connections were established with referring physicians to facilitate the process and an electronic 'tickler' was established to alert staff of any records outstanding 72 hours before the appointment, both of which vastly reduced the internal processing time.)

The "questionable" five percent of appointments were scheduled, but an alert was routed electronically to a nurse practitioner who was responsible for reviewing these appointments, and discussing situations (through an electronic form created solely for this purpose) with the otolaryngologist to determine if the patient would be better suited to see another provider. If that was the case, the nurse practitioner would initiate contact with the patient and/or see the patient in the office, answer questions, discuss the physician's recommendation, and arrange for an alternative provider. If applicable, the nurse practitioner would cancel the patient's appointment to close the loop. The internal process time plummeted from a high of 85 minutes to an average of 10 minutes, while the patient wait time dropped to an average of five days.

As with any new process, proceed with your initiatives knowing full well that there may be significant resistance to change. Be aware also that the resistance may be just as strong to relatively small changes as it is to large-scale changes. Expect that the change management truism, "I'm all in favor of progress, it's change I don't like" will apply. Once the task of revising a process begins, don't make the mistake of leaving out those who opposed the change; doing so may only harden their opposition. While including the opponents of change in the process is helpful, it is also important to make sure those who will be affected are involved in working out the details and providing feedback that can help you fine tune the new process for success.

STEPS TO GET YOU THERE

The PDCA cycle: Plan–Do–Check–Act

Here's how to propose process change using the "plan, do, check, act" (PDCA) cycle of lean thinking:

- Plan: Establish the goal for a change and the steps necessary to achieve it
- Do: Implement the proposed changes
- Check: Analyze the results in terms of the performance of the process
- Act: Based on the results, standardize and stabilize the change by incorporating it in the process or start the PDCA cycle again.

WORDS OF WISDOM

Try "Trystorming"

Don't let the PDCA cycle get bogged down in deliberation. Instead of always carefully planning and pre-testing every idea, "trystorm" the new idea. Put new ideas into practice rapidly, try them out for a short time, and quickly assess and adjust to make them work.

Focus on the people

To eliminate waste and redesign flow, everyone must be involved. Traditionally, organizations designed systems that broke processes down into the smallest components so that low or unskilled labor could perform the repetitive tasks while professionals were responsible for higher-level work. The unskilled workers were not allowed to modify, eliminate, or, in some organizations, even comment about their tasks or functions, as the focus is solely on the production of volume.

Translate this scenario from the noisy factory of yesteryear to your practice and you'll see actual parallels to the operations of a modern medical practice. Your personnel are tasked with rooming patients, answering calls, scheduling procedures, and so forth. You expect them to do as they are told, do it quickly, and without push-back or complaint. The result you expect is productivity. But is that always what you get?

Womack and Jones write, "[Lean production] transfers the maximum number of tasks and responsibilities to those workers actually adding value to the car on the line, and it has in place a system for detecting defects that quickly traces every problem, once discovered, to its ultimate course."

Lean thinking teaches us that we have just as much to learn from the unskilled laborer as we do from the physician. I consider the many visits that I've had to practices where the receptionists are the first to pull out their lists of ways to improve – while the physician is often the one who comments that "everything works just fine."

In a lean-thinking environment, managers become mentors and enablers, not just foremen who keep after workers to get their tasks done on time. In an empowered environment, all providers and staff become a part of the process redesign effort, and lean thinking actually relies on their input to facilitate change.

Technology is powerful, but not nearly as powerful as the people behind it. Although technology can enhance the process of redesign, it is not the solution in and of itself. Lean thinking harnesses automation but does not rely upon it. Instead, it draws upon what the customer wants, and from the people who perform the work.

When introducing lean thinking, your practice may wish to promise no layoffs to assure morale is not decimated by the changes to come. Job security will be at the top of many people's minds and this guarantee can allow the ideas to flow while staff feel secure that they are not designing themselves out of employment with your organization. What you cannot and should never promise is that no one's job will change. As people redesign processes, it means changing the way they work.

Stopping the line: How it applies to medical practices

To truly make lean thinking work, your staff and providers must be able to "stop the line" if they see waste. "Stop the line" refers to halting the production line in a factory when a defect is detected or suspected. A factory worker signals to stop the line, typically by pulling a cord or lever, and the production line stops until the defect is corrected. The theory is that mistakes are inevitable, but reversible. Correcting them as they occur is faster, easier, and less likely to cause harm.

Or course, your practice doesn't have a production line, but it does have patient flow, which we can define as the process of providing the best patient care in the optimal flow that drives out waste. Also unlike a factory, you would be ill advised to "stop the line" when a snag appears in the daily patient flow. Yet, you do end up slowing things down many times a day as you or your staff attempt to solve small problems, such as finding missing paperwork.

Even if you don't actually stop the line, the goal should be to place everyone on alert for performance improvement opportunities. Foster the ability to take ideas and put them into action (almost) immediately. If it is not possible to hold those discussions immediately, then at the very least make sure to recognize and discuss solutions at the first huddle after the discovery of the muda, or waste in a process. (More on huddles in Chapter 8, "The Patient Encounter.")

Many practices find it efficient to encourage staff (not just physicians or managers) to record waste when they spot it and allow them a forum in which to present their observations. Buy-in from the highest level of the organization is critical to the success of this process. It should include reminders to seek out waste, formal and informal recognition of those who do so, time set aside at staff meetings for discussion, empowering of mid- and lower-level managers to remedy situations of waste, and reporting of results (both successes and failures). Most important of all is the commitment of executive leadership to prompt action and transparency about efforts to root out waste.

This book, I hope, will inspire you to make a careful evaluation of all of the processes in your practice. Finding much of the waste in your current processes won't take extensive consultations, but rather just common sense. We overlook these opportunities because they are often tied into the way we run our practices. In other words, it's time to start questioning the "way we've always done it."

Opportunities for a medical practice to stop the line on waste and error might occur when:

➤ The physician realizes that he or she is waiting three or four minutes every morning for the exam room computer to boot-up so the physician adds starting computers to the clinical assistant's morning assignments.

➤ The receptionist realizes that nearby road construction will delay patients for the next three months. The lean-thinking team implements a telephone script for schedulers to advise patients to allow extra time to get to their appointments, posts the information to the practice's Web site, and includes it in the practice's greeting and on-hold telephone messages.

➤ A biller discovers that one of the physicians has ordered MRIs for dozens of patients with a diagnosis code for unspecified back pain. The biller gathers examples (all of which include a substantiated diagnosis in the office notes), prints out payers' local coverage determinations for MRIs, and types up a succinct but informative memo regarding coding. The biller then integrates an alert in the charge-capture system that the diagnosis will not be supported and cannot be used. The biller diplomatically acknowledges in the memo that human error can occur but also deploys technology that forces users to correct their coding errors.

➤ A clinical assistant notices that two physicians have just asked for help in finding an ophthalmoscope, and this seems to occur several times a month. The clinical assistant suggests the practice install a special cradle that will fit only an ophthalmoscope in a visible location in each exam room. Confirmation of the proper location of the ophthalmoscope is added to the equipment checkout steps on the practice's daily exam room preparation list.

In none of these examples was it necessary to form a special task force or call a supervisor to implement the change. Instead, the changes were made the next day. Let's stop and acknowledge that in the real world, not every suggested change goes smoothly. Sometimes another defect in the system is exposed. When that happens, an additional change is made. The lean-thinking process continues even when the team is not in session. Thus, lean thinking becomes part of operations – not a one-time exercise – and changes are embraced and expected.

If these seem like minor process changes, they are. There is no magical solution to optimizing your patient flow. The key is that the changes you make will add up to a tangible redesign that will improve the value your practice provides to patients. Once people are empowered to look for ways to improve, you'll be pleasantly surprised by what they find. They'll start to believe that it's their responsibility – their duty – to find, expose, and resolve problems.

While this book focuses solely on the operations to support the care provided, consider the implications for patient safety. Your team should look at processes in terms of how to deliver the best work flow to the patient but also from the viewpoint of how best to incorporate patient safety into the redesign of any process.

Despite their best efforts, managers cannot identify and make all the changes needed in the workplace. It's not that you are unwilling or disinterested in change. It's simply that you cannot know and see every step of every process in your practice because you're not the one who carries all of those processes. Thinking lean must come from within. The benefit of doing so is that once improvements are made, the energy and passion to make things better for your patients catches on and becomes a passion that all staff see as their duty to pursue.

Using benchmarks

Industry data offers little assistance in lean thinking. The benchmarks, upon which many practices rely for measuring the success of their operations, are simply reflections of current processes – often, wasteful processes. Benchmarks can become just another way for an organization – or an entire industry – to tell itself "this is how it's always been done" and that "we're doing just fine."

Benchmarks are often used as a justification making the changes needed to perform up to industry norms, but they offer no insight into a process or how to improve it. Indeed, benchmarks often drive people to engage in inefficient behaviors just to improve the metric. This reward for wasteful practice occurs frequently in patient flow as practices strive to beat industry benchmarks by laying off staff to beat a staff-per-physician benchmark. Yet, research has proven that practices with more staff per physician are more profitable.[3]

Management must replace benchmarks with new ways to evaluate and measure the functions of staff, the tools and resources they use, and the workflow that is built around those staff and tools.

Just because it's the industry norm doesn't mean that it's the right way to do it. Wise managers seek to map processes and look at the many steps of each process to determine where value is added and where it is not. Then, instead of using the old way of staffing according to benchmarks, the organization determines how much time it will take to perform a function. The timing is called in the lean thinking parlance "takt time" *[pronounced "tact-time"].*

To facilitate your efforts, I'll introduce average per-function times related to each step of the patient flow process in this book. Although the guidance is offered, every practice is unique. It pays to focus not only on the data, but on the right way – that is, what's best for your patients – to perform every function.

The Five S's

A critical step in eliminating waste, and one of the pillars of lean thinking, is formulated by the Five S's. With a goal of minimizing the waste of time, the Five S's represent a visually-oriented system for organizing the workplace through steps of:

1. Sort: Clear the work area;
2. Set in order: Designate locations;
3. Shine: Clean the work area;
4. Standardize: Everyone doing the same thing, with everything in the same place; and
5. Sustain: Ingrain the process in the organization.

Perhaps you can see the application of the Five S's in a manufacturing plant or even in straightening out your messy garage or cluttered desk. It may be a bit more difficult to apply this concept to your practice, but it is possible.

To illustrate, let's use the example of the clinical workstation in a medical practice, which typically houses the clinical assistants, nurses, as well as their communications to physicians and work tools, such as forms, computers, and reference materials. Consider that a clinical workstation is often the most visually chaotic area of a medical practice. Take a look at the one in your practice and you may see stacks of paper, sticky notes stuck to almost every available flat surface, and supplies scattered about (if they aren't missing altogether). In addition to the unpleasant visual clutter, this all-too-typical workstation could also be the nexus of waste occurring in the many processes that intersect here.

Lean thinking espouses the following when tackling the problem of the disorganized clinical workstation:

Sort the tasks and functions of the workstation. Identify the tasks and organize papers, supplies, and other resources in clusters based on the task or tasks for which they are used. Tasks and functions may include medication renewal requests, urgent questions for the physician, forms for the physician to complete, completed charge tickets, surgeries to schedule, referrals to make, patient education brochures, physician and other providers' continuing education brochures, and so forth. Remove all unnecessary equipment, supplies, and resources. Do not make a bin for every single task. Instead, select the eight to 10 most important – or most frequent – tasks performed here and create work spaces for each. The special space for the task may be a shelf, a bin, a spot on the counter, or even a separate folder in a file bin, but it must be distinct and identifiable. Identify supplies or resources needed to complete each task, and incorporate as many as possible of these supplies in the workstation. Mark clearly a specific area of the station where the physician can work during clinics. Notably, your process review should delineate what steps of the process should occur before a task is routed to a physician. For example, when a patient requests a Family and Medical Leave Act (FMLA) form, staff should fill in the patient's demographic information, the practice's demographic information, and a chart number or account number for reference before giving it to the physician. Forms should be completed consistently. Any attachments should always be in consistent formats and placed in the same order. Ultimately, the most efficient way to organize, clearly identify, and share tasks is through the use of electronic information technology.

Designate and label. Whether it is a physical location like a workstation or a virtual workstation in an electronic file, it is important that legible signage point to a location for each task and the function. For example, at a workstation make a list of the related supplies and where they should be placed. If there are multiple workstations, make sure supplies and task areas are consistent between at all locations.

Keep the work area clean and orderly. Do not allow incoming work to pile up in a general in-box, nor allow completed work to pile up in an out-box. Similarly, in an electronic filing system of tasks, be sure to archive old files and folders.

Standardize the layout of the tasks and functions, and maintain the space consistently. Determine what and how many supplies are needed, and identify the placement of the supplies.

Determine a consistent approach and protocol for each function or task performed at the workstation. This may include, but not be limited to, how triage calls will be handled when a physician is not in the clinic, or how a medication renewal is handled for a patient who has not been seen in the previous 12 months.

Pool the staff's collective knowledge of the inbound work, and decide how it could be standardized. Constantly evaluate the prevention of piles of paper or variations on the workstation's protocols. Initiate discussions around the tasks associated with the work, the resources required, the staff assigned, or the necessity of asking more people to handle the work.

Break old habits of the staff and providers who allow work to pile up in stacks to work on later. Codify expectations through performance evaluations, protocol handbooks, and checklists. Make good work habits an expectation – instill those expectations as part of the culture.

Applying the Five S's is more than a clean-up exercise. The waste that a disorganized or poorly planned clinical workstation generates will regenerate throughout the practice, causing numerous other inefficiencies. A workstation that has been improved by the application of the Five S's will:

1. Force incoming tasks to be reviewed and then acted upon immediately to completion. This contrasts with reviewing the task and placing it in a pile, only to be reviewed again later in the day to determine the next step. Often, incoming work is reviewed two or three times, by two or three people, before someone begins to work on it. The multiple review time is a waste. The new layout of the workstation will force the commencement of the process by requiring someone to process the work.

2. Allow everyone who works at the station to see instantly the location and status of any tasks and its related resources. This will eliminate the often-asked question, "do you know where such and such is?" Although this is certainly easier to accomplish with an electronic "workstation," a paper-based practice can use basic organizational techniques, such as initialing and dating, pre-made stamps and other simple means to help keep track of work in progress more effectively.

3. Establish a designated "go to" area. This will please busy staff and providers who likely have only a few moments of time between patients to do a task. Precious time is wasted when those few moments are spent looking for, instead of doing, the task.

4. Allow staff and providers to come and go from the task area separately without losing time or effort. In other words, no one has to "know" where the nurse keeps the messages; the uncompleted messages are always in the proper spot. Chaos does not erupt when the personnel change from one work station to another.

5. Offer a portrait of cleanliness and organization that positively reflects the practice to its customers (see Exhibit 1.2). This contrasts with the clutter and disorganization that often

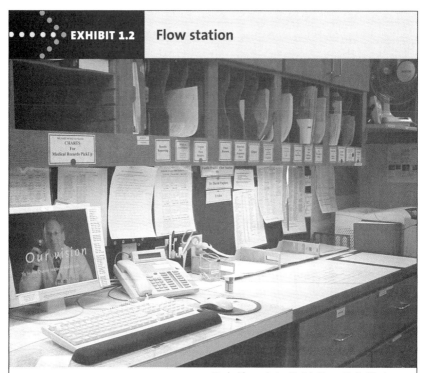

EXHIBIT 1.2 **Flow station**

Used with permission, Virginia Mason Medical Center

"Providers also have standard work. For example, indirect patient care occurs throughout the day, not batched at the end of a clinical session. This way, non-visit activities are handled quickly, with no need for staff overtime to process them. We have created flow stations. The medical assistant functions as 'flow manager,' setting up indirect care to be done between each visit. Providers follow a sequence of steps each time they exit an exam starting with completion of documentation, answering a message, signing a prescription, one test results, one mail item and then to the next exam. The flow manager does external set up of each provider task by completing all necessary information so physicians need only review and approve. This system saves time, and medical assistants feel more engaged, working shoulder to shoulder with providers. Elimination of waste has reduced time patients spend in the clinic from 72 to 46 minutes (36 percent reduction)."

—Dr. Brian McDonald
Chief, Virginia Mason Satellite Clinics
Virginia Mason Medical Center
Seattle, Washington

results in our patients justifiably questioning our management of the information and tasks related to their care. In other words, when a test result is not in yet, the patient will not automatically assume that your practice misplaced the paperwork.

WORDS OF WISDOM

Don't wait for an external change, like a new computer system or a new building, to begin changing work flow. Make design and constant refinement part of your practice's value stream.

Focus on the organization

Medical practices form operational departments, such as reception, billing, scheduling, etc. Each department depends on others to some extent to get its work done. Trying to optimize the processes of these various departments within a silo – disconnected from consideration of other organization processes and needs – will often have a detrimental effect on work flow.

Think about the impact of redesigning the registration process without considering the repercussions on the whole organization. Say, that a medical practice adds more computer capability to its registration process. The goals are to ensure that patients' insurance coverage is active and that benefits for services are always verified before rendered to the patient. A few hours are spent training staff to use the new software. Unfortunately, the practice soon finds that its great ideas to enhance registration efficiency actually increase the amount of time that front-desk staff must spend per patient by an average of 2.5 minutes. For some, including new patients, the process drags out to 10 minutes. Because this practice always schedules its new patients at the beginning of the day, office hours frequently started 10 minutes late. Patients with late morning appointments had to wait, the employee's lunch break ran later or was skipped to remain on time and, the daily clinic often ended late. Assigned staff to stay through the final patient of the day was causing overtime costs to add up. This practice optimized its registration, but not its patient flow. It failed to look at the bigger picture before changing the process.

To master patient flow, it's important to consider the many processes and tasks your practice performs from the patient's perspective, not just the viewpoint of the unit or department.

An intentional effort to redesign the core processes of your practice to focus on the patient will keep the focus on taking better care of patients, and you'll spend less time trying to dance to someone else's tune. That's why today's savviest physicians are using lean-thinking techniques to master patient flow in their medical practices.

 BEST PRACTICES

Make your practice "small"

As a medical practice grows in size, it becomes more difficult to see the operations of the whole practice. It should be no surprise that larger practices face steeper challenges in trying to successfully optimize the functions of one department without having a negative impact on the whole practice.

To avoid this problem, make your "practice" as small as possible conceptually. Consider the potential for greater efficiency if you were able to see and hear an entire process. That's just what many practices are trying to do in new buildings or renovations; they build pods designed for a small number of physicians and their teams. Gone are the days of the 10-employee front desk sitting adjacent to a large waiting room. Decentralizing those employees into 10 pods offers more value to the patient and the practice.

There will be less noise and chattiness inherent in a large reception area adjacent to a large number of staff. Plus, the smaller work units will allow each front desk to integrate into its practice team.

WORDS OF WISDOM

Learn from others

To learn from others, without the cost of a large consulting fee, contact a manufacturer in your community or region that has studied lean thinking (which most have). Ask if they would be interested in switching management teams for a day or two to see if ideas can be shared across industries to the benefit of both organizations. Start with a tour, and let the discussion about new ideas — new ways of mapping the value stream — flow from there.

KEY CONCEPTS

Lean-thinking terms

Continuous flow: Producing one product or service at a time or in small batches, as opposed to large batches, with each process step making just what is requested by the next step. Also called single-piece flow. Examples include an internal medicine practice where lab draws are performed in the exam room, versus a central lab draw station, and an orthopedic surgery practice where casts are removed and placed in the exam room, versus a separate cast room with a separate process.

Cycle time: Length of time to complete a process as timed by observation. Measure to determine your current state, and evaluate opportunities to reduce non-value added steps or replace with value-added steps. Examples include the time from the patient's check-in to the patient's departure, or an intermediate step, such as the time from ordering a lab to its completion.

Just-in-time: Producing a product or service when it is needed and in the right quantity. A common manufacturing term, just-in-time (JIT) applies to products. In the service industry, it applies primarily to supplies. Because supplies must be stored, often can expire, and may be rendered obsolete by new technology, stockpiling is discouraged. Instead, JIT delivers supplies based on the organization's needs.

Kaizen: Improving a system or process step to create more value with less waste. Examples include redesigning the reception and arrival function of a patient by eliminating the front desk and sign-in list and escorting patients directly to the exam room, which inherently performs the receiving and arriving functions and automating coding directly from the physician's documentation with a direct and seamless interface to the billing system.

Kanban: A signal or sign that offers direction to pull work in when – and only when – a resource is needed. Although applicable primarily to manufacturing, service businesses have used the concept of the sign to perform a similar function. The sign can be used as a clear alert in a process flow. Examples include tasks clearly marked for a clinical assistant to perform when rooming a patient or written orders upon completion of the encounter, a card inserted in the stack of gauze boxes on top of the par level to signal reordering and a red sign delineating an urgent message (with details) for the physician to attend to while in clinic.

Non-value added steps: Process steps that add no value to the customer or the organization. Typically introduced at some point in history but no one has reevaluated the need for the process since then. Often, these can be spotted when the response questioning the process is: "that's the way we've always done it," or a similar response. An example is requiring staff to photocopy a patient's insurance card three times and to file it in date or alphabetical order for the use of multiple parties, instead of scanning it into the information for rapid retrieval.

Plan, Do, Check, Act: The cycle of proposing a change in a process. Also known as the PDCA cycle, or the Deming Cycle for W. Edwards Deming who originated the concept in the 1950s. The PDCA cycle has four stages:

➤ Plan: Establish the goal for a process and the steps necessary to achieve it;

➤ Do: Implement the proposed changes;

➤ Check: Analyze the results in terms of the performance of the process; and

➤ Act: Based on the results, standardize and stabilize the change by incorporating it in the process, or start the PDCA cycle again.

Poka Yoke: Mistake proofing a process rather than blaming people for errors. This involves removing the human element, where possible, from job functions. Examples include requiring a registration field, such as the patient's date of birth; or establishing a container for a supply in the exam room that only fits the supply that is needed in that particular place.

The Five S's: In Japanese, seiri, seiton, season, seiketsu, and shitsuke. Translated into English, the Five S's are: sort, set in order, shine, standardize, and sustain. (Notably, translations may vary.)

Takt time: A measurement of production based on a balance of the customer's demand and the organization's production. Examples include determine how many inbound telephone calls occur per hour, rather just by day. By knowing the number of calls per hour, the practice can then deploy the correct number of staff to handle the volume.

Value stream: Non-value and value-added processes required to deliver a product or service from origination of the request to the customer. Mapping the process both as it exists and as it is proposed to change are important steps in the "plan" stage of the PDCA cycle. Examples include listing all steps in scheduling an appointment, from the patient's phone call to the completion of the scheduled appointment.

Waste or muda: Activity that creates no value (safety, efficacy, speed, convenience, etc.) for the customer but consumes the resources of the organization. For a litmus test, ask patients if they would want to pay for it. If the response is "no," it's likely a waste. Examples include using voice mail to screen patient calls and requesting patients to sign in on a list before they can be greeted.

References

1. James P. Womack, Daniel T. Jones, Daniel Roos. *The Machine That Changed the World: The Story of Lean Production* (New York: Rawson Associates, 1990).

2. James P. Womack and Daniel T. Jones. *Lean Thinking* (New York: Simon and Schuster, 1996).

3. Medical Group Management Association, *Performance and Practices of Successful Medical Groups*, editions: 1997 through 2006.

CHAPTER 2

The Physician's Time

Key Chapter Lessons

➤ Recognize your physician's time as the practice's greatest asset

➤ Understand the applicability of leverage to your practice

➤ Categorize your physician's time

➤ Discover how office design and technology can save time

➤ Learn to maximize productive time by reducing waste and time that can be delegated

➤ Identify the value of co-location

➤ Analyze the contribution of productivity improvement to earnings

➤ Calculate your average value of a customer (AVC)

➤ Implement strategies to manage physician time better

➤ Identify steps to improve personal time management

Your most valuable asset

Before we leap into examining the patient's experience with your practice, let's explore a fundamental concept behind your operations. Take this little test to see if you understand the value of your practice's most important asset.

Who can bill for a service in your practice?

    a. Telephone operator

    b. Medical assistant

    c. Physician

    d. Biller

    e. Office manager

Of course the answer is "c," the physician. The vast majority of the revenue produced by your practice is a function of the physician's time[1].

In an environment where an insurance company or patient is responsible for the invoice, the physician must bill for the service to get paid. In a capitated environment, inefficient use of a physician's time can translate into a smaller patient panel that, in turn, reduces the group's per-member, per-month (PMPM) payments. The name of the game is to leverage your physicians' time so that they are as productive as possible in contributing to your patients' care – and your bottom line.

Don't fall into to the trap of thinking that your physician's time is just another resource of the practice. The physician's time *is* the medical practice (see Exhibit 2.1). It's what patients really want from you. It's the asset that every other resource of the practice must support to provide maximum value to patients. Designing your operations to surround this valuable asset is more than a wise business approach, it's also the critical step in creating the patient-centered approach and mindset that patient's value. That approach will become more important in coming years as pay-for-performance plans, quality measures, and other initiatives become perhaps permanent fixtures of the reimbursement landscape. Most importantly, however, it's the *right* approach to take. In thinking lean, it's our goal to design our operations around the patient. Optimizing the physician's time with the patient is value – pure and simple.

Physicians are the medical practice's key to providing value to patients. They also are the practice's most costly resource. The

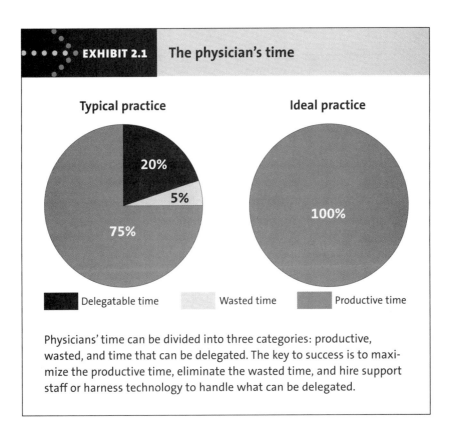

EXHIBIT 2.1 — The physician's time

Typical practice — Ideal practice

- 20% Delegatable time
- 5% Wasted time
- 75% / 100% Productive time

Physicians' time can be divided into three categories: productive, wasted, and time that can be delegated. The key to success is to maximize the productive time, eliminate the wasted time, and hire support staff or harness technology to handle what can be delegated.

critical question is, can physicians (or nonphysician providers) bring in more money to the practice than it must spend on the fixed costs of supporting their activities?

As you take steps to improve patient flow, view the usefulness of the improvements you make in terms of whether or not they optimize the physicians' time to care for patients.

The physician's minutes add up

At first, redesigning the patient flow process may seem like a lot of work for little return. There is no magical solution that equates to an "ideal" operation. Most suggestions in this book equate to a minute here and a minute there. What's the use of freeing up just a minute or two of the physician's time per patient visit? Multiply those salvaged minutes or fractions of a minute by the number of patients your physicians see each day, week, or month. You can see that saving a minute here and there can add up to hours over the year. These are the hours in which the physician is delivering *value*.

Fortunately, for those involved in managing a medical practice, the value to the patient mirrors the benefit to the practice's bottom line. Since the primary customer value and the financial driver of profits in a medical practice is how the physician's time is used, that asset – the physician's time – is where to focus many of your efforts to smooth patient flow. Don't make the mistake of devoting hundreds of hours of staff time and, perhaps, hundreds or thousands of dollars on top of that, to improve a process that doesn't help the physicians become more productive in terms of time. Think in terms of what can help the physician and patient work better together.

Examine the physician's non-clinical tasks

The best way to quickly maximize the amount of time the physician can spend with a patient is to look for ways to reduce the amount of time the physician has to spend on non-clinical administrative tasks before, during, and after a patient visit.

Do you see your physician spending time to track down test results, filling out long forms, or going through a medical staff directory to find a referring physician's telephone number?

 KEY CONCEPTS

Capitation: A methodology of payment for physician services that is based on a flat fee to manage the care of a patient. In contrast to fee-for-service, which you are paid a fee for each service, capitation transfers the risk of care management to the physician. That is, if the patient covered under capitation never sees or communicates with the practice during the year, the payment is all profit. However, the next patient could require a monthly visit to monitor his or her condition, plus supporting telephone time.

Consumer-driven health care (CDHC): An approach to health insurance that features insurance portability and tax advantages for beneficiaries but requires higher initial out-of-pocket costs from insureds. CDHCs are frequently linked to health savings accounts (see below), but the term is ubiquitous with any plan that increases the patients' responsibility to pay. Because patients bear a higher financial responsibility for their own health care, CDHC subscribers are more likely to make inquires about the costs of physician services.

Contribution margin: The revenue generated by an additional volume of services minus the variable costs to produce the volume equals the "contribution margin." For example, an in-house lab generates $20,000 in revenue and incurs $5,000 in variable expenses to perform an additional number of tests. Thus, the lab has produced a contribution margin of $15,000 to help cover fixed expenses. In general, when the contribution margin is positive, performing additional services is a good financial decision.

Health savings account (HSA): A tax-advantaged, portable account, regulated by the U.S. Department of Treasury, that individuals with high-deductible health plans can use for qualified medical expenses. Unlike other flexible health spending plans, HSA tax-deductible contributions, whether from individuals and/or their employers, can accumulate and grow tax free. HSAs and high-deductible health plans are intended to make patients into more cost-conscious consumers.

Leverage: The ability to use a resource to increase the value of an asset. For example, leveraging a physician's time by having a nurse return a portion of the calls allows the physician to spend more time with that day's patients. While the nurse answers the telephone calls, the physician can generate more revenue by seeing the next patient. *(This definition simplifies the twin issues of operating and financial leverage. Operating leverage refers to the extent a business commits itself to higher levels of fixed costs. Financial leverage refers to the extent to which a business gets its cash resources from debt as opposed to equity.)*

Panel: The number of active patients that a physician manages. Typically defined as the number of patients seen in the past 36 months, panel sizes run as low as 500 to a high of 6,000, depending upon the physician and the specialty. Panel size is sometimes used to describe the workload of the practice because having more active patients in the panel means more visits, more telephone calls, more prescription requests, etc.

Pay-for-performance: Enhanced or supplemental reimbursement for achieving standard quality measures established by an insurance company to foster quality outcomes for their beneficiaries. To qualify for the bonus payments, the practice must be able to record, monitor, and report these quality outcomes.

Per-member, per-month (PMPM): The amount of payment made in capitated relationships (see "capitation") for physician services. Insurance companies make a monthly payment ($0.50 to $20) on behalf of each of their covered beneficiaries for physicians to manage the care of that patient.

Relative value units (RVU): The work unit of the Resource-based Relative Value Scale (RBRVS), which is the methodology chosen by the Health Care Finance Administration (HCFA) to pay physicians for Medicare services. There is an RVU associated with each current procedural terminology (CPT®) code, and the scale of all of the codes is published each fall. RVUs are used by many practices as a measurement of productivity because the scale is based on the work, practice expense, and malpractice associated with each code. Moreover, the scale is identical across the country, making benchmarking easy.

● ●

Is there a relatively modest change that can be made in your facility's floor plan or can a nurses' station or computer terminal be moved or redesigned so it will save the physician a few extra steps? The cost to make such changes can be recouped several times over if doing so makes more efficient use of the time of a physician.

Check with vendors to see if there's a way to shorten or simplify the way physicians interact with the practice management system or electronic health record (EHR). Easy-to-access electronic templates for progress notes, electronic prescriptions, desktop-based fax or electronic transmission of test orders, consult requests, referrals or other forms can expedite workflow. If that saves time for the physician, then it's a good option to explore.

If possible, spend a half a day observing your physicians as they interact with other staff before and after patient visits. Take notes of what tasks they perform, how long each task takes, and how long it takes for them to walk to or prepare for the next task. Note times by the minute. You might quickly see a way to improve a simple process that is eating up your physician's time, such as waiting to transfer paperwork from the back to the front office or chaperoning patients from one area to another.

STEPS TO GET YOU THERE

Put a pedometer on physicians, providers, and staff before making changes to your practice's spatial arrangement. Ask participants to record their mileage for a day under the old scheme. Then, ask them to wear pedometers for a day after the changes are implemented, and note the results. If your redesign worked, they are walking fewer miles per day, or they are getting more done in the same number of steps.

The role of space in productivity

Research proves that the bigger a medical practice gets, the more operationally inefficient it becomes. Why? One significant reason is that physicians and staff must walk more steps in a larger practice. It sounds trite, but it's true.

The offices of a solo physician who has barely 1,000 square feet of office space may feel cramped but can get from the front office to an exam room and back again in mere seconds.

On the opposite end of the scale are the physicians who build an expansive suite of offices that feature long, wide hallways, spacious exam rooms, and physician offices located on a separate floor. In these practices, a walk from the front office to the farthest exam room seems to take 10 minutes. While that facility may look pretty, those extra footsteps gobble many additional minutes a day. And the cost of those extra minutes will add up to real money very quickly, especially if physicians are the ones who have to make these hikes.

THINGS TO CONSIDER

Extra steps reduce physician efficiency

Suppose your practice is one of those where the physicians walk each patient's encounter form to the front desk out of fear that the patient will wander off with the form and never be seen again.

Now, suppose it takes each physician 60 seconds to complete the walk to and from the front office.

A physician who saw 30 patients a day would spend an additional 30 minutes a day just carrying forms back and forth. Of course, the physician would start batching some of the errands whether you wanted it or not, but that would still add up to enough time at the end of the day for him/her to see one more patient, or at least catch up on other tasks and go home on time and little less stressed.

If this practice had 10 physicians, then the revenue lost due to those extra steps would cost the practice significant income by the end of the year.

In most practices, physicians spend way too much time walking around. Consider this: Is there a CPT code for walking an encounter form to the front desk? What about accompanying a patient to the exit, or escorting patients to the bathroom? Of course not. (Notably, this doesn't mean that patients should be wandering aimlessly through the practice. Good navigation means that the physician can be sitting in the next exam room with the next patient delivering value while the patient who is ready to go can easily find the way out.)

The most efficient physicians consider their suite of exam rooms – usually, three – to be their "playing field." Unless there is an emergency, they remain on the field. This not only saves steps – and time – but it keeps them focused. Put a piece of tape on the ground around your physician's "field." Spend a day shadowing the physician to measure how much time is spent on the field and off. You'll be amazed that the answer is often more time is spent off the field than on it. Change this, and you'll improve your efficiency – guaranteed.

Co-location

What can you do to make your office space more efficient for the physicians as well as the staff? For starters, review the processes that make physicians take too many unnecessary steps between work areas. Then, try "co-location," which is bringing the right people and resources together strategically to perform their jobs faster and more efficiently. Use rearrangement of workspace, better adaptation of technology or both to achieve optimal co-location.

The 1990s and early 2000s were the decades of centralization and compartmentalization. Everything from business offices to telephone operations was combined and given its own physical space. Although this achieved some economies of scale, efficiency was compromised because employees were separated from each other and, often, from the resources they needed to do their jobs and the communication that was essential to getting the job done.

A good alternative to the compartmentalization trend is physical co-location. Staff and physicians work together in workstations where they can perform all functions as a team. This type of grouping tends to occur naturally in very small medical practices.

These "care teams" work well because communication between the team members is direct and everyone has a pulse on how the day is going. Messaging delays are decreased because the person who takes a message can quickly find the answer or locate someone who does.

Scheduling is optimized because the scheduler understands the ebb and flow of the day. Clinical staff know the patients and can more easily assist them. With an EHR, the care teams have access to patients' medical records at their fingertips. Add a printer, scanner, and fax (available in an all-in-one version as well), and the team can function totally on its own.

Many medical practices use secure instant messaging, cell phones, pagers, personal digital assistants, two-way radios, walkie-talkies, colored lights, personal pagers, and other electronic tools to help staff communicate to each other within the practice. Some practice management systems and EHRs have options that can improve internal communication, such as arrival notification or patient flow modules. The more notification about where patients are and what they need, the better the day goes for everyone.

Today's technologies allow information to be transmitted on a real-time basis. Technology-based co-location can be more efficient than physical co-location if it empowers staff to communicate with each other without taking any steps.

Why pay your staff and your physicians to walk the hallways? Saving them steps pays off in better use of the physician's time, which, as we explore elsewhere in this book, is better off spent with patients, not getting exercise.

 YOU KNOW...

You know you're wasting physicians' time when...

...you see them walking around looking for something or somebody to help. If your workflow forces physicians to walk forms, messages, or even patients up and down long hallways then you are losing money. Take a day to watch how many steps they take.

Watch for muda

Spend a day – even a half day will do – to carefully track each physician's steps and actions. As you do, ask the following questions to root out waste:

Do physicians walk patients to the exit as they leave? It's always a nice touch but no patient is going to discuss serious medical issues in the hallway and it certainly isn't acceptable according to the Health Insurance Portability and Accountability Act (HIPAA) as it's not in the best interest of preserving the patient's privacy. Even if they are willing, since these conversations are usually not documented, they cannot be considered when coding for the visit. Thus, you can't bill for this "escorting." Instead, guide physicians into giving patients a kind goodbye as they leave the exam room. If patients tend to get lost in your facility trying to find their way out, consider improving navigation by placing more (or better) signs in the hallways or ask a staff member to escort them. Place signs at the patient's eye level, and use colors (e.g., a large red patch of carpet in front of the lab) to enhance navigation.

Do physicians often leave the exam room to look for missing forms or supplies? If so, compile a list of everything that physicians use in the exam room. Keep an inventory. Inspect and stock the rooms daily. Remember, a physician will find supplies much faster if every exam room is set up exactly the same. (See Chapter 8, "The Patient Encounter" for more ideas about preparing for the visit.)

Do physicians leave the exam room because information is missing that is needed for the patient encounter? If test results, hospital discharge summaries, or consult notes are missing, implement a chart preview process. Even with an EHR, it's still important to verify that these documents have been received. (See Chapter 8 for more ideas.)

Do physicians fall behind schedule because they slip away to do other business? Are they going to their offices between patient visits to return a few telephone calls, and then start surfing the Internet or tending to other tasks and lose track of time? If so, convert an old supply closet or other small space near the exam rooms into a private workstation where physicians can quickly make telephone calls.

These and other common, time-consuming habits can easily be changed once you recognize the impact on physician productivity. Eliminate unnecessary steps, and physicians will spend more time doing what they love – seeing patients.

For more tips on physician efficiency, see Chapter 8, "The Patient Encounter."

CASE STUDY

Small volume increase brings big profit boost for Dr. Smith

Solo pediatrician, Dr. Smith, desires $15,000 a month for physician income, plus $15,000 per month to cover fixed costs, for a total of $30,000 in monthly expenses. The practice receives $80 per visit, but has to spend $5 to pay the variable expenses of each visit. That leaves $75 to pay for fixed expenses per visit, plus what the physician wants to receive in income.

Seeing 4,048 patients a year (22 patients a day, 46 weeks per year, four days per week) gets Dr. Smith to specific goals, but what if two more patients could be seen each day? (Notably, the physician can either add two more slots, *or* decrease the no-shows accordingly.) The practice would now take in $27,600 (two patients times 46 weeks times four days per week times $75 per visit) to contribute directly to the bottom line.

Do the math:

Net revenue per visit ($75) x patient volume (368 patients) = total revenue ($27,600)

Over the course of a year, that additional profit could support meaningful improvements to equipment, facility design, or staffing for Dr. Smith.

Dr. Smith, by adding only two patients a day, can invest the profits, or increase his income. Either way, even an uneducated observer can identify the value of a physician's time.

For more on how operations relate to finances, see Chapter 13, "Fundamental Financials."

Productive physicians are happier physicians (and so are their patients)

The less productive the physician is, the more the physician will have to work to produce the volume needed to cover the practice's fixed costs. The more inefficient the physician is, the greater the risk of burnout or bankruptcy, or both.

The productivity of a physician is directly related to time. Time, of course, is finite.

The physician only has so much time in which to care for patients. The more time the physician has to care for patients, the more revenue he or she can generate for the practice. It sounds simplistic but don't forget that other concept: time is finite. The practice must consider allocating some of its resources to help its physicians use their practice time to create practice revenue. The three minutes it may take a physician to walk down two hallways of the practice to find a nurse to complete the patient visit and then to dig through a file drawer for a referral form is not time spent producing volume – it's just time wasted!

This isn't a chapter on staffing, but it should be pretty clear by now that a practice must consider allocating some resources on the fixed cost side (such as non-clinical staff time and information systems) to maximize the time of its greatest assets – its physicians.

The positive impact that certain fixed cost resources (staff, technology, and so on) can have on the productivity of the practice's assets (physicians and nonphysician providers) is why most medical practices have clinical assistants perform intake functions like blood pressure checks, weigh-ins and certain other routine assessments after a patient checks in.

When expressed in terms of salary cost, the five or so minutes it takes a clinical assistant to do these functions costs a fraction of the physician's five or so minutes. The physician could be generating revenue for the practice by spending that five or so minutes with another patient while the clinical assistant prepares the next one. In coming chapters, we'll move beyond this basic timesaving step to look for other ways to make the best use of the time of physicians and the patients.

As you review the options and ideas explored in the next sections of this book, keep asking yourself, "Would this change improve the value that my physicians deliver to patients?" If the answer is "yes," then the next question is, "How much fixed cost increase (if any) can I absorb to make this improvement work?" Finally, ask yourself if an increase to your fixed costs will generate at least the same amount of revenue. Unless there is a compelling reason to spend the money, don't do it. If new costs will not create similar or greater amount of offsetting revenue, then reconsider. The best costs to add are those that not only offset the costs, but also increase revenue above and beyond the costs.

Remember that not all investments pay off immediately. Investing in patient service leads to long-term rewards in retaining patients and generating the best marketing – word-of-mouth.

Strategic considerations

There are a great many financial considerations in understanding how to make the best use of a physician's time, but there are many strategic considerations as well.

Yes, a physician's time is your most valuable asset, but simply increasing work hours should not be the sole solution. A good work/life balance with adequate personal time is the key to a happy and productive person (see "best practices"). And, yes, we also recognize that increasing fixed and variable costs should be done carefully after considering all of the financial ramifications. But don't forget, patient service is always a consideration. Spending money to create better service is an investment, too – in creating loyal patients.

 BEST PRACTICES

Ten personal time management steps that work

The new information technologies of the 21st Century can improve efficiency and save time or they can torpedo efficiency while robbing you and your staff of precious time. Fortunately, there are ways to regain control over personal time in this technological era. Make a pledge to take the following steps:

1. Keep a realistic to-do, jot-down list in the same place and in a consistent format. Keep phone calls, follow-up tasks, shopping lists, and reminders in the same place (paper or digital). Log all phone calls so you'll know which calls you've returned and what's pending. Make a strike mark through completed tasks.

2. Maintain a calendar that displays an entire month at a time. It will help you visualize and balance your many time commitments. Put professional and personal commitments on

the same calendar. Block out time to work without interruption on critical tasks.

3. Keep important contact numbers (e.g., school phone number, spouse's cell, operating room, etc.) in a single portable location so you can find them immediately: a cell phone, portable digital assistant, or a small paper notebook will do.

4. Create and vigilantly maintain a clutter-free, organized, and functional workspace. Use a filing system that allows you to prioritize: (1) active projects (e.g., this week); (2) inactive projects (e.g., future or on hold); and (3) reference material.

5. Eliminate technological disruptions. Unsubscribe from less-than-critical e-mail forums and e-newsletters. Establish no more than two places where people can leave your professional messages, such as one voice mail box and one electronic communications (e-mail box). Don't be afraid to turn off a phone's voice mail function.

6. Get rid of intrusive technology. If you find yourself checking your Blackberry as you drive your kids to school, enough is enough. Get a mobile Internet service that requires you to log in to your laptop to get e-mails.

7. Teach practice support staff how to review and help handle your messages (e.g., before you ever see a message from a patient who wants a medication renewal requiring a pre-authorization, your staff should confirm the last renewal date, the pharmacy's contact information, and fill out the administrative portions of the pre-authorization forms).

8. Establish a new e-mail "mantra": touch only once. Decide immediately upon receipt whether to handle the message (an urgent matter that has an impact on operations, customer satisfaction, or quality of care), file it (a non-urgent issue but one that requires future action), forward (delegate to someone else), or trash. When delegating, give specific instructions about what you want done and ask for confirmation of completion. Add a note to an e-mail subject line if

necessary so that anyone who sees it can instantly determine what it's about without opening it.

9. Set ground rules for e-mail and voice mail. Squelch the urge
   to send e-mails about the superfluous ("Has anyone seen
   my favorite blue coffee cup?"). Never use a "group list" or
   "reply all" unless absolutely necessary. Don't feel compelled
   to respond to every e-mail. Skip e-mail altogether and talk
   directly about sensitive matters (personnel issues, patient
   issues, etc.). Only use voice mail when you cannot get to the
   phone; never use it as a screening device.

10. Learn to say no. Figure out what does not add value to your
    life – and then drop it. That measure of "value" may not
    always be monetary because not even money can undue the
    damage that stress causes.

Average value of a customer (AVC)

What is a patient worth to your practice? We've talked about the
value of a physician's time but what happens if you forget about
the patient's time? Unfortunately, many physicians and adminis-
trators do just that when they look at their already-full waiting
rooms and do not consider the impact on operating costs from
dissatisfied patients.

When a patient leaves before seeing the physician, the practice's
costs for that patient's appointment – nurse's time, building space,
utilities, equipment leases, and so on – do not walk out with that
patient. Every dime of that patient's cost to your practice's overhead
stays behind. Those costs are subtracted from the practice income
that, in many medical practices, is the physician's compensation. To
illustrate to your physician the impact of losing patients, try calculating the average annual value of a patient.

This analysis should not replace a detailed cost accounting study, of course. Instead, it can be a quick and easy way to determine the "value" of each customer to your practice. Practices of all types can use their own data to develop similar measures for each of their physicians.

CASE STUDY

What's your AVC?

In order to calculate the AVC, NeuroAssociates had to first calculate its Average Revenue per Customer (ARC), as shown in Exhibit 2.2. To do this, NeuroAssociates divided its net collections (revenue) by its patient panel (unique patients) for the year. The result was a $240 ARC.

Don't confuse "patient visits" with patient panel in the "All Patients" column. A patient may visit a physician several times, but in column one, we are looking only for the value or revenue per patient, not per visit.

However, the values in the "Surgery Patients" column (column two) do represent unique visits since the surgeon performs only one surgery on the patients. If your practice's physicians often do more than one surgery or procedure per patient, then adjust column two accordingly.

The charges, revenue, and volume number in the "Surgery Patients" column can be obtained by having the practice management system report all CPT codes for surgeries performed by the practice's surgeons.

NeuroAssociates figured its ARC at $240 for all patients and $545 for patients who have surgery. However, the ARC does not

EXHIBIT 2.2	Calculating ARC and AVC

NeuroAssociates of anytown		
	All patients	Surgery patients
Total gross charges	$1,000,000	$500,000
Collections	$600,000	$300,000
Patient panel	$2,500	*
Surgeries	*	$550
ARC/Year	$240	$545
Calculation	($600,000÷2,500)	($300,000÷550)
Overhead rate	45%	15%
AVC/Year	$132	$463
Calculation	[$240 x (1–.45)]	[$545 x (1–.15)]

*Not applicable

account for costs the practice must incur to serve its patients. NeuroAssociates applied its 45 percent overhead rate (total practice revenue divided by total fixed and variable practice costs) to the ARC, and determined that its AVC is $132. That is, each patient the practice served during the year contributed an average of $132 to the income of NeuroAssociates' physicians. Because the practice's overhead for its surgery patients is so much lower (15 percent), the AVC for each surgery patient is $463.

If a physician member of NeuroAssociates saw an average of two fewer patients a week – either by cutting back on contact hours or having the patients walk out because they got tired of waiting – the impact would be a $12,144 loss in annual income

(that is, 46 work weeks a year, times 2 patients per week, times
$132 in average value of the customer). Assume that some of
those patients would have needed surgery that the physician
would have performed and the annual loss would amount to
much more.

• •

The average value of a patient of a primary care practice measures
the "lifetime" value of that patient. Unlike specialists, primary care
physicians are likely to have the customer (patient) over a period of
years. They manage their patients' health until the patient moves
out of town, changes insurance companies, becomes dissatisfied
with the physician's service, or leaves for other reasons. As described
in the case study of NeuroAssociates, a neurosurgery practice, the
value of the customer to a surgeon is largely based on episodic
care, not a long-term relationship. Given this assumption, you
can calculate the AVC for a primary care physician using the
following formula:

AVC =

Cumulative retention rate *
(profit contribution margin – acquisition cost per customer –
retention cost per customer)

Sample AVC of a family practitioner =

85% * [($45 contribution margin per visit * 3 visits per year *
15 years) – ($100 advertising and screening cost per patient) –
($2 per visit per year * 3 visits * 15 years)]

= $1,600

This analysis assumes the practice's patients present an average of
three times per year for 15 years. The practice's acquisition costs per

patient are $100, while the practice spends $2 per visit to retain the patient (beyond the cost of the office visit itself). Eighty-five percent of the practice's patients remain as patients from year-to-year, and the practice makes a $45 contribution margin per visit. According to the practice's data, each of its patients is "worth" $1,600.

The principle of the average value of a customer (AVC) is the same for the specialist and the primary care physician. Because the primary care physician loses a "lifetime" of a patient versus an episode, the average value of their customers is higher. However, specialists have a lot more to lose in volume because their patients turn over much faster given the episodic nature of their practice. Either way, when you lose a patient, you lose income. Maintaining practice operations geared to patient service is not only valuable to your patients, it is valuable to you ... in real dollars.

The greatest asset

No matter how you look at it, the goal of a medical practice should be to focus on delivering value. To provide value to patients, referring physicians, and the practice's bottom line, focus on your physician's time as your practice's greatest asset. Do that and you'll be well on the path of enlightenment and ready to reduce waste and initiate change!

References

1. Not all practices rely on physicians as the sole billable providers. Many function with nonphysician providers, such as nurse practitioners, physician assistants, nurse anesthetists and other clinicians. Instead of listing each profession when discussing the role of a billable provider, this book will refer to a "physician." It is important to note that if your practice employs billable providers other than physicians that their profession can be substituted for "physician" throughout the book.

CHAPTER 3

Telephones

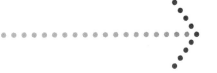

Key Chapter Lessons

- ➤ Familiarize yourself with key telephone concepts
- ➤ Calculate your "Telephone IQ"
- ➤ Develop a thorough analysis of your current system and future needs
- ➤ Learn about valuable telephone reports
- ➤ Recognize steps to change telephone demand
- ➤ Create a "mystery telephone patient survey"
- ➤ Understand the pros and cons of telephony applications for your practice
- ➤ Find tips for voice mail, automatic call distributors (ACDs), and auto attendants
- ➤ Recognize steps to select or change your telephone system
- ➤ Learn about staffing your telephones – and what to watch out for

Learn to handle telephones; or they will handle you

There are many ways to help physicians manage their time and their patients but one of the most important influences on how patients move through the practice is a low-tech, often-overlooked tool – the telephone.

Before patients come in for appointments they generally call. That's your first opportunity to impress them with good, efficient service and get the information that will make life easier for your practice.

After their appointment, patients call – and call again and again. While welcoming the calls you need, question the calls that neither the patient wants to make nor which you want to handle. Lean thinking suggests we consider why so many patients call to clarify medication dosages or care instructions. These calls are the norm, not the exception. They should not be unexpected because most patients leave the office with nothing but what they've heard during the exam. Often, the patients who come bearing notepads to take notes are looked upon as "troublesome." Calling about test results, of course, is another common reason for incoming calls but these, too, are not unusual considering that we probably told the patient to call. "If you don't hear from us in a couple of weeks, be sure to call us" really means "we've lost your test results." With patients' confidence waning, it's no wonder that practices are flooded with more calls than they can handle.

Let the patient drive the value. The patient wants you to deliver timely and accurate information without having to call and wade through the telephone system, leave a voice mail message, and play a game of phone tag.

The telephone is your friend, honest

What's happening with the telephones in your practice? Do patients complain about busy signals or long hold times? Do referring physicians complain that they can never get through? Do staff members spend too much time chasing down answers to questions from callers who just want to renew routine prescriptions or get test results? If so, then your telephone system and how you use it both need an overhaul.

Telephone demand is what you make it

When tending to telephones demands more staff time or patients can't get through, the traditional solutions have been to add more telephone lines, buy new equipment, and/or hire another telephone operator. These steps may be necessary but there are other options. Before adding to your practice's current telephone infrastructure, look for ways to *reduce* telephone demand. Consider changing how you handle scheduling, prescription renewals, referrals, and other processes. Maybe your practice is unintentionally causing many of its current telephone problems. You may have plenty of telephone lines but perhaps you are driving patients to use them too often.

Take a few minutes to assess the general state of the telephone system in your practice by completing the "What is Your Telephone IQ?" test (see Exhibit 3.1). Did you score above 75? If so, keep everything just as it is. You also have permission to skip this chapter and consider moonlighting as a telecommunications consultant because your practice is among the very few that have no major telephone issues.

For the rest of the world, please read on to learn how to assess your telephone system and discover ways to change the processes that may be artificially stimulating high telephone demand.

START | **GETTING STARTED**

Changing telephone demand

➤ Track call volume.
➤ Perform mystery shopper surveys and review results.
➤ Gather data from the telephone system and/or by observation.
➤ Ask staff to collect data on inbound call topics.
➤ Analyze outbound calls to find patterns.
➤ Analyze the current telephone system's pluses and minuses.
➤ Determine which telephone calls could be avoided altogether, handled at the encounter, or migrated to the practice's Web site.

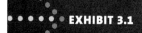 **EXHIBIT 3.1**   **Telephone IQ worksheet**

What is Your Telephone IQ?

DIRECTIONS: *Read each question carefully.*

Being as honest as you can, mark whether your practice is:

5 = Excellent – Keep as is;

4 = Above average – Opportunities still exist;

3 = Average – Improvements need to be made;

2 = Fair – Needs attention; or

1 = Poor – Below acceptable standards for our practice.

When you finish, consider the areas you marked with a 1 or 2. Decide how and when to improve those areas. If you don't know the answer to a question, be sure to find out!

_____ 1. The number of incoming lines is adequate to handle both peak and low times.

_____ 2. Callers are not kept on hold for more than two minutes.

_____ 3. We ask every caller's permission before putting him/her on hold.

_____ 4. Everyone in the practice who answers the telephone uses his or her name and the practice's name.

_____ 5. Specific backup personnel are scheduled so the telephones are answered promptly.

_____ 6. Everyone has been trained thoroughly on the telephone equipment.

_____ 7. We have up-to-date equipment with the latest time-saving features.

EXHIBIT 3.1 *(continued)*   **Telephone IQ worksheet**

_____ 8. Periodic telephone training is provided to fine-tune telephone skills.

_____ 9. Callers don't complain about busy signals when they call our practice.

_____ 10. Callers don't complain about being put on hold excessively.

_____ 11. Callers are not disconnected quite often when we transfer calls.

_____ 12. Callers don't complain about the complexity of the system.

_____ 13. The telephones are always covered (during regular working hours).

_____ 14. All calls are answered by the third ring.

_____ 15. Voice mail messages are kept current, are helpful, and sound pleasant and friendly.

_____ 16. Callers don't complain that their messages go unanswered.

_____ TOTAL

76-80 = You are the Gold Standard! Congratulations.

60-75 = Opportunities still exist. Explore staffing, system, and functional changes.

45-59 = Start making changes to improve the system and process.

<45 = Get right on it! Your patients and referring physicians need you to make improvements so that they can access your practice.

Modified from work of ©University Physicians, Inc., Baltimore, MD, 2007. Used with permission.

Inefficient telephones costs money

What are the consequences of an inefficient telephone system? Consider this: the telephone is your physicians' main link to the outside world. Without it, patients don't get scheduled, referrals are not made or received, patient triage is delayed or doesn't happen, after-hours questions from patients don't get handled, prescriptions don't get renewed, claims can't be followed up, and so on. With all of this at stake, why do so many medical practices turn this vital lifeline over to the lowest paid, least trained and, often, least experienced employee? In addition to reengineering what and how you handle the telephones, be sure to look carefully at who you hire to answer the telephones. Your operator represents your patient's first "moment of truth" with your practice, and determines whether patients' questions or concerns are routed to the correct function – or not. Investing in this critical position cannot be overlooked.

GETTING STARTED

Pay attention to workers' needs

Start enhancing your telephone system by improving working conditions for your telephone operators. Discuss equipment needs with staff. Do they need hands-free headsets? Better chairs? You may avoid future workers' compensation claims by paying attention to ergonomics and buying good quality equipment.

Even if you've hired the right operator, instead of hiring more operators or adding telephone lines to try and make telephone problems go away, look for ways to redesign patient flow processes. By redesigning processes, demand for the telephone is actually reduced instead of simply redirected. Demands that cannot be eliminated can be shifted to the most appropriate stage of the patient flow process and to the most appropriate person. Remember, let patients pull the value. They don't want to be mired in a long trek through your telephone system anymore than you want to spend all that extra time answering their calls.

Warning: These time- and money-saving ideas to change your telephone demand may involve changing resource allocations, altering telephone triage systems, implementing new technologies, relearning current technologies, and changing staff responsibilities.

Tracking call volumes

Most automated telephone systems can produce reports that show the volume of calls that come in each hour, day, or week, as well as how many rings before calls are answered and the amount of time callers wait on hold. In addition to knowing the number of calls processed per hour and by which operator, it is important to know your practice's call abandonment rate. In other words, how often are incoming calls not processed?

SupportIndustry.com's "2006 Service and Support Metrics Survey" measured average telephone call abandonment rates at several large companies and found that 21.4 percent of survey respondents claimed an average contact abandonment rate of less than 1 percent and that was an increase of 3 percent over 2004 figures. How does your practice stack up?

If you aren't sure whether your current automated telephone system can produce these reports, contact your vendor or dig up your system's instruction manual and read it. Newer systems should be able to produce these reports with very little hassle. Ask the vendor how you can get the reports. You can also invest in software that monitors all of these important statistics regarding calls.

When buying your next telephone system, don't consider one that doesn't put important volume and other reporting capabilities at your fingertips.

Why are these reports so important? Because they are the first place to look when trying to solve telephone issues. These reports can tell you if your attempts to change telephone demand are working.

THINGS TO CONSIDER

Telephone system reports

➤ Time on hold report

➤ Time of day report

➤ Calls per day report

➤ Number of calls processed

➤ Amount of time on each call

➤ Abandonment rate

Track inbound calls first

If your telephone system cannot produce reports (or you wish to supplement them), you can track the inbound calls manually with an "inbound call-tracking form" (see Exhibit 3.2). Understanding the nature of inbound calls will help the telephone system assessment process.

Give a tracking sheet to the practice's operators and other staff assigned to handle inbound patient calls. Ask them to track the calls they receive within each hour block for a minimum of three consecutive days. Remind the call trackers each morning and several times throughout the day. It may take a couple of attempts to get a complete enough record. Although you are not looking for statistical perfection, it's important not to underestimate the volume of inbound calls or miss an important category.

EXHIBIT 3.2   Inbound call-tracking form

Name: _____

Date: _____   Phone extension: _____

	Prescriptions	Scheduling	Billing	Referrals	Test results	Nurse/ Physician	Other	Total
8 to 9								
9 to 10								
10 to 11								
11 to 12								
12 to 1								
1 to 2								
2 to 3								
3 to 4								
4 to 5								

Modify the tracking form based on the most common reasons for inbound calls and the timeframe in which your phones are open. Copy the form and distribute to staff responding to inbound calls.

INSTRUCTIONS FOR USERS: Place a slash mark "|" for each call. If the patient calls back, place a dot on the top of the slash mark, or another designated method to identify repeat calls.

To make the job easier, provide a form that allows call trackers to check off the most common topics. Be sure that your call trackers mark any calls that are repeat calls – that is, callers have called once (or more) previously without getting resolution to their questions. To do this, ask call trackers to make a special mark on the log whenever patients indicate that they have already called about the issue.

The value of this exercise is that you might learn, for example, that 30 percent of your incoming calls concern test results, 10 percent are for prescription renewals, and five percent are for directions to your new satellite clinic.

Of course, you'll want this survey information to be gathered only at the point of the practice's first live contact with the patient's inbound call. Placing these survey forms at telephones in the back office could cause transferred calls to be counted two or more times, depending on how many times the patient is transferred.

After you've looked at the categories, calculate the percentage of the total calls that were repeat calls. In many practices, as many as 30 percent of the total incoming calls are repeat calls (see Exhibit 3.3, "Sample Telephone Analysis").

YOU KNOW...

...you're having telephone problems when...

...the number of walk-in patients starts increasing. This can occur when patients feel they have pressing problems but cannot get through to the scheduling desk or to anyone else to triage their questions. Frustrated by your telephone tie-ups, these patients will show up unannounced (and probably get more frustrated if your practice hasn't taken action on the tips in Chapter 4, "Scheduling"), or worse, they'll find someplace else to go.

EXHIBIT 3.3 Sample telephone analysis

Type of call	Total	Repeat percentage
Prescriptions	32	28.1%
Scheduling	30	0.0%
Test results	35	2.9%
Nurse/Physician	45	33.3%
Billing/Referral	12	33.3%
Other	16	0.0%
Total	170	26.5%

Repeat calls are 26.5 percent of incoming volume in this example.

Telephone analysis results: Total calls and repeat calls

No matter how you accomplish it, make sure you know why your patients are calling before making significant changes to any processes. You may discover inadequacies in other processes, such as patient education, prescription renewals, test result notification, referrals, or scheduling. Areas in which there are a high percentage of repeat calls are prime opportunities to improve your practice. Target those areas first for your performance improvement initiatives.

Distribute the results of your incoming call analysis and engage staff and physicians in discussions of what might be sparking these patterns. Further analysis may show that a physician is telling patients to call back the following day to get their test results when, in fact, those results take more than 24 hours to be returned. Or, you may discover that you need to do a better job of promoting your new clinic's location or instructing patients to call their pharmacy, not the medical practice, for routine refills.

Break down each category of inbound calls. Develop action items and associated time frames and persons responsible for each category (see Exhibit 3.4). Don't do everything at once, or you'll surely fail. Nor will you be able to monitor your success if you act on a dozen things at once. Monitor the same criteria – call volume, abandonment, etc. – before and after implementing changes.

(Find more ideas about prescription management in Chapter 9, "Prescriptions.")

WORDS OF WISDOM

An informed staff reduces risk

Make sure that:

➤ Administrative staff know basic medical terminology. Everyone whose duties include answering a telephone must be able to spell important medical terms that describe chief complaints, diagnoses, medications, etc. Indecipherable messages force you to call back patients, pharmacies, laboratories, or other physicians to figure out what they said. That's just more work for you.

➤ All staff recognize patient emergencies and have guidelines to handle extenuating circumstances with referring physicians. This includes anyone who would ever answer your telephones – even the medical records clerk working after hours. The

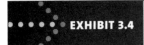

EXHIBIT 3.4   Action items related to prescription calls

Opportunity identified	Recommended action	Date	Person responsible
1. Patients call in for refills.			
	Action: Educate staff and patients about the difference between renewals and refills.	1/15/2009	RJW
	Action: Educate patients to contact their pharmacy directly regarding refills.	1/15/2009	RJW
2. Patients call in for renewals.			
	Action: During a scheduling call, request patients to bring in medications.	2/15/2009	JCH
	Action: Integrate discussion regarding medication renewals during rooming process.	2/16/2009	KIJ
	Action: Physicians to write down protocols for triage nurse regarding out-of-office renewal requests, to include medications and timing.	3/1/2009	RWB
	Action: Physicians to approve maximum time frame for which renewals can be made without patient being seen in the office. Recommendation: 12 months.	1/15/2009	RWB
	Action: Establish a communication alert between physician or clinical assistant and check-out staff regarding renewal timeframe so that follow-up appointments can be made within time frame.	2/15/2009	KIJ
3. Pharmacies call in for clarification of prescription and formulary.			
	Action: Review e-prescribing vendors, with criteria that solution must alert physicians at the point of care to formularies.	4/1/2009	JCB
4. Patients can self-serve through a Web portal.			
	Action: Review Web portal vendors. Discuss opportunities for other process improvement (e.g., test results management) with stakeholders. Gather information about pricing, functionality, user-friendliness, and references. Test idea with patient focus group.	12/31/2009	JCB

records clerk doesn't need to become your triage nurse but you never know who will be around when a crisis occurs. An informed staff means an efficient office. It's good risk management and good patient service.

Outbound calls can be opportunities to improve

After organizing your internal call reports, staff observations about incoming calls and the results of your mystery patient survey, analyze outbound calls to find patterns. A form similar to that used for inbound calls may help. Don't confuse staff by doing the inbound and outbound surveys at the same time unless the inbound calls are received by a different individual (e.g., telephone operator) than the one who places them (e.g., the triage nurse who only makes outbound calls). In this case, give the inbound tracking form to the telephone operator and the outbound form to the nurse.

If it seems that the percentages of outbound calls by topic match up with those of inbound calls, then there may be some room for improvement in the process related to that topic. For example, a high volume of inbound and outbound calls dealing with test results may indicate that your staff and patients are spending too much time playing phone tag when other, simpler communications solutions might work.

BEST PRACTICES

Set call volume goals

➤ Industry standard for call volume: four to five inbound calls per patient appointment.

➤ "Best Practices" goal for call volume: one inbound call per patient appointment.

Let's break it down: The ratio of telephone calls from patients asking questions about prescriptions, test results, or medical issues to actual office appointments per day ranges from 4:1 to 5:1 in the typical medical practice. If your practice sees 100 patients a day, then your call volume likely ranges from 400 to 500 calls per day. A best practice is to strive for a 1:1 ratio between inbound calls and appointments; namely, an initial call to schedule the appointment. How? Reduce the need for the call and replace as many inbound calls as possible by anticipating patients' needs and contacting them before they can call you. It's much more efficient to communicate to patients than having them call you.

Let's look at some examples. You take care of each patient's prescriptions during the office visit and use an electronic tickler system to remind clinical staff to call patients soon after their visits if you suspect there could be any concern about the dosage, delivery, side effects, or efficacy of the medication you've just prescribed.

Reinforce the habit of making these follow-up contacts with newly prescribed patients by discussing with your clinical team the most common questions you tend to get. When patients are scheduled for procedures or hospitalizations, schedule staff to call before and after the visit to check on their welfare as well as to seek out any questions. Be sure to set appropriate and realistic expectations about when test results will arrive, and call patients promptly when results arrive. Schedule post-operative appointments when you schedule the surgeries. These are only a few of many improvements you can make in your practice; you'll find other examples throughout this book.

In sum, the best practice is to anticipate what the patient will need – and deliver it. Don't make the patient call you. Design your telephone processes around the "best practice" goal of hitting the golden ratio of one incoming call per visit.

Mystery telephone patient survey

To supplement your internal analyses of your practice's telephone performance, try a mystery telephone patient survey (see Exhibit 3.5). Ask friends or colleagues to call your practice and note how often they get busy signals, how long they wait on hold, what they hear while on hold, and their impression of the courtesy of the staff answering the telephones (who should **not** be told that the survey is being conducted).

If possible, have the surveyors attempt to call the practice during each hour block, that is, 7:00 to 8:00 a.m., 8:00 to 9:00 a.m., etc. You may be surprised – and not always pleasantly – by what happens when people call in during the lunch hour, immediately after the practice opens in the morning, or just before closing. The mystery telephone patient survey will not give you all the answers you need to fully assess your telephone system but it will give more credibility to anecdotal information you may hear from patients. Mystery telephone patient survey reports can be combined with reports produced by your telephone system and with other observations to give a clearer picture of what's going right and/or wrong with your telephone system.

 BEST PRACTICES

The mystery telephone patient survey in action

Mystery telephone patient surveys can be used to assess telephone service, as well as reception and registration service. Whether you choose to do the survey by telephone or with a live visitor, here are some tips:

➤ **Set a goal.** With a goal in mind (Is our staff courteous? What's our waiting time? Do we project a professional image?), you'll quickly see ways to make the best use of the results. Mystery patient survey results can be particularly useful if delivered as part of a performance improvement initiative, a strategic

EXHIBIT 3.5 Mystery telephone patient survey

Pick one of these sample questions:
1. Can you give me directions to your office?
2. Can you tell me something about Dr. _____?
3. Do you accept _____ insurance?
4. How long would I have to wait to get a physical exam with Dr. _____?

Practice name: _____

Caller: _____

Call date: _____

Call time: _____

Overall impression
☐ Exceeds standards   ☐ Meets standards   ☐ Does not meet standards

Number of rings: ☐ 1 ☐ 2 ☐ 3 ☐ More than 4

Courtesy of person answering telephone
☐ Very pleasant   ☐ Pleasant   ☐ Rude or hurried

Did the person answering the telephone give you his or her name?
☐ Gave name clearly   ☐ Gave name   ☐ Did not give name

Did the person answering the telephone give you the practice's name?
☐ Gave name clearly   ☐ Gave name   ☐ Did not give name

Did you get put on hold?
☐ Never put on hold
☐ Briefly put on hold after being asked if OK
☐ Put on hold without being asked

If you were put on hold, how long did you wait?
☐ Less than 30 seconds   ☐ 30 to 90 seconds   ☐ More than 90 seconds

Level of knowledge of person answering telephone
☐ Extremely knowledgeable; gave complete, correct information immediately
☐ Knowledgeable; gave correct information
☐ Gave incorrect information

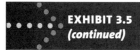

EXHIBIT 3.5 *(continued)*   **Mystery telephone patient survey**

Were you transferred to another individual who ultimately answered your question?
☐ Not transferred; call handled by first person
☐ Transferred once to correct person with appropriate explanation
☐ Transferred more than once, transferred to wrong person or transferred without appropriate explanation

Was a message taken for someone to call you back?
☐ Message not taken; call handled by first person
☐ Message taken appropriately; received call back in specified time
☐ Message taken inappropriately; call not returned in specified time

Courtesy of person answering question
☐ Very pleasant   ☐ Pleasant   ☐ Rude or hurried

Did person answering the question give his or her name?
☐ Gave name clearly   ☐ Gave name   ☐ Did not give name

Did you get put on hold by the person who answered the question?
☐ Never put on hold
☐ Briefly put on hold after being asked if OK
☐ Put on hold without being asked

If put on hold by this person, how long did you wait?
☐ Less than 30 seconds   ☐ 30 to 90 seconds   ☐ More than 90 seconds

Knowledge of person answering question
☐ Extremely knowledgeable; gave complete, correct information immediately
☐ Knowledgeable; gave correct information
☐ Gave incorrect information

Level of concern of person answering question
☐ Demonstrated high level of genuine interest in caller
☐ Demonstrated interest in caller
☐ Demonstrated little or no interest in caller

Comments to support ratings exceeding or not meeting standards:
_____
_____
_____
_____

planning session, or in a kaizen (process improvement) exercise (see Chapter 1, "The Lean-Thinking Revolution").

→ **Prepare the survey.** Use the mystery telephone patient survey or redesign one used for live visitors. The telephone survey (see Exhibit 3.5) should include questions like, "How many rings before staff answered your call?" and "How would you rate the customer service exhibited by the staff member who answered your call?" Use the same survey for your evaluations. Although having one mystery patient call is a start, it's best to have a sample to draw from. For example, it's recommended that mystery telephone patient surveys run for a period of one month, with a minimum of 30 calls observed.

→ **Find the mystery patient(s).** Depending on the purpose of the project, find a patient volunteer, ask a family member or colleague to help, or hire a consultant. Unless you're hiring an experienced professional, set expectations clearly.

→ **Receive feedback from patients directly.** If you're intimidated by having a mystery patient program, or simply don't want to find one, consider getting feedback from patients directly. Choose a small but interested cohort of patients from your active population and ask them to meet at your practice once a quarter. Although it changes the dynamics of the group, you may wish to include the human resources director from a local employer, an office manager from a referring physician, or another non-patient who may hear a lot of feedback about your office from your patients because of his or her job. Feed the group lunch, ask some questions, listen carefully, and take lots of notes. In addition to providing invaluable feedback, a patient advocacy group can improve the impression that your community has about you based on your dedication to improve.

When asked to provide feedback, mystery patients — or your own patients — can be wonderful resources to your practice as you seek to improve service, access, and operations. Don't always rely on your impressions; let the voice of the customer speak loud and clear.

Responsiveness

When SupportIndustry.com measured the average time it takes businesses that offer telephone-based support to answer calls and the
average time their callers spent on hold, they found that 19.3 percent of respondents took less than five seconds to answer a call. The
largest percentage was the 28.1 percent of companies whose telephone staff took between 5 and 15 seconds to answer a call. As for
hold time, 26.3 percent of companies say their customers experienced no waits for service, while 31.6 percent put clients on hold
for less than a minute and another 35.1 percent put them on hold
for between one minute and two minutes.

Sure, your practice doesn't have the resources of the large service
companies reporting in this national survey but the fact is your
patients expect you to do at least as well. Or perhaps they expect
you do better because as a medical practice, your "customers"
call you because they are feeling ill, not because their televisions
won't work.

No matter what measurement tool you have used, it is more than
likely that you've concluded that performance improvement is
needed, if not essential. There are many ways to change the
processes that can spur telephone demand. The following sections
spotlight strategies to help you improve performance.

Stop playing "pass the caller"

Does this happen in your practice? The receptionist transfers a
patient's call to the scheduler, the scheduler cannot determine if the
patient is sick enough to deserve one of the practice's precious few
slots for acute appointments, the patient is transferred to the nurse,
the nurse puts the patient on hold to consult with the physician,
and, finally, the patient is transferred back to the scheduler. What's
the accumulated time for all of these transfers? It can be up to 30
minutes. The amount of value-added time to the medical practice?

Maybe, three minutes. The amount of value for the patient? None. They just wanted an appointment.

The lesson of this all-too-frequent game of transfer tag is that you must develop internal processes to combine tasks and limit telephone transfers. Don't waste your patients' time. Don't tie up your telephone lines so other patients can't call for appointments. Staff your telephones with personnel who can help the patient or route callers to staff who can get the entire job done.

Allowing the appropriate staff to get the job done without all of the transfers is perhaps the greatest asset that an electronic health record (EHR) can offer to your operations. With the patient's information close at hand, the needs of many callers – from patients to referring physicians – can be handled more expeditiously. If you have an EHR, make sure you take advantage of the tools that maximize your practice's ability to get the job done, thereby eliminating the many inefficiencies of playing "pass the caller."

Learn from the experts

Why do some employees have a knack for handling even the toughest, most complicated patient telephone inquires? Here are the lessons you and your staff can learn from these telephone mavens:

Be happy (or at least act happy). You can sense someone's attitude through the telephone. Patients will hear it in your voice if you are smiling as you speak into the telephone. Try putting a mirror on the wall in front of your telephone operator and asking the operator to smile sincerely when answering each call, just as would be expected in a face-to-face encounter.

Know your stuff. Patients call for so many reasons that locating the correct staff member can be a chore. Give each telephone operator a daily list of everyone's whereabouts. It will save precious time in looking for people and it will lessen callers' time on hold. There also are many common questions each day so script responses that the operator can use to get right to the point. Directions to the office or referred testing sites should always be handy. If you can anticipate some of those questions, post them with the correct responses on your practice's Web site in a frequently asked questions section.

Guide callers. Some people have a hard time getting to the point, so help them along by politely asking, "What can I help you with?" Try role-playing during a staff meeting to show employees how to help patients get to the point without being pushy.

Some people have a natural gift for handling telephone inquiries. Listen to how they do it, and turn their skills into training so you can start improving everyone's telephone efficiency and service quality.

Training tips to improve telephone manners

Maybe you can't significantly reduce the volume of incoming calls – this is a service business after all – but you must refuse to tolerate poor telephone service from your staff. Appropriate telephone call handling tactics should become part of your practice's essential staff training. They can improve the service your practice delivers.

Keep writing tablets near all phones. As soon as the caller states his or her name, write it down. Otherwise, you may forget the name as you listen to the details of the request, forcing you to ask for the caller's name again at the end of the conversation. They'll wonder what other information you missed. After you have the name, use it as often as you can during the conversation. The name offers a connection to the patient, and demonstrates that you are listening and attentive.

Use a consistent greeting. For example, say: "Nephrology Associates, this is Jan speaking. How may I help you?" Don't let your staff or providers deviate from the script. It's a small but important step that will ensure each caller gets a consistently high level of service.

Avoid abbreviations. It may be quicker for your receptionist to say, "Hello, Surg Onc" (as opposed to "Hello, Surgical Oncology Associates") but you'll lose time in the long run as callers pause and wonder if they reached the right place. Everyone who answers a telephone should say your practice's name with as few abbreviations as possible. It makes a more professional impression and ultimately contributes to a higher level of service.

Watch non-verbals. A bad mood or lousy attitude seems to leap through the telephone. Watch inadvertent non-verbal communications, such as sighs or moans. Beware of talking too rapidly or loudly as well as using a condescending or inappropriate tone. Make a point of smiling as you speak. Patients will sense that smile even over the telephone.

Maintain a calm demeanor. If the caller has a beef with your practice or is simply taking out a bad mood on you, don't absorb the caller's emotions. Suggest that staff post a quote, photo, or some other calming focal point at their workstations. It will give staff something to focus on when difficult situations arise.

Prepare for rough spots. Script a few statements for difficult situations for your staff to use as lead-in statements. These might include: "I'm sorry that we didn't meet your expectations, Ms. Jones." Remind them to use the patient's name in the conversation; it will demonstrate that they are listening. Have them write down the caller's comments to verbally summarize at the conclusion of the conversation. It will indicate that they took the complaint seriously. Many callers just want to be heard. They should be sure to state the next step that they will take with the complaint, such as giving a note to the physician or nurse. Patients who want an answer should be given realistic expectations about response times.

Conclude calls with a bang. Tell staff to use the patient's name – "Ms. Jones," "Mr. Smith," etc. – at the end of conversations. Stating the patient's name tells them the problem is being handled by the physician's competent staff. They should also thank patients for choosing your practice, particularly if scheduling an appointment. Wrap up calls by asking the caller if there is anything else needed. For example: "Thank you for choosing the Cardiovascular Group, Ms. Jones. Is there anything else I can do to assist you?" If performed consistently, you'll leave a positive and memorable impression on every caller.

 YOU KNOW...

Get the answer the first time

Discuss information needs with staff. Do they need access to instant messaging to alert the triage nurse that a patient is calling back again? Do they need access to the EHR to identify whether a task, such as test result notification has been completed in order to inform the caller? Do they need access to the 'on-call' list for communication from the hospital? Determine what resources you can deliver to your operators, and you will gain the operators' buy-in to assist with other practice duties.

Avoid unnecessary repeat calls

If you don't have the ability to process the calls as they come in, set a policy in your practice regarding a timeframe for returning calls to patients, referring physicians, and other callers. I recommend no more than two hours to return a call because it is courteous to patients who are often sitting by the telephone waiting for your call. If you cannot resolve patients' question within two hours, call patients back to inform them about the status of your response.

Accrediting organization URAC sets expectations for nurse call-backs in 30 minutes. See Words of Wisdom for more information on URAC's standards.

This helps prevent the person from calling back – again and again – asking the same question. Repeat calls tie up staff time unnecessarily and foster caller frustration and even anger.

WORDS OF WISDOM

Washington, DC-based URAC, and independent, nonprofit organization that accredits and certifies health care organizations, establishes the following expectations for response times for phone-based nurse triage:

Health care call center (HCC) 13 requires a nurse to respond to a message from a patient within 30 minutes. In addition to a message, HCC13 also notes that phone nurses can accept clinical calls directly or via a transfer from non-clinical staff.

HCC11 sets 30 seconds as the standard of average speed of answer for calls from patients.

Bonnie Sturges, RN, Nurse Accreditation Reviewer

BEST PRACTICES

Set expectations

There's nothing more frustrating to a customer than unmet expectations. If you tell the patient to expect a test result in five days, deliver the result within those five days. Better yet, tell them to expect five days and deliver in three days. Delight patients by setting expectations appropriately. Develop reasonable expectations that you can always beat by discussing the common timeframes that you give to patients for test results notification, prescription renewals, surgery scheduling, referral processing, physician or nurse callbacks, etc. Distribute the expectations to providers and staff and incorporate them in patient materials and your practice's Web site. Never set an expectation you can't beat. Exceeding your own expectations will create delighted customers. Not meeting them is a recipe for disaster.

Decentralize scheduling

How many calls does your triage nurse answer per hour? How many of those calls end up with the patient needing an appointment scheduled?

More than likely your triage nurse is not trained to schedule appointments. No wonder your scheduling staff is so busy. No wonder patients are upset: they likely had to wade through a telephone tree, wait on hold to get to the triage nurse, then wait on hold again to get an appointment. Is this delivering value to the patient? No way. By training whoever handles triage to also schedule patients, you shift that demand away from other staff. More important, you score points for good customer service.

 WORDS OF WISDOM

Don't deflect demand

Consider the time your practice's staff spends on the telephone deflecting appointment demand. Triage nurses are important components to a successful practice but too often they turn into gatekeepers. The resources expended in deflecting demand can be tremendous.

I even had a pediatrician ask me, "You mean we're allowed to ask the parents if they want their child to be seen when we pick up the telephone? My nurse doesn't have to approve their request?" Although I was shocked at her comment, I realized that many practices have gone down the approval path a bit too far. The irony is that rarely, if ever, does the process result in the patient's (or parent's) request being declined. So, why do it? It's muda or waste, and we can attack it!

Many medical practices are re-engineering their appointment schedules to create more access ... and to reduce the time that staff spends on the telephone to deflect demand – an expense that adds no value. (See Chapter 4, "Scheduling" for more information.)

BEST PRACTICES

Appointment scheduling by all

Train *all* physicians and staff in the practice to schedule appointments for established patients. Yes, even physicians, though that should be an exception rather than a rule. Spreading out scheduling chores gets patients to the service they need and gets them – and your staff – off the telephone faster. It can help in situations, such as trying to schedule an appointment in the exam room for the mother of a child screaming from the pain of a shot, or it may help if other staff must step into handle some front office chores when the receptionist is on leave. Think of scheduling appointments as sales: everyone should help you sell!

Post-visit services

Traditionally called "check-out", medical practices are embracing post-visit or practice services at the convenience of the patient or their families. We'll expand on practice services in Chapter 11, but recognize that how the physicians and staff handle closure with the patient can have a positive – or negative – impact on telephones. A patient well-informed about an upcoming test won't need to call back about preparatory instructions, directions, or inquires about how to obtain the results. Indeed, anticipate your patient's needs and deliver it before they have to call back to ask.

Create appointment templates that cover a minimum of three months. Past three months, patients may become even more forgetful or commit to other obligations that conflict with the appointment time. And that means they will have to call back to reschedule, which adds to your daily telephone volume.

Evaluate the percentage of the patients with appointments that were scheduled 90 days or more in advance who end up rescheduling, canceling, or just not showing up. Also count those whom your practice bumps to another time slot because the provider's schedule changes. If you determine that more than 10 percent of your patients fall into these categories, establish an electronic recall list by date. According to the follow-up protocol dictated by the provider, place patients into your recall list 30 days before their requested appointment.

Rescheduling: Avoid the bumps

A physician changes clinic hours. Your staff goes into high gear to quickly contact patients to reschedule appointments. Of course, you never seem to get most patients on the telephone on the first try, so you and your staff must leave messages or resort to sending certified letters. And, of course, every one of those patients has to call back to reschedule.

The administrative tasks pale in comparison with other ramifications like the fact that many patients may be in the middle of a course of treatment – and are now being seen weeks later than they should – or the fact that many of those patients will need medication renewals as they await another appointment date.

Don't let physicians create this extra work. Wise medical practices ask physicians to commit to communicating clinic schedules six weeks in advance and sticking to them. They limit rescheduling to emergencies.

Read more about bumps in Chapter 4, "Scheduling."

Reminders can reduce telephone demand

How else can you reduce telephone call volumes? Try sending out reminders to patients four to five days in advance of their appointments, or calling patients two days in advance. Yes, it will increase your costs. But that small additional cost will likely be offset by a great savings in the amount of time that staff must spend handling incoming calls from patients who can't recall the exact time or day of their appointment. It may also produce cost-savings by reducing no-shows or late arrivals.

Many practices are automating reminder telephone calls to patients. These systems can work well and can be integrated into most practice management systems. Just make sure the calls are friendly sounding and do not breach patient confidentiality.

Let schedulers schedule

Too many practices do not allow their schedulers to schedule. You can tell these practices almost at a glance. They are the ones where the staff answering telephones must constantly leave their workstations, and hunt down physicians, nurses, or other providers for permission to schedule an appointment. Just one or two physicians in the practice who insist on approving all appointments in advance can cost dearly in terms of staff time.

When schedulers have to continually ask permission to do their jobs, patients are left on hold and incoming lines are tied up. Or, worse, schedulers must play a completely unnecessary game of phone tag with patients.

If you're a subspecialty practice with an appropriate need to screen appointments, see the section on pre-appointment screening in Chapter 4, "Scheduling" for more information.

Prescriptions

Most encounters with a physician include a medication – an initial prescription, a change of medication, or a refill. There are several steps that you can take to better handle prescriptions – and consequently, reduce your telephone calls. Calls from patients about routine prescription matters contribute significantly to most practices' in-bound call volumes. See Chapter 9 "Prescriptions," for an in-depth discussion of how handling the prescription process better can significantly reduce telephone volume and related staff time to handle those calls.

In summary, these tips include:

- ➤ Transmitting prescriptions to pharmacies electronically;
- ➤ Writing legibly whenever faxing a prescription or delivering it manually;
- ➤ Instructing patients to call the pharmacy instead of your practice for routine refills;
- ➤ Renewing prescriptions during patient encounters;
- ➤ Carefully timing follow-up visits in conjunction with prescription periods; and

➤ Establishing efficient prescription renewal protocols such as creating written guidelines for telephone renewals and documenting all medication renewals.

Manage patient-to-physician calls better

"I only want to talk to my doctor." Ever heard a patient say that? If you are hearing it a lot, then it's time to consider taking a team approach to health care delivery. Patients who consistently see one clinical assistant or nurse each time they visit their doctor are much more likely to open up to this individual. Your verbal support for that nurse is critical. Tell the patient that the nurse is an important member of your "team." Reinforce your nurses' credibility by printing business cards for them. It's a small investment that creates greater credibility, and better patient access.

BEST PRACTICES

Manage message flow

➤ Recognizing the importance of managing the flow of messages from inbound telephone calls, high-performing medical practices spend extra time to train staff how to handle messages. It may seem like common sense but you can leave nothing to chance to make sure the act of taking a message is done consistently. Tell your staff that when taking telephone messages, they should: Respond to patients who ask to speak with physicians or providers by asking if there is something you can do to assist the patient. The patient may just need to schedule an appointment.

➤ Make sure to ask the patient for the information the physicians and providers say is needed. Physicians must establish protocols about what information they want to see in patient messages, including what facts from the patient's record must accompany the message.

➤ Make sure all telephone messages include who took the message, when, the name of the patient or caller, the nature of the call, the urgency of the situation, and if there is permission for the provider to leave a voice, text message, or e-mail response, if applicable.

➤ Look up the patient's account before the message is handed to the physician or provider to make sure the patient is in the system and the information can be pulled up easily.

➤ Keep messages on active status until the issue is resolved. Don't delete the electronic message or file it in the patient's record (or elsewhere if about a non-medical issue) until the matter is handled.

Finally, high-performing practices have message stations. See Chapter 1, "The Lean-Thinking Revolution" to see a workstation used by a practice – and why it works so well.

Follow-up calls

Historically, surgical practices would always place a telephone call to their patients on the day following discharge. This activity still occurs but it is no longer common practice. In addition to leaving an indelible impression on the patient, these calls can also have a positive impact on practice operations.

Proactively calling a patient can prevent a medical problem from increasing in severity. Complications drive up telephone calls, medication requests, and office visits as well as the obvious negative impact they have on the patient's care.

If you're a surgical practice or perform procedures, try calling your patients one or two days after the service. Review medical instructions, evaluate the patient's improvement, adjust medications if appropriate, and reinforce discharge instructions. In addition to preventing future telephone calls, this one call may be your best marketing technique and it helps your patients get better faster.

Managing test results

Many medical practices still tell patients: "If you don't hear anything from us, everything is okay." That may make it easy on the staff but it is hardly considerate of the patient. Patients may want to know their exact cholesterol levels, how they compare to last year's test, and what the physician thinks about it. Often, keeping patients in the dark will just spur them to call in to get the information, which can tie up your staff.

The several ways to manage test results better described in depth in Chapter 10, "Managing Test Results" will also reduce your practice's volume of incoming telephone calls. Tips for doing so that are described in that chapter in more detail include:

➤ Being proactive about notifying patients of results instead of telling them to call your practice after a few days to check;

➤ Setting realistic expectations about when patients should expect to hear about results;

➤ Assessing patients' expectations about how they would like to be notified about results;

➤ Improving communications and coordination with referring physicians who also may communicate to patients about their laboratory, imaging, or other diagnostic testing;

➤ Implementing an automated telephonic- or Web-based test result retrieval system for patients to securely access their results; and

➤ Integrating the test results notification process with patient education to head off many patient questions.

No matter what the system, make sure that you employ a staff that understands the importance of results – and why it's critical not to miss any. A staff that recognizes the implications of results falling through the cracks is the perfect addition to any test results management system you deploy.

Reduce unnecessary clinical calls

Looking for ways to reduce unnecessary follow-up telephone calls from patients without alienating them? Do a better job of anticipating – and answering – patients' questions before they leave the office.

Rural physicians and physicians who cover call on weekends or evenings are not the only ones who spend too much time answering telephone calls about non-urgent clinical questions. Studies show that up to half of the calls a medical practice receives about clinical matters come from patients who were just seen in the office. Many times, these patients ask for information they should have received – and probably did receive verbally – during a recent office visit.

Use the sample Incoming Clinical Calls Log (see Exhibit 3.6) to track incoming clinical telephone calls for several weeks. The information from this log will help you improve patient-physician communications, reduce the volume of incoming clinical telephone calls to your practice, and enhance patient education.

 STEPS TO GET YOU THERE

Follow these steps for best results:

1. Ask everyone in your practice who handles clinical calls to use the Incoming Clinical Calls Log.

2. Record the general purpose of each patient's call, the date of the call, and the date of the last appointment.

3. Keep the logs for a few weeks, then review the entries in the "Reason for Call (Summary)" column. Group the frequently

EXHIBIT 3.6   Incoming clinical calls log

Incoming clinical calls log

Date	Nurse initials	Time	Date of previous appt (Ask patient or look up)	Was the patient's appt within the last week? (Y/N)	Reason for call (Summary)

asked questions into basic categories. For example, a surgical practice may be able to group patient questions into:

➤ Preoperative instructions: "Can I take my hypertension medication the day before surgery?"

➤ Postoperative wound care: "What do I do if it's been three days since the surgery and the site is still tender?"

➤ Logistics: "What time should I be at the hospital?"

➤ General questions: "Can I drink a beer with this medication?"

4. Count the patient questions in each category.

5. Note the time elapsed since the patient's last appointment and highlight those received within one week of the patient's last appointment.

6. Review the results with the physicians and clinical assistants. Look for patterns. Note which categories had the most questions and which questions are asked most often.

7. Discuss how your practice can proactively educate your patients about the frequently cited categories and pay particular attention to the questions asked by patients who were just seen in the office.

8. Perform the call logging exercise biannually and look for other trends.

9. Seek solutions such as:

➤ Placing the answers to frequently asked questions on your practice Web site;

➤ Directing patients to your Web site for test preparations, preoperative instructions, and other common, standard information;

➤ Asking patients during or at the end of the appointment if they have questions about the visit and the care provided;

➤ Developing a "Q&A" for the diagnoses or services provided most frequently to your patients;

➤ Purchasing or developing videos or brochures that describe the treatment plans your physicians use most often;

➤ Offering patients a handout with Web sites, support groups, or other resources that you recommend;

➤ Proactively addressing side effects of medications, procedures, or treatments; and

➤ Developing an action plan for patients regarding the treatment and presenting it to patients in a notebook that includes a log for patients to use to record details about their care.

It may seem impossible to ask your clinical staff to spend more time teaching patients but improving in-office written and verbal communications will reduce incoming call volume. You could see the results in just a few weeks. Your patients will be better educated and more medically compliant, and your practice will operate more efficiently.

What time is your callback?

If patients need to speak directly with the physician and you can't accommodate the time in your schedule, consider scheduling patients for their telephone callbacks. Designate time each day that your physician will be available for telephone consultations. This will maximize the physician's time and improve the relationship with patients. Plus it helps everybody avoid the annoying game of phone tag.

Only implement this process if you've exhausted the possibility of creating face-to-face access.

Billing and referrals

How can you reduce telephone calls from patients with billing questions? Review your billing statements. Can you understand them? Your statement might read, "insurance pending." *You* know that means you've sent a claim into the patient's insurance company but the patient is left with the impression that the insurance coverage may be in jeopardy. Assuming their coverage is "pending," confused patients will call. If you can't understand your own statements or realize that they could easily be interpreted incorrectly, rest assured that your patients are having problems. Revising statements for better clarity will reduce the number of information gathering, non-collection telephone calls to billing staff, and help you redirect your staff to improve collections.

Give your billing and referral department their own telephone numbers. Print those numbers on billing statements so patients can call them directly. Set up an e-mail account (billing@yourpracticename. com) to improve access to your billing staff.

Establish bill payment online for patients to be kept informed of their balances and submit payment.

Anticipate general information requests

The time that your staff spends on the telephone with new patients who need directions to the practice can be reduced by directing patients to your Web site. Include a map of driving and parking directions in the languages that accommodate your patient population. As patients can be late or totally lost with inaccurate directions, be sure to have several people unfamiliar with your location test your directions before posting them. And don't forget to include information about public transportation if needed.

Your Web site should also display hours of operation, financial policies, locations, directions, services, etc. Patients who have easy access to this information won't need to call you for it.

Take it up a notch

Don't stop with general information requests. Use your Web site to deflect other types of telephone calls:

➤ Appointment scheduling: Allow your patients to schedule directly online through software integrated with your scheduling module, or to make requests;

➤ Appointment reminders: In a secure environment and with the patient's permission, e-mail reminders to patients, enabling you to get requests for reschedules and cancellations with ease;

➤ Test results: With the patient's permission, post normal test results on a secure Web site to which you can direct patients;

➤ Prescription renewals: Accept requests for prescription renewals from patients via your secure Web site; and

➤ Forms: Automate your registration and medical history forms. Direct patients to your Web site to complete them, and integrate the forms' submission with your practice management system or simply allow them to be submitted electronically to your staff who will then manually review them.

Direct other tasks to the Internet. You will have the information you need to manage the task, and in writing, it's easier to distribute. Plus, you can perform these tasks during a slow period of operations.

Unnecessary clinical calls

You may be receiving calls about issues that need not be addressed via the telephone. For example, if you round at an assisted living facility, your practice may receive dozens of calls each week from the facility's staff reporting minor injuries that are not emergencies but which must be reported. Evaluate your "frequent callers." Maybe there's an alternative form of communication you can use that would still fulfill your obligation to be informed but would not require the synchronous communication of a telephone call.

Alternative forms of communication may include text paging, e-mail, or fax. In this example, ask the facility to fax or securely e-mail the non-emergency injury reports to you. Better yet, give physicians or nonphysician providers a way to access your EHR from the facility so they can instantly review, handle, and document the reports while they're at the facility itself (e.g., the assisted living facility). If you maintain patients' records on paper, store those records at the facility and assign a physician or nonphysician provider to review, handle, and document the calls at the facility. Either method will eliminate the administrative demands on the office staff to manage those messages.

You can't get rid of all of these inbound calls – don't even think that you can just tell patients not to call – but you can reduce the number of calls somewhat with a little effort.

Reduce the rework

There are many steps you can take to reduce telephone demand and improve your telephone operations, but the most important step of all is to actually do the work and do it right the first time.

Incorporate the idea of a "virtual" exam room into each physician's schedule. Using this concept, physicians do not go more than four encounters before they address any outstanding messages, required documentation, and paperwork. Visit this virtual exam room several times an hour; don't leave all of this work until the end of the clinic or at the end of the day.

If you make the virtual exam room concept part of your day, you will reduce the amount of recall and rework time that is now likely part of your evening ritual after the office closes. It puts an end to patients calling your practice multiple times and your staff spending all that time recording, filing, batching, and organizing messages and paperwork.

For more information about the virtual exam room, see Chapter 8, "The Patient Encounter."

By attacking the work before it attacks you, you allow your staff the opportunity to better help your patients and efficiently and effectively support the physicians as they see patients.

Inbound vs. outbound calls

Many of this chapter's recommendations won't eliminate communication with patients, but they can turn an inbound call that the patient (or other caller) initiates into an outbound call (one your practice initiates). Let's look at why changing the way the calls are made makes sense for patient flow.

Inbound call traffic, which is what we've come to rely upon, is more difficult to manage than outbound traffic. To understand why, consider three facts. First, you can rarely get the correct person right away to answer the call. This fact necessitates installing technology (automated attendants) and/or a live operator(s) to process and distribute calls. Either way, you are spending a pretty penny just to handle – not even answer – the call. Second, inbound calls cluster during times that also happen to be peak volume times in the clinic. Thus, rarely can resources be matched with the work (the call) without a significant opportunity cost. In fact, most practices end up dedicating more resources to manage inbound calls because it's too difficult to balance both. Third, the inbound calls must be processed blindly. Thus, when the call is received, staff must often pull a paper record or query an electronic record to determine the proper context of the call. Either way, there's a time delay – and a cost – to understanding the context of the call (and importantly, having the means to document it). Many practices have integrated EHRs just to decrease the handling time but either way, the person taking the call must take the time to review the context.

Before we identify which is better, consider an outbound call. The three challenges of the inbound call are now decreased to just one challenge – getting the patient on the line. A practice doesn't need an automated or manual telephone operator to place an outbound call. Outbound calls can be made during low times of work and you already have the information at hand. Outbound calling is efficient because you're in control of the work; an inbound telephone call controls you.

This is not to discount the challenge of reaching the patient but consider that most patients now carry their phones with them (cellular phones, that is).

Most importantly, what do our patients want? They want timely and accurate information. It's difficult to deliver those wants using our current processes. Wouldn't patients prefer that we call them before they have to call us?

If you don't make any outbound calls, your patients will surely call you. Get started on turning more inbound into outbound calls. It's more efficient – and better for your patients – for you to call them.

THINGS TO CONSIDER

Summary of strategies to reduce telephone calls

➤ Establish office workflow so that transfers are unnecessary to avoid non-value-added time for you and your patients.

➤ Set a policy regarding the timing of callbacks to avoid unnecessary repeat calls from callers waiting for a response.

➤ Train your triage nurse to schedule appointments to avoid sending the caller back to the scheduler.

➤ Schedule follow-up appointments within a reasonable timeframe at surgery scheduling and checkout to reduce future appointment calls.

➤ Don't reschedule clinics to avoid the administrative work of rescheduling appointments.

➤ Make appointment reminders to reduce calls from forgetful patients asking about an appointment's date and time.

➤ Allow your schedulers to schedule without needing to get every appointment approved.

➤ Manage the prescription process to reduce calls from patients and pharmacists.

➤ Promote your clinical team to patients so they can respond to their needs over the telephone.

➤ Place a call to patients after a procedure or surgery to proactively handle questions.

➤ Manage test results by effectively communicating to patients.

➤ Reduce clinical calls with proactive steps to educate patients before they call.

➤ Schedule callbacks to reduce telephone tag.

➤ Clarify billing statements and offer online bill payment to reduce billing calls.

➤ Anticipate general information requests to reduce calls about directions and policies.

➤ Handle information from frequent callers through other communication vehicles to reduce unnecessary calls.

➤ Enable your practice's Web site with a secure area to handle more functions, such as registration, appointment reminders, test results notifications, routine prescription renewals, and so on.

Technology and telephones

If you still find yourself frustrated by the inability to handle your call volume, it's an opportune time to evaluate your telephone system and its components. Your telephone information system may need new features or you may need to learn more about its existing features. A multitude of functional options is now available to practices to employ; let's review a few of the most popular.

KEY CONCEPTS

Telephone systems

Auto attendant: System that answers and routes calls after prompting callers. For example, "Hello, you've reached Anytown Medical Associates. If you know your party's extension, please dial it now. Please dial 1 for appointments, 2 for the nurse, 3 for prescriptions, and 4 for billing and referrals. Dial 0 or hold for the operator."

Automatic call distributor (ACD) or uniform call distribution (UCD): Software products that help telephone operators better manage incoming calls by distributing calls evenly to staff, pointing callers to specific functions (appointments, prescription renewals, etc.), and placing callers on automatic hold – "in queue" – until a staff member is available to take the call. ACDs or UCDs can be used in place of, or as a backup to your receptionist.

Call accounting: Software programs that capture, record, analyze, and organize call data. The information is stored in a database that can be queried for operator productivity, call abandonment rate, and other analyses.

Call forwarding: Allows you to program the system to ring elsewhere if a station is busy or a call is not answered within a predetermined number of rings. Some systems permit external forwarding; some forward only within the system.

Call hunt: Bounces incoming calls automatically to the next available (not busy) line.

Call park: Allows you to place callers "in orbit," removing them from general telephone traffic in order to alert employees that a call is waiting.

Call transfer: Allows calls received from internal or external callers to be sent from one telephone to any other within the system.

Caller identification (ID): Allows you to identify the caller's registered name and number.

Capacity: The number of telephones, lines, and software that a telephone system can handle. For example, a 24-port system can handle a combination of 24 lines and telephones.

Cellular telephone: A wireless telephone that can be transported with the user away from the docking station.

Central processing unit (CPU): The main cabinet that houses the system's intelligence and controls its activities.

Custom call routing (CCR): Enables you to design custom routing points for callers – a big plus offered by some auto attendants. For example, a caller can leave a message in a mailbox and then be routed to specific locations within a business.

Direct inward dialing (DID): Enables a caller to bypass the receptionist and go directly to the desired extension. DID trunks are assigned through the telephone company. Each trunk ordered has 24 associated telephones, each of which can be assigned to individual staff.

Integration: Combining telephone, fax, and e-mail functions into a single system.

Interactive voice recognition (IVR): Software that prompts callers for information by asking them to use their telephone keypads or, in some systems, utter certain phrases in response to automated questions. IVR improves staff efficiency by routing callers to the appropriate staff based on information the caller provides.

Intercom: Enables you to ring another telephone within the system and talk internally without tying up an outside line.

Port: Point of connections in a system. Consider this the interface point at which programs are routed into the telephone system. A two-port voice-mail system enables two activities; a four-port voice-mail system allows four; an eight-port, eight. Ports are avenues that are open for travel once connected to a CPU.

Predictive dialer: A computerized system that automatically dials batches of telephone numbers for connection to staff. These systems adjust the calling process to the number of staff it anticipates (or predicts) will be available when the calls being placed are expected to be answered. The predictive dialer discards unanswered calls, engaged numbers, disconnected lines, answers from fax machines, answering machines and similar automated services, and only connects staff to the calls that are actually answered by people.

Remote notification: A pager or cell telephone notifies the user that there is a voice-mail message.

T1: A digital transmission link with a capacity of 1.544 Mbps (1,544,000 bits of data per second). T1 normally can handle 24 simultaneous voice conversations or data links over two pairs of wires, each one digitized at 64 Kbps. This is accomplished by using special encoding and decoding equipment at each end of the transmission path to multiplex one circuit into 24 channels.

Telephony: The use or operation of an apparatus or device for the transmission of sounds between distinct, separate points (can be with or without connecting wires).

Traffic: The number of users on a call.

Trunk: A line or telephone number.

Voice over IP (VoIP): Also referred to as IP telephony and Internet telephony, technology that enables routing of voice conversations over the Internet or any other IP network. The voice data flows over a general-purpose packet-switched network, instead of the traditional dedicated, circuit-switched voice transmission lines.

Wireless telephone: A portable telephone that can fully integrate into your system, but which can be used from anywhere in your office.

Voice mail: Use it – don't abuse it

Used correctly, voice mail is a wonderful tool that speeds work flow, saves time, and makes maximum use of human resources. But if you aren't careful, voice mail can waste staff time, frustrate patients and referring physicians, and destroy your practice's service reputation.

Is voice mail a time-saver or time-waster in your practice? It's likely the latter if this 12-step scenario sounds familiar:

1. A patient calls your practice.
2. The receptionist who answers asks the caller to briefly describe the problem or question.
3. The receptionist transfers the patient to the correct staff member.
4. Unfortunately, that staff member is elsewhere so voice mail answers the call.
5. The caller again describes the inquiry to the voice-mail box.
6. Sometime later in the day, your nurse finally dials into the voice-mail system.

7. The nurse enters a password.

8. Then, the nurse wades through a menu of options, such as, "Press 1 for new messages" and "Press 2 to hear saved messages."

9. The nurse listens to the patient's inquiry (often, a lengthy message) and takes notes.

10. The nurse writes down the patient's telephone number usually given at the very end of the message and then saves or deletes the message from the system.

11. Then, the nurse calls the patient (add at least one more step if the nurse decides to assign the callback to someone else) but the patient is not at the callback number. The nurse leaves a message.

12. Eventually, the nurse gets the patient on the line and the entire inquiry is repeated. By now, the patient has thought of a few more questions to ask.

Now, consider this alternative: the patient calls, asks a question, and you answer it. Sounds impossible but thousands of medical practices are handling patient inquiries in real time every day. Here's how they keep their voice mail from becoming a source of practice inefficiency.

Don't let staff use voice mail as a secretarial service. They may be on other calls but more likely they are just in the middle of another task or don't feel like responding. Some might even use voice mail to screen calls. Make a simple rule: Pick up the telephone if you're not already on another call; use voice mail only when you're not available. Using voice mail for time-shifting – batching return calls to be made on your own time – doesn't increase efficiency. You just end up busier than ever.

Set patients' expectations. Tell callers what information you need for each work process. Voice-mail greeting messages at referral desks, prescription lines, or wherever else you use voice mail to help handle volume spikes should clearly tell callers what information they need to leave.

Route calls into secure electronic messaging instead of voice mail. Instead of inviting patients to leave rambling voice mails, have operators take messages and route electronically to the correct staff for reply. Because the messages can be printed out or displayed on screen as text, they can be more easily shared and reviewed. In other words, you won't have to sit and listen to the entire voice message again just to review the facts.

Put the right staff on the telephones. Hire medical assistants (MAs) as operators. They won't replace your triage nurse but with protocols, scripts, and directions on how to take messages, MAs can be efficient screeners.

As you can see, voice mail doesn't always increase practice efficiency. Think of it more as a back up mechanism during peaks of heavy volume or special circumstances. Make voice mail work for you, not against you. Start answering the phones and start enjoying the benefits of getting work done in real time.

If voice mail is not designed and used properly, your loyal patients and referring physicians may quickly steer business away from you. If designed and used properly, it's a great way to improve the operation of your practice for certain functions.

Implementing voice mail the right way

If you are considering adding voice mail, first determine the needs and uses for it. Look at each area of your practice (billing, referrals, scheduling, staffing, etc.). Callers leaving a voice-mail message often expect a near-immediate response, especially if the question is urgent. Therefore, you may decide to give your billers voice-mail boxes, but not your nurses.

When choosing a voice-mail system, consider its reporting abilities. Sample activity reports should include the number of messages recorded, total length of messages, and average time before the message is deleted. These functions will help you monitor how your staff responds to messages from patients and referring physicians.

Also, consider how a voice-mail system indicates that a message is waiting. Is there a blinking light, an liquid crystal diode (LCD) display, or other visual cue to tell you that there's a new message in the system? Be sure that your system includes clear and succinct voice prompts that are user-friendly to internal staff members as well as to your patients and referring physicians.

Make sure that the system's port size and storage capacity are adequate for your needs. For example, how many messages can the voice-mail system hold? How long of a message can callers leave? What happens when the system is full?

Training is as important as the system itself. Is the vendor's training comprehensive yet quick and simple? You don't want your staff spending days and days trying to learn the system; the transition should be seamless.

WORDS OF WISDOM

Train, train, train

Training on your telephone system is just as important as training on your practice management system. Be sure to allocate enough time to orient and train new employees, as well as to educate everyone in your practice about system upgrades and other changes.

Of course, not everyone loves voice mail, even if you have the best intentions and it's installed properly. Like an auto attendant, a complex system can easily frustrate callers, especially if they are given too many options but not offered the option to reach a live operator.

Choose an integrated voice-mail system or one with interactive voice response (IVR) software that recognizes and adapts to usage patterns. Sophisticated IVR systems can route calls from one of your top referring physicians, for example, straight to your head nurse.

Callers and internal users should be able to locate their destinations easily in just one or two steps. Avoid a non-integrated system because it will not allow users to return to a menu after they leave their voice-mail message. As with a misused auto attendant, a non-integrated voice-mail system will bounce users from an extension where no one picks up, back to the greeting message, back to another unattended extension, back to the greeting, and so on – a potentially endless cycle, and one that could drive away patients and others.

In general, voice mail works best for the non-clinical functions of your practice, or at least those where there won't be an emergency that may lead to a bad outcome. These non-emergent uses for voice mail include billing, prescription renewals, referrals, and office management. Although calls to these areas should be answered promptly, setting them aside for a short period should not lead to a risk-management problem.

 WORDS OF WISDOM

Voice-mail tips

➤ Use voice mail to back up staff who are on the telephone or otherwise unavailable.

➤ Always offer a "live" operator option so patients and others can get immediate assistance if needed.

➤ Check voice-mail boxes frequently to ensure fast response.

➤ Consider voice mail more appropriate for billing, referral requests, and prescription renewals.

➤ Prevent risk management issues. Don't use voice mail to triage clinical calls.

THINGS TO CONSIDER

Don't send callers to telephone jail

Great management tools like telephone auto attendants can turn into weapons if you are not careful. I called a practice recently and heard this after the greeting:

Press 11 if you are a physician

Press 9 if you want to speak to the billing office

Press 16 for a referral

Press 15 to schedule an appointment

Press 7 to leave a message for the nurse

Press 19 if you need test results

Press 12 if you need a prescription refill

If you know the extension of the person you wish to reach, you can press that at any time

Press 10 to speak to an operator

What impression does this give a patient? Does it say that your practice is a warm and caring place? That the staff are efficient? Or does it say that visiting your practice is going to be like standing in line all afternoon at the Department of Motor Vehicles?

Auto attendants

Another telephone feature to consider is an auto attendant. An auto attendant is a call processing system that answers calls and assists callers. Callers can route their calls by choosing options such as, "Press one for the triage nurse," "Press two for the business office," "Press three for appointment scheduling," and so forth.

If unmanaged, auto attendants can backfire. Sometimes physicians react to the negative responses of what is often a small, but vocal, subset of patients by giving out their direct or "back line" telephone number. Before long, the "back line" becomes a main line. Thus, the cost savings of the auto attendant are never realized as the practice struggles to manage multiple points of telephone entry.

Although patients expect to encounter auto attendants when calling credit-card companies, banks, airlines, and government offices, they place higher demands on their physician's office. Patients interact with their physicians on a much more personal level than they do with their banks and are disappointed when it sounds like a computer is answering their physician's telephone.

Practices in rural areas and those with a large elderly patient panel overwhelmingly reject this technology because their patients feel it is impersonal and difficult to use.

If you decide to use an auto attendant, deploy it with caution. Though potentially helpful for improving office workflow and saving money, the technology has some drawbacks for medical practices that must be carefully considered.

First, analyze the investment that you are about to make in the product. Solicit feedback from your entire practice, as it will affect everyone from the receptionist to the physicians, as well as your patients. Ask: Will it save us money? Will it make our practice more efficient? Will it increase our response time to patients? Will it improve our ability to provide value to patients? If the answers to these questions are "no," then don't invest in an auto attendant.

Second, map your practice's workflow to ensure this new technology is used efficiently. Ensure that your callers will be responded to in a timely manner.

Third, carefully select the product and the vendor. Study the vendor's track record. Talk to several other practices that use the product. Negotiate a trial period to test the product, and don't skimp on service. Are all of these cautions really necessary? Yes! Your patients will never forgive you for losing their calls, and you'll put yourself into a risk-management situation.

Fourth, integrate the product. From day one, test it out yourself. Is it working? Spend a few minutes each day in your reception area asking patients for their opinions. Seek feedback from physicians and staff. Is it effective? Has it saved you money? Has it made your practice more efficient? Has it increased your response time to patients? Is your "return on investment" positive? Expect to use the system for at least six weeks before you see any impact.

If you have determined that the technology isn't right for your general number, consider its application for certain situations, such as in the business office, as a "back-up" for busy operators, for personal calls to employees, or for reaching a referral specialist.

Voice mail can be integrated with an auto attendant, allowing callers to leave a message at their chosen option if the requested staff member is unavailable. Essentially, the auto attendant takes the place of a receptionist routing calls to staff. If you choose this option, make sure it's user-friendly and allows your callers to choose "0" to reach the operator because some people prefer to speak to an operator or don't know which option they should choose.

WORDS OF WISDOM

Use auto attendants wisely

List no more than five options so callers don't loose track and patience.

Example:

1. Schedule an appointment
2. Speak with a nurse
3. Discuss your bill
4. Renew a prescription
5. Speak with an operator

Number options "1" through "5" and list in order

➤ Always provide the option of a live operator and make sure there is a live operator

➤ Before listing options, tell callers what to do if it's an emergency

➤ Don't use an automated voice, ask a staff member to record

➤ Deliver custom messages about your practice to callers while on hold or being transferred

➤ Use a system that allows you to see how long calls are waiting

➤ Test your system weekly

➤ Offer options to non-English speaking callers, depending on your patient population.

Automatic call distributors

An automatic call distributor (ACD) – or a product with similar functionality called a uniform call distribution (UCD) – system can serve as a mechanism to distribute calls more effectively within the practice. The ACD software recognizes busy lines and places callers in waiting lines, distributing the calls to specific lines when they come free. Essentially, an ACD creates the opportunity for you to better route, handle, and categorize calls. Be sure to understand the storage capabilities of the system and what happens to overflow.

WORDS OF WISDOM

What to look for in an ACD

➤ Expandability

➤ Flexibility

➤ Wallboard support (displays incoming calls on a visible LED)

➤ Operators can attach callers to an auto attendant

➤ Callers can opt in or out of "queue"

➤ Silent monitoring

➤ Operators can log in and out

➤ Report generator

Telephony applications

Telecommunications software products (referred to collectively as "telephony" are now readily available for use in a medical practice. These software products integrate with your practice management system and/or your telephone to replicate or back up services that your staff currently provides. For example, you can purchase a product that integrates with your practice management system (the scheduling module, in particular) to use the schedule for the following day to remind patients of their appointment – the software finds the telephone numbers associated with each patient's name.

WORDS OF WISDOM

Try these computer telephony applications

➤ Appointment reminders and confirmation

➤ Lab results reporting

➤ Patient account balances

➤ Patient educational material requests

➤ Pre-recorded patient instructions and explanations

➤ Prescription requests

➤ Staff notification

➤ Patient satisfaction survey

GETTING STARTED

Selecting or changing your telephone system

➤ Learn telephone system terms and procedures. Like health care, the telecommunications industry is full of acronyms and technical terminology. Knowing these terms will keep you on equal footing with your potential vendors.

➤ Learn the basic telephone equipment structure. Knowing the system's parts and features will help the process.

➤ Define your practice's needs. Review your existing system, as well as the features of the potential new system. Do you want voice mail, an auto attendant, automated call distribution, etc.?

➤ Involve your employees. Speaking with all of your staff to discuss specific needs, functions, and ideas for functionality will help you choose the right system for your practice.

➤ Gather information and proposals from vendors. Select three to five vendors to submit a request for proposal (RFP) for your telephone system. The more specific you are, the more information you will garner from the proposals.

➤ Deal only with quality vendors. The telephone is your main communication portal to external customers (patients and referring physicians), as well as your internal network. Taking risks on an inexperienced vendor is foolish and may cause harm to your practice.

Don't let your telephone system compromise patient confidentiality

If your practice provides services that may be considered sensitive (psychiatry, obstetrics, and infectious disease are a few that come to mind), consider blocking your practice's "caller identification (ID)" when calling patients. When you call patients to remind them of their appointment or report that their test results have arrived, your practice's name and number may appear on the recipient's caller ID display. This identification could compromise the patient's confidentiality if others in the household or business see it.

In addition to caller ID, consider answering your phones with the names of your physicians instead of the name of your specialty. For example, instead of using "Infectious Disease Consultants" in your telephone greeting, answer, "Drs. White and Smith." This will protect your patients' confidentiality in the case of "curious" family members or associates who redial your number from the caller ID.

While this concern may not be applicable to all types of medical practices or to all patients, keep in mind that some patients have higher demands for confidentiality. They may want to keep all of their medical affairs hidden from their family members as well as co-workers. If this is the case in your practice, be sure to ask your patients how best to handle communication from your practice. Put the request(s) in writing, with easy visibility in their chart. If you ask, you must be prepared to deliver without any mistakes.

No matter what features or applications you consider, keep in mind the needs of your patient population. Pay special attention to the design of an automated system if large numbers of patients are not used to dealing with automated telephones or do not speak English. Remember to look at your current processes first to change telephone demand, followed by enhancing your operations changes by employing technology to help you and your patients.

HIPAA and telephones

The Health Insurance Portability and Accountability Act (HIPAA) – requires that a "reasonable" effort be made to protect patient health information. HIPAA does not specifically address the role of telephones in a medical practice but does give guidelines that can be applied to the situation.

General: Base telephone policies on sound business practices, common sense, and the use and disclosure of the minimum protected health information required to perform the specific task.

Position of operators: Move telephone operators and triage nurses away from locations where other patients may easily overhear private information.

Reminder calls: Your Notice of Privacy Practices should include a statement that you may want to place appointment reminder calls. Considering including a consent form for reminder calls in new-patient registration materials. If a patient declines to allow you to make any reminders by telephone, respect this request. If patients agree to allow reminder messages to be left on their voice mail or answering machines, make sure staff know what information is to be included. HIPAA rules instruct us to limit information to the minimum necessary; but do not specify what should be included or excluded. Industry practice has been to limit the information to patient's name, date, time, and physician's last name. An example is: "This message is for Jane Doe. You have an appointment with Dr. Jones on Tuesday at 2 p.m." Do not include the specialty of your practice or the nature of the appointment.

HIPAA encourages physicians to be in communication with their patients and allows physicians to communicate minimum necessary information to family members or other caregivers as they see fit.

If your reminders are communicated through the mail, use these same guidelines about minimal information.

E-mail: You can send e-mail to patients, pharmacies, referring physicians, and others, but it should be encrypted. That is, both users will need to use the same encryption software and have a personal digital identification number. For most medical practices, a secure Web portal is the most manageable option. This option sends an e-mail to the patient that a message awaits, but the patient must log into a secure section of the Web portal to obtain the content of the message.

Text messaging and instant messaging: Experts do not consider either of these technologies fully secure in most environments. Avoid using either to communicate with patients.

Test results: Again, HIPAA doesn't specifically address test results, but sound business judgment would mean that you do not leave test results on a patient's voice mail, answering machine, or e-mail account without written permission obtained in advance.

Revisit these important issues on a quarterly basis to make sure that your telephone operations keep up with federal and state regulations.

Staffing your telephones

Your performance improvement initiatives and a better telephone may help you better manage your phones, but they won't ever end the volume of telephone calls – nor should they. Indeed, you'll always need staff to respond to calls. How many you need is the real question.

Before you add to your triage nurse staff, use the Incoming Clinical Calls Log to evaluate where calls could be avoided altogether by improving patient education while patients are in the office. Further, scrutinize the calls regarding issues that may have been better handled in the office face-to-face with a clinician. As patients seek more "telephone medicine" and only a handful of insurance companies reimburse for it, your practice is being stuck with the overhead. If the patient would be better off coming in, then go ahead and make the appointment.

STAFF BENCHMARKS

Practice operations task	Workload range
Telephones with messaging	300–500 calls per day
Telephones with routing (electronic system) only	1,000–1,200 calls per day
Telephone triage	65–85 calls per day

Forget trying to staff your telephones based on how many physicians they serve. The number you need depends on how many telephone calls need to be answered.

The workload range depends on patient population, information system, level of automation, and work processes at the practice. The more information you gather and/or deliver during each call (thus, the higher the transaction time), the lower the productivity you should expect.

Given the multitude of variables, measure the time it takes your staff to handle each telephone call and apply that transaction time to reach your practice's ideal workload range.

Estimate your staffing needs based on how you have configured your telephone operations and the benchmarks listed above. Don't ever take benchmarks at pure face value – if an operator must walk from the desk to deliver every message to the nurses' station, for example, then adjust the benchmark accordingly.

A warning about staffing your phones: telephone staffs, like all of us, have a tendency to pace their work to match the demands of the moment. For example, a busy orthopedic surgery practice looked for ways to reduce staff. During its telephone analysis, the practice realized that the volume of incoming telephone calls was much greater on Mondays, then decreased as the week went on. However, on Fridays, even though the call volume was lower, the operators' time on the telephone was higher per call. Staff complained that they needed more help. But when the orthopedic practice analyzed the situation, the results were surprising. As the phones rung less, the staff talked longer. The operators spent 25 percent more time per call on Fridays because they expanded their efforts to match the demands of the moment. Since there were more moments (and fewer calls), there was more talking (see Exhibit 3.7).

This is a natural phenomenon, but it's often hidden. Even the manager thought that the practice needed another operator. You can't do much to prevent the expansion-of-effort phenomenon, but don't let it lead you to increase overhead unnecessarily. In this example, the orthopedic practice simply hired another operator to work on Mondays, thus saving more than 80 percent of the cost of a full-time employee because the part-time worker did not receive benefits.

After-hours telephone protocols

Most medical practices contract with an answering service to manage after-hours calls. If you do, be sure that your service's message taking is exceptional and that your practice receives all communications in writing as a record in a timely manner.

EXHIBIT 3.7 **Staffing to call volume**

Day of week	Operator time (mins)	Phone volume	Seconds per call
Monday	1,149	1,200	57.5
Tuesday	677	700	58.1
Wednesday	512	650	47.3
Thursday	479	620	46.4
Friday	701	589	71.4

Orthopedic Surgery Consultants

Operator time (mins)   Phone volume   ---■--- Seconds per call

You aren't, however, legally required to have an after-hours service. (Notably, this advice isn't applicable to some specialties, such as trauma surgeons and emergency medicine physicians, for obvious reasons.) Record a message to your patients that your office is not open. Encourage them to leave a voice mail message if they want your staff to have some information the following day. Offer your cell telephone number for use with emergencies only. Most physicians find their patients very respectful of their time, and the cost savings is indeed significant.

A final word on telephone management

Managing telephone demand is not a one-time solution. It's continuous. Evaluate technology and staff costs each year. Improving the management of the processes that drive telephone calls will cut the volume of unnecessary ones, reduce your overhead and staffing costs, and increase patient satisfaction.

If the telephones were cited as a satisfier for patients, we'd have no compelling reason to change. But when practices reach out to the voice of the customer, the voice rings clear: "I hate your phones." Although we often blame the system itself; it's time to recognize that it's not just the system. It's the processes that we've set up, and it's time to change them.

CHAPTER 4

Scheduling

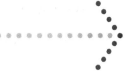

Key Chapter Lessons

➤ Evaluate your scheduling process

➤ Learn common scheduling methodologies

➤ Identify scheduling bottlenecks to make improvements

➤ Extend your hours to improve patient access and your bottom line

➤ Discover the benefits of group visits

➤ Use your Web portal to perform online visits

➤ Evaluate same-day appointment requests

➤ Use advanced access to make your day run smoother

➤ Integrate staff resources with your appointment schedule

➤ Understand scheduling fluctuations and how to measure them

➤ Recognize the root causes of "no-shows" and how to reduce them

➤ Examine "bumped" appointments and their financial effect and how to avoid them altogether

➤ Learn to conduct the surgery and procedure scheduling process more effectively

➤ Identify the steps to facilitate appointment recalls and appointment reminders

Scheduling: the key to better patient flow

Here's a quick quiz based on chapters one through three of this book: what's your practice's most valuable asset? It's your physicians. Or, to be more precise, it is their time.

One of the most critical components to managing clinical office time well is your appointment scheduling process. So, in addition to embracing the concepts of lean thinking (Chapter 1), cleaning up your time management act (Chapter 2), and handling your telephones better (Chapter 3), take some time to conduct a thorough evaluation of your appointment scheduling system. Poor scheduling can cost your practice money: fewer patients are seen and the physician's valuable time is wasted.

Figure out if your scheduling process is maximizing your time or wasting it . . . and frustrating patients – and you.

GETTING STARTED

Do you need to rethink your scheduling process?

➤ How many staff members must patients speak to when trying to schedule appointments?

➤ How long must patients wait on hold when they call to schedule an appointment?

➤ How many times are patients trying to schedule appointments put on hold and transferred to other staff?

➤ Do schedulers have to ask nurses or physicians for permission before scheduling patients?

➤ Do last-minute cancellations and no-shows continually play havoc with the practice's daily schedule?

➤ Do physicians run on time some days but get completely behind on other days for no apparent reason?

➤ Do you have trouble making room for patients' acute requests?

Scheduling methods

To start, let's get the basic scheduling methodologies down. Medical practices use three general methods of scheduling: single interval, multiple interval, and block (or wave) intervals. In brief, these methods operate as follows:

Single intervals: Each visit receives the same amount of time on the scheduling calendar, regardless of the type of visit (new or established) or chief complaint (health check or asthma). An example is scheduling all appointments on the quarter hour.

Multiple intervals: The intervals between appointments depend on the type of visit or the patient's chief complaint(s). For example, an acute care visit with a single complaint would receive 15 minutes on the scheduling calendar while a new patient visit would be given 30 minutes.

Block (wave) intervals: There is a single block of time for multiple appointments regardless of the type of visit or the patient's chief complaint. For example, all 12 morning appointments are asked to present at 9:00 a.m. and are seen in some predetermined order until the end of that morning's clinic.

THINGS TO CONSIDER

Communicating to your new patient

When patients call for an appointment, that's your chance to introduce your practice – and make the best impression.

Take the initiative and consider:

➤ Asking patients who referred them

➤ Indicating the length of time a patient can expect to be at your office for the appointment (overestimate and never offer this information if you can't beat it)

➤ Mentioning the contingency plan for contacting patients if the physician must tend to an emergency (and make sure you get the their contact information)

➤ Asking patients how they would like to be addressed at your practice

➤ Reminding patients of any dietary or other preparations for the visit

➤ Describing the practice's policy regarding patient payments at the time of service

➤ Telling patients that you look forward to seeing them at their upcoming visit

➤ Directing patients to your Web site or portal for more information about the practice

➤ Thanking patients for choosing your practice

Getting these points across early helps reduce misunderstandings and, ultimately, helps patients get more value from their visit to your practice.

Simpler scheduling

Your practice probably has different types of appointments that run different lengths. Some medical practices take this multiple-interval approach to scheduling to an unnecessary extreme. They have dozens – if not hundreds – of appointment types. Their staff spends precious minutes trying to determine if the patient fits into a "return-acute long" or a "return-acute medium" slot. A colleague of mine visited a practice that had appointment slots for "short," "short-short," "short-short-short," "long," "long-long," and "long-long-long" appointments. Of course, when the patient adds more detail to the complaint or comes up with a new complaint, the patient no longer fits neatly into one of these categories and the day's scheduling house of cards topples.

A practice with a scheduling system that is too complex soon learns that patients are good at gaming the system to get in. They don't want to get a short timeslot or be rejected altogether, so they learn the buzzwords to get past the staff-gatekeepers and in to see the physician. This nonsense is not only frustrating to the patient, it's costly to you. Your clinical staff cannot prepare appropriately for a patient encounter based on a misleading chief complaint.

Our complicated system of appointment types also creates extra overhead that adds little to no value to the practice. What does the patient care if the appointment is a "long" or a "long-long-long?" The patient doesn't – and just wants to be seen. So, why spend hours developing, maintaining, and training staff on appointment types that rarely accomplish the goal of predicting the length of the appointment? It makes no sense.

Release your practice from the burden of a complicated scheduling template. Simplify the scheduling model. Limit appointment types to as few as possible. Many physicians are scheduling office appointments in three basic categories:

➤ Short (usually for established patients);

➤ Long (usually for new patients and complex established patients); and

➤ Procedures.

There may be exceptions to this simplification, but don't let the exceptions take over the process.

If you adopt a simple schedule, you'll see more patients, reduce your staffing costs, and have less frustrated staff.

THINGS TO CONSIDER

Too many appointment types

I visited a practice that had 1,100 different appointment categories. Seriously! The schedulers had thick notebooks with instructions about each appointment type that they had to consult with every time a patient called. The system never worked as planned because few schedulers stuck around for very long. Not only were the salaries low but schedulers had to bear the brunt of physicians' and patients' frustrations when the scheduling process inevitably broke down.

Make sure that you haven't given your schedulers an impossible job.

Modified wave

Some medical practices combine a simple section with a twist to block (or wave) scheduling by using a modified wave approach.

In this approach, a long or complicated patient visit is scheduled at the same time as a visit of shorter duration. This intentional double booking can allow the physician to begin performing the short visit while the clinical assistant prepares the longer visit. For example, scheduling a well-woman visit and a sore throat patient to both begin at 9:00 a.m. allows the patient getting the well-woman check-up time to undress, weigh in, and do other intake activities under the direction of the physician's clinical assistant. Meanwhile, the physician handles the acute visit patient whose visit is shorter.

The modified wave approach helps when a practice is plagued by patients who fail to show for appointments. It could schedule several patients at the top of each hour. (If the practice usually saw one patient every 15 minutes, then four or more patients could be scheduled at the top of the hour, depending on the practice's no-show rate.) If one of those four or five patients didn't show up, there would be no negative impact on the physician's productivity at all. Even the patient seen at the end of the hour would have waited only 45 minutes, perhaps less. Although that long of a wait is not enviable, it is often the *average* wait time seen in practices that are struggling with high rates of no-shows.

During some hourly blocks, the physician may be able to get ahead of schedule to start using the "virtual patient" concept described in Chapter 8, "The Patient Encounter," or even see one of the patients from the following hour who happened to show up early.

Try modified wave scheduling (or any of the other techniques described in this chapter) for a month. Like many operations improvement initiatives, if it doesn't work – if it isn't producing value for patients and providers – you can always go back to the way you've always done it.

THINGS TO CONSIDER

Treat your schedulers well

It may be time to take a hard look at your schedulers' working conditions. Do they:

- ➤ Work in a crowded, unpleasant space?
- ➤ Have to get up every five minutes to ask physicians for permission to make appointments?
- ➤ Struggle with an inefficient scheduling system or outdated software?
- ➤ Receive disrespectful treatment from physicians and staff?

If you answered yes to any of these questions, then get to work to improve your most valuable scheduling resource: your schedulers. They are the *sales representatives* of your practice. Give them appropriate pay, a respectful work environment, and the tools they need to perform their jobs. They'll stick around longer – and keep your practice on track.

Clustering

Some specialists supplement their scheduling methodology by clustering patients with similar complaints or services. A surgeon performs post-operative clinics; an obstetrician sees prenatal patients; or a multidisciplinary team of specialists treats transplant patients. Clustering promotes efficiency by using the same processes, supplies, equipment, and often, mindset.

Clustering makes good sense for many practices, but make sure that it doesn't limit your availability to patients. If your post-operative clinic is only held on Tuesday afternoons, you may have difficulty accommodating many of your patients.

Clustering makes great sense when there are multiple providers that a patient needs to see in concert. A liver transplant patient, for example, may need to see a transplant surgeon and a hepatologist; a breast cancer patient may need to see an oncologist, breast surgeon, and radiation oncologist. To the extent possible, these appointments should be coordinated – commonly called "complex scheduling" – not only to give more convenience to the patient but also to facilitate communication about the patient's care.

Group visits

Take a creative approach to scheduling. One way to boost both collections and patient satisfaction is to try group visits. During group visits, physicians can see six to 12 patients at once. Instead of a traditional 20-minute encounter with one patient (four hours to see 12 patients), a physician can see 12 patients in just 60 to 90 minutes. Of course, you'll need a practice site with a room large enough to comfortably accommodate 10 to 15 patients. Because group visits are especially successful when held outside of traditional office hours, you'll also need a building that is accessible in the evenings or on weekends.

Group visits work well for certain types of patients who need partic- ular services. But look around. There may be many of these patients in your practice. In a group visit for diabetic patients, the physician can explain the condition to 10 patients at once instead of 10 differ- ent times during the week. This leaves additional time for patients to discuss more individualized issues during one-on-one visits with the physician.

Since group visits can include nonphysicians, such as nurse practi- tioners, dieticians, or counselors, patients can get more education from different experts. Many patients find group visits supportive because they are with others who have similar complaints or condi- tions. Sometimes, the supportive environment allows physicians to address sensitive concerns that a patient might feel too embarrassed to bring up during a one-on-one visit.

Rightly so, group visits may raise concerns about patient privacy, as well they should. Since patients may ask questions or provide com- ments in a group – and other patients will hear about their medical condition – make sure that your practice has a confidentiality waiver agreement in place.

 WORDS OF WISDOM

Confidentiality in group visits

Patients have expectations of privacy and confidentiality when they visit your practice, regardless of whether it's for a group visit or a one-on-one visit with a physician. Even though you ask group-visit patients to sign confidentiality waivers, advise them that your practice respects patient privacy and they should, too. Tell group-visit patients that they are not expected to share with the group any personal information that they would want only a doctor – and no one else – to know.

Explain to group-visit patients that anything they learn about individual group members should not leave the room. Remind patients that respect for the privacy and opinions of others are what make the group visit work. Finally, and most importantly, never force a patient to have a group visit in lieu of a one-on-one visit. Offer it as an option and let the patient make the choice.

KEY CONCEPTS

Drop-in medical group appointments (DIGMAs)

The DIGMA is a variation of the group visit and is based on a concept developed by Edward B. Noffsinger, PhD, at Kaiser Permanente in the 1990s. The visits are set up by appointment and scheduled weekly or twice monthly. Unlike group visits, which may focus on one disease or condition, DIGMAs tend to be open to patients with different diagnoses. These visits often run 60 minutes, instead of the 90 minutes or more, typical of the group visit, and can more easily be held during regular hours and in smaller facilities.

To set up a DIGMA, invite patients to "drop-in" for an office visit at a specific time. The only criterion for participation is to be on the physician's panel. In this approach, a physician and another nonphysician health professional lead the visit. Since the group meets at the same time and day each week, patients may drop-in when they choose. However, ask patients to register in advance so that their charts are reviewed before they arrive. This type of visit works well for patients with chronic diseases that have a great need for information and support.

Group visits are easy to schedule. Choose a common condition –
asthma, diabetes, arthritis, chronic obstructive pulmonary disease,
obesity, to name a few – shared by many of your practice's patients.
Or select a type of mandatory checkup such as nine-month well-
child visits. Ask 15 to 20 patients if they'd like to have their next
visit in a group setting; expect five to 12 positive responses but stop
asking when you reach your pre-determined limit. Explain the concept to them face-to-face, in a brief phone call, or write a statement
detailing the benefits of a group visit. Emphasize how they can benefit from interacting with other patients and, if applicable, the other
clinicians who will assist.

The group visit should be offered as an option or an enhancement
to one-on-one care. Ask interested patients to sign a statement
describing the visit's protocols and return the form to you to indicate they will attend the session.

Some practices target high-risk patients on the theory that the additional support will be helpful. However, if these patients are at risk
because they are unmotivated or have other issues that reduce their
medical compliance, then don't expect all of them to attend group
visits. Likewise, transportation problems, distance, hearing difficul-
ties, or language comprehension may cause some elderly, rural,
needy, or foreign-born patients to avoid group visits. Consider these
issues if group visits do not perform as expected.

Register patients prior to the visit, and review their charts ahead of
time. During the sessions, which might last up two or more hours
on a weekday evening, ask two clinical assistants to record each
patient's vitals and chief complaints privately in nearby exam
rooms, just as they would during a regular patient visit.

Next, gather the patients in a conference room to hear the physician
present a 5- to 10-minute presentation on relevant medical issues.
Then, clinical assistants escort the patients to exam rooms one-by-
one for their physical exam by the physician.

While patients wait their turn to see the physician, they can ask questions of an educator – your dietician, for example – or talk to other patients who have similar problems. A clinical assistant can take blood or complete other orders during this time, too.

After completing the physicals or exams, the physician returns to the group to answer patients' general questions and wraps up the session.

There's no easy way to bill for your group visit services. Establish a dialogue with the insurance companies with which you participate to discuss coding and reimbursement for group visits.

Many practices find that serving a light, healthy meal helps improve evening attendance, so they charge a modest fee to cover the catered food.

Group visits are a "win-win" for your practice and your patients. It doesn't hurt to try them – it only takes a little time and effort for your practice to test the concept.

 GETTING STARTED

Group visits

- ➤ What will the criteria be for the group?
- ➤ When will the group be held?
- ➤ How will we inform our patients?
- ➤ How will we make the appointments?
- ➤ Where will we hold the group visit?
- ➤ Do we need adjoining exam rooms?
- ➤ Who will "host" the visit?
- ➤ Will guest speakers attract patients?
- ➤ Can we serve a light meal?

➤ When and how will we review patients' charts?

➤ How and when will we register the patients?

➤ How will we document the visit?

➤ How will we code and bill for the visit?

. . . .

Extended hours

Another value-added scheduling technique is a simple one: open your practice beyond what are considered regular office hours. Extend office hours into the evening, weekends, or open early in the morning. Extended-hours care has been met with appreciation from patients (and parents) who can receive care without missing work.

Practices in urban areas often find patients respond enthusiastically to an early start time, evening hours, or weekend clinics. It helps patients reduce their time off work and avoid rush hour traffic. Many physicians and staff also eagerly switch to earlier or later hours just to reduce commute times.

Plus, if structured correctly, these odd hours can allow a full-time physician or staff member to work 40 hours a week but also have a half-day or even a full day off.

In addition to providing access for patients, the practice can benefit financially from after-hours clinics.

Extended-hours care can result in physicians receiving fewer non-emergency calls in the middle of the night or on weekends. The practice increases revenue because physicians usually cannot bill insurance for giving advice over the phone, no matter how late at night it is. With extended-hours clinics, patients can be seen face-to-face. In addition to being a billable event, patient care is improved because there is physical contact with the patient.

Seeing patients early in the morning, during the evening, or open-ing on weekends doesn't result in an additional rental fee from your landlord. You've already paid for the facility, so keeping it open doesn't cost a dime extra for building expenses. Extended-hours care enables a practice to use the space it already has, and many other fixed costs (i.e., malpractice, information systems, etc.), which have already been paid.

If your practice is constrained by or running out of space, extending hours is a proven solution to "create" more space. (Of course, don't forget that scheduling through the lunch hour allows your practice to take advantage of often-empty exam rooms.) Extended hours offer the opportunity to increase your per-visit revenue. Several bill-able procedure codes relate to extended-hours care; evaluate the opportunity for your practice to be reimbursed an additional fee over and above the normal office visit allowable.

In sum, patient visits billed during extended hours have a higher contribution margin.

Extended hours aren't just for primary care practices; they can work for many other specialties. It's another way you can make it possible for patients to pull the value to them based on their needs and preferences.

To run a successful extended-hours clinic, you must carefully match your practice's physician supply with your patient demand – a diffi-cult task. Above all, you must remain flexible.

Measure demand for extended hours. Do a rough estimate of your patient population's demand for an extended-hours clinic, the num-ber of staff you'll need and the hours the clinic should remain open to achieve its full potential.

> ➤ To estimate demand, log the appointment requests you
>   receive during regular office hours that you cannot accommo-
>   date. Include any calls that you resolve via telephone triage

but could be done in person had there been a slot. Since many patients won't call because they know you're not open, you'll have to estimate how many other requests you might receive. Include your patients in your fact-finding process by asking if they would use your extended hours.

➤ Multiply your practice's average revenue per encounter by your volume estimate. The result is the estimated daily revenue from the extended hours. To get your average revenue per encounter, take your collections from the year prior and divide this number by your encounters for that year. It will likely be in the range of $50 to $200 per encounter.

➤ Contact the insurance companies with which you participate to determine their policy regarding reimbursing the after-hours fees, which are typically $25 to $35 in addition to the visit itself. Add the additional fees, if applicable, to the volume you estimate the insurance company will represent.

➤ Use the volume estimates to determine the hours and staff for your extended-hours clinic. If you estimate that only two patients will show up, start by extending your schedule one morning or evening a week. Staff a clinical assistant and receptionist to come 15 minutes before the first appointment (or stay through the last appointment). If you think that 100 patients will take advantage of an extended-hours clinic, you may need more days, staff, and physicians. Replicate your staffing from the "regular" day, but don't overstaff the extended hours. Encourage cross-training and try using staggered staff and physician schedules so you can operate the clinic with little to no additional overhead.

➤ Market your services. Send a postcard to all patients, or perform a target mailing to those who might be interested in your extended hours. Stuff an announcement in all patient statements, and post the fact on your Web site. Offer extended hours to patients scheduling follow-up visits. Don't be surprised that it will take a month or two for the word to get out that you're open. Re-evaluate after a month. If demand is higher than you estimated, then consider expanding hours or increasing the number of physicians.

Flexibility is key to the success of extended hours. There will be days when the schedule is full – or light.

The best part of extended hours is that you can try it once, and return to your normal hours if it doesn't work.

CASE STUDY

After-hours express clinic

Noticing an increase in same-day appointment requests during the winter months, Northeast Pediatric Partners initiated a fast-track clinic. The daily session, which they called "KidsExpress," was held each morning from 7:30 to 9:00 a.m. from January through March, and featured 10-minute appointment slots. One physician and one nurse practitioner handled each morning's session. The arrangement allowed parents to bring their children in for urgent problems. The rotating assignments allowed the physicians and nonphysician providers to work more flexible schedules. In addition, the physicians on night call received fewer calls from parents because they knew they could bring their child in the next morning. Finally, the burden of these sick visits, which are predictably higher during the winter months, didn't result in long waiting times and frustration for everyone during regular office hours.

Online consultations

To supplement face-to-face care, your practice can offer the option of online consultations, often called "virtual care", to patients. Consider one-time consultations, popular for specialty practices to offer to patients seeking second opinions. Or, develop a model for virtual office visits for your own patients to supplement your face-to-face encounters. Deliver care through a subscription-based model for patients who wish to have ongoing access to you, or provide one-time online visits. Online visits allow you to extend care when your practice's appointment schedule is otherwise full. Handle or triage minor-acuity, non-emergent problems or perform follow-up care. Supplement online care with video conferencing, recognizing that the user (patient) must have the capability on his end.

Although some insurance companies reimburse for virtual care, many consider online consultations to be non-covered services. Structure your payment mechanism appropriately, according to your contracts with the insurance companies with which you participate. If you collect from patients, be sure to do it upfront.

Regardless of the structure, make sure you are clear about how the service works and what's needed to complete the visit. For second opinions, it is likely that you'll need images, interpretations, pathology reports, and so forth.

Don't just dabble in virtual care. Develop the online consultation through a secure Web portal, with appropriate alerts about the timeframe for you getting back to the patient. Follow through on all requests.

Supplementing your in-office care with virtual visits differentiates your practice, extends a service to patients who are increasingly turning to the Web for their personal needs, and has the potential to improve your bottom line.

For more information on online consultations and other services a Web portal can offer, see "Chapter 12, Technology."

Same-day appointments

We'd like to give patients the swift service that our digital, instant access economy is conditioning them to expect. Although online consultations provide access when you're busy, don't consider that option as a substitute for face-to-face encounters with patients presenting with acute problems. To accommodate these patients, many practices do hold a portion of each day's slots until the day before or until the same day to accommodate last-minute requests for appointments. A few slots may be kept open in each physician's schedule and accommodated by a nurse practitioner or physician assistant or handled by the physician who is designated the "doctor of the day."

Assigning one physician as the "doctor of the day" – or the acute caregiver – is not an efficient way to make same-day appointments available. The inefficiency stems from the fact that physicians are now seeing someone else's patients and having to read someone else's notes, test results, treatment plans, and so forth. Depending on the specialty, the "doctor-of-the-day" may have to tell the patient to schedule another appointment with the regular physician because the fill-in doctor was only able to address the patient's most acute need. Many practices find that the "doctor-of-the-day" model simply delays when the patient sees his or her own physician; it doesn't actually satisfy the patient's demands.

No matter how you accommodate your appointment requests from patients with acute needs, you must consider the paramount question: How many appointment slots should I hold open each day to handle acute appointment requests?

Conducting an analysis of appointment requests and fulfillment will help you to determine how many appointment slots your practice needs to hold open. The analysis works for both the doctor-of-the-day model and the open access to all physicians model.

Use your practice's own data. How many requests for same-day appointments do you really have? How many of these requests does your practice fulfill? Track the number of each using a request and fulfillment analysis tracking form for at least a month (see Exhibit 4.1).

Track the peak days of the week and the month, as there is often variability among these. For example, practices often see an increased demand for acute visits on Mondays. Track requests by morning and afternoon, as they may vary as well.

You may notice seasonal trends. Pediatricians, family physicians, internists, allergists, and other specialists may need to adjust the number of walk-in and same-day slots seasonally to account for flu and allergy seasons and back-to-school physicals.

Use the 80-percent rule of thumb to dictate the number of slots to be held open. If the practice averages five same-day appointments a day, then hold four slots open during the day. Cancellations and no-shows can often create the additional slot that you will need. If your practice never has cancellations or no-shows, ignore the 80 percent rule and simply hold open exactly the number of slots you've determined in your analysis of demand. Be sure to repeat the analysis every year to make sure you're keeping pace with patient needs.

Also, look at how many same-day appointments you are contractually obligated to schedule. Some insurance companies may stipulate that their patients must be seen within 24 hours of request. Calculate the percentage of your practice's patients that fall under such rules. If it is 10 percent of the practice's patients, and each physician sees 30 patients on a normal day, then you may need to hold two or three slots open per physician. Consider the patient demographics of that payer, too. Average age will have an impact on the expected utilization.

EXHIBIT 4.1   Appointment request and
fulfillment analysis tracking form

Name: _____

Week: _____

Morning

	New patient			Established patient		
	Requests?	Fulfilled?	Percent	Requests?	Fulfilled?	Percent
Monday						
Tuesday						
Wednesday						
Thursday						
Friday						

Afternoon

	New patient			Established patient		
	Requests?	Fulfilled?	Percent	Requests?	Fulfilled?	Percent
Monday						
Tuesday						
Wednesday						
Thursday						
Friday						

In the "Requests" column, mark all requests for appointments by day of the week. Be complete; include requests you handled via telephone triage and referral to urgent care/emergency department. In the "Fulfilled" column, mark requests that you were able to accommodate as face-to-face appointments. Next, calculate your fulfillment rate – how many requests were fulfilled – by dividing the fulfilled column into the request column. If your rate is less than 100 percent, your practice has an opportunity to add value to patients by reducing barriers and improving access.

Advanced access

If you are frustrated by calculating the exact number of slots to hold open or if you find yourself trying to protect the last remaining slot from patients who don't "deserve" it, then you'll want to consider advanced access.

YOU KNOW...

...you are just protecting, not managing, the schedule when you tell patients:

➤ "Let me transfer you to the nurse who can help you with your [medical] problem over the phone."

➤ "Sounds like you need to come in, but let me check with the doctor."

➤ "Just how sick are you? How red is the blood? Is it really red, or is it brown? If it's brown, then it's old and we can see you tomorrow."

➤ "We can't see you, but you need to be seen, so go to the emergency room." [Of course, after seeing your patient, the emergency medicine physician often declares, "Call your regular physician to make an appointment about this issue!"]

Most often, there is little value to be gained from spending energy and time protecting your physicians' schedules. Do you think that an insurance company or a patient values this protection? Think again!

Advanced access is leaving your entire appointment schedule – except previously scheduled new patient and follow-up visits – open to patients who call with acute needs and want to be seen in short order. Patients see their own physician or, at least, their own care team, not a designated "doctor of the day." Advanced access can make your practice more accessible to patients, get new patients in faster, reduce no-show rates, and make the entire scheduling process run smoother.

Although it seems quite daunting for practices that routinely book appointment weeks – even months – in advance, advanced access is business as usual for many specialties. Consider what happens at an oncology practice. When a referring physician calls the oncologist with news that a patient has a large mass in her breast, does the scheduler at the oncology practice respond, "It'll be six weeks before she can get into see us"? Or, would a trauma surgeon ask the emergency medicine physician to hold the motor vehicle accident victim in the trauma bay for a few more hours? If they did, they'd be out of business – and may even have some malpractice cases on their hands. The point is that advanced access is a fancy term, but it simply means being able to accommodate patients when they – or their referring physicians – desire.

Advanced access, however, is more than just a scheduling methodology. It's a change of attitude, work style, and even culture. Practices with backlogs often carry the same backlog over time. If measured on January 1st, for example, the backlog of appointments is six weeks and measured again on July 1st, it's still six weeks. If the backlog is consistent, then the laws of supply and demand would empower us to say, why can't it be *zero weeks*, thus eliminating the backlog altogether? (See Exhibit 4.2.)

When a practice matures, the backlog of appointments often goes unchallenged. When a backlog becomes just part of the landscape:

- Staff spend more time attempting to determine whether patients who call in with acute needs "deserve" an appointment;
- Staff spend more time giving medical advice over the phone; and
- Staff have less time to assist the physician.

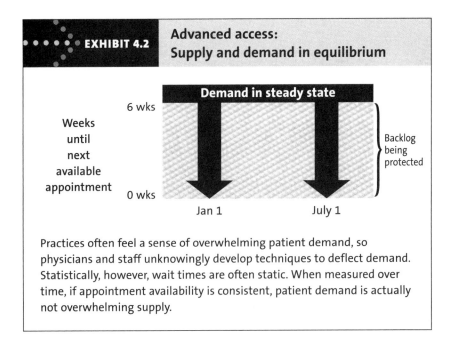

EXHIBIT 4.2 Advanced access: Supply and demand in equilibrium

Demand in steady state

Weeks until next available appointment

6 wks

0 wks

Jan 1 July 1

Backlog being protected

Practices often feel a sense of overwhelming patient demand, so physicians and staff unknowingly develop techniques to deflect demand. Statistically, however, wait times are often static. When measured over time, if appointment availability is consistent, patient demand is actually not overwhelming supply.

Some practices even revel in their backlogs, taking pride in lengthy appointment availability.

The activities resulting from backlogs are not reimbursed by our current payment systems; that is, neither insurance companies nor patients pay you for maintaining a backlog.

Of course, you welcomed those acute appointment calls when you first opened your practice but many practices shift focus as the practice matures. And that shift significantly hurts access, efficiency, and profitability.

As the waiting time grows, so too do your staff's attempts to control demand. The process of controlling demand consumes precious nursing resources in particular (in many practices, consuming all of them). Soon, patients become frustrated and no-show rates climb.

If you've moved from welcoming patients to protecting physicians from patients' demands, advanced access may be the solution for you.

Advanced access principles

The four principles of advanced-access scheduling are:

1. The continuity of the patient/physician relationship is fundamental to fulfilling the patient's needs;

2. Processing work on a real-time basis is critical to cost-effectiveness and efficiency;

3. Success in creating timely access requires a balance between physician supply and patient demand; and

4. When physician supply and patient demand are in equilibrium, the practice can accommodate all of today's appointment requests today.

Principle One: Continuity of the patient/physician relationship. This continuity is fundamental to fulfilling patients' needs. The disconnect occurs when patients who want to see "their" physician for acute visits are frequently scheduled to see a covering physician. Many patients end up seeing their chosen physician a minority of the time. If patients can see their own physicians, their demand for additional appointments often decreases. Moreover, patient satisfaction increases significantly.

Principle Two: Processing work on a real-time basis. Real-time processing is critical to cost effective and efficient operations. Delays create unnecessary expenses. Here's a way many practices cause unnecessary delays: patients' telephone messages are taken by an operator, the record is retrieved electronically or manually, evaluated by a medical assistant, reviewed by a physician, and return calls are made by a nurse. Often, the cycle repeats again and again before the patient's question is answered sufficiently.

This messaging process may take an hour, an entire day – or even multiple days – to complete.

Because it is difficult for patients to get timely access to care, or even get their telephone calls returned in a timely manner, many try alternative routes to get the care they want. Now, the practice has the additional burden of managing the alternative routes patients use to get care. More practice resources, including a great deal of administrative and clinical staff time, are spent on fulfilling patients' interim needs and deflecting their demand.

It is usually more efficient to schedule appointments when patients call rather than routing their requests through so many channels. Hand-offs and forms reduce the time that staff can productively spend in patient care (and billable activities). It is more efficient to spend time on patient visits instead of finding ways to keep them out of the practice.

Principle Three: A balance between physician supply and patient demand. In order to meet patients' demands, there must be a reasonable supply of physicians. If the physician's capacity is full, then supply and demand are out of balance. When the physician is at capacity and average wait times lengthen, a practice should consider ways to reduce demand or improve supply, such as improving efficiency in the office or recruiting an additional nonphysician provider or physician.

Principle Four: Accommodating today's appointment request *today*. When physician supply and patient demand are in equilibrium, the practice can accommodate today's appointment requests today. When demand truly exceeds supply, the amount of time to the next-available appointment increases over time. However, at many practices these access gaps remain consistent. That is, it took 45 days to see a new patient last March and 45 days this March. If the time of delayed access remains static (that is, demand is *not* growing faster than the supply of appointments), then process changes – not adding physicians – can reduce the time to the next-available appointment to zero days.

For more information on supply and demand, see Chapter 5, "Patient Access."

Backlogs develop over time and, in a way, provide comfort to many physicians because they perceive long wait times as indications of their popularity. Statistically, backlogs should be unnecessary if wait times are stable.

THINGS TO CONSIDER

Advanced access for specialists

If your specialty practice relies on getting referrals and needs authorizations before providing services, you may have to modify the concept of advanced access. Referral-dependent practices often need two or three days to get insurance companies' authorizations for referred patients. If so, consider those two to three days the equivalent of zero days when measuring the time to the next-available appointment.

Integrating advanced access scheduling

Educate stakeholders. Patients, physicians, and staff must believe in advanced access. Patients will be surprised to learn that they can be seen the same day they call for an appointment. Physicians will be anxious about having an open schedule when they walk in every morning. Staff may instinctively try to deflect demand for appointments to other days, thinking that this helps keep physicians' schedules open.

Work through the backlog. Your practice must first eliminate its backlog of patients waiting for appointments. If your time to next-available appointment is five weeks, it will take your practice at least five weeks, but possibly six weeks, to accomplish this objective.

WORDS OF WISDOM

Scheduling backlogs

Here are some tips to work through your scheduling backlog:

- Contact patients whose appointments are several weeks away, and open up an evening or two a week or on a Saturday to accommodate patients sooner.

- Try online visits. Determine if patients could be treated "virtually" and extend care through a Web portal for your practice.

- "Max-pack": Pull work into the day – if you see a patient who has a physical scheduled in two weeks, handle it today.

- Evaluate the scheduled follow-up appointments to find patients whom you could call and touch base with over the telephone instead seeing in the office.

- Look at what other members of the team could do. Could a physician assistant see some patients? Can a nurse screen patients over the phone before their visits? Can a follow-up appointment be replaced by an e-mail discussion?

- Consider group visits. A group visit will allow you to see more patients and achieve higher satisfaction in less time. (See the section on group visits.)

Whittling down your backlog takes physician and staff dedication but it can be done.

Develop an effective process for record retrieval. Because many patients are scheduled on a same-day basis, your records staff must be able to fulfill requests rapidly. An electronic health record makes this step easy.

Prepare for variability. Physicians and staff may have to stay late once in a while.

Plan for contingencies. What happens if patient demand exceeds physician capacity on some days? Do you have a back-up plan? Ask nonphysician providers to backup physicians when demand exceeds the availability of appointments. If your practice does not employ these clinicians, can a physician agree to take on the rare day when all of the physicians are overloaded? If you predict demand with accuracy, you won't need to access your contingency plan very often, but it's still good to have one.

Schedule patients with their chosen physicians. The continuity of the patient-physician relationship is essential to advanced access scheduling. Ask part-time physicians to team up to function as a full-time physician. Tell patients that the part-time physicians are now a team.

Empower staff to meet patient needs. For example, manage telephone messages on a real-time basis, instead of just handing callers off to other staff. The more times a patient is handed off, the greater the chances of miscommunication.

Speed internal communications. Invest in better communication systems and take other steps to improve communication between the front desk and the back office. Maybe you can rearrange space to put clerical and clinical staff in closer physical proximity, or collapse the two functions into one fully cross-trained team.

Eliminate appointment distinctions (i.e., routine versus urgent). Simplify the appointment template; the multitude of appointment types becomes irrelevant under advanced access.

Plan for the visit. At the time an appointment is scheduled, ask patients if there is anything that they need taken care of during the appointment. Seek accurate information at the point of appointment scheduling (e.g., liquid nitrogen to remove a skin tag). Ask, "Ms. Jones, to help Dr. Smith be prepared for your visit tomorrow; can you tell me what you are coming in for?" Look in the chart for needed preventive care, medication renewals, and so forth. Do tomorrow's work today; pull that work into today.

Complete the visit. Don't deflect work until later in the day. Dictate the note, finalize the paperwork, send the referral, or transmit the prescription to the pharmacy at the time the request or need arises. Consider the length of your appointments. Maybe you need to increase the spacing of appointments (for example, from every 15 minutes to every 20 minutes) if paperwork is included. Because real-time work is more efficient than batching work, you may actually reduce the total time you spend on paperwork by incorporating some of that time spent on paperwork into the patient's visit. In other words, do some of the paperwork with the patient in the exam room. It might just reduce the length of your workday.

Don't cluster follow-up visits. Schedule patients' follow-up visits as needed but if Mondays are busy days, then schedule follow-up visits on other weekdays.

Let patient demand manage physician supply, not the other way around. If 1,000 new patients sign up with your practice, seek temporary help immediately while you recruit a permanent physician to meet the increased demand. Schedule vacations in a similar fashion. The majority of your physicians should not go on vacation during the weeks or months that patient demand predictably peaks for your specialty (e.g., flu season for a primary care physician). You'll know there is an imbalance between your physicians' capacity and your patients' service demands when you see time-to-next-available-appointment numbers increasing.

Spread the word. Greet patients with information about your new advanced access scheduling policy so they won't be surprised when they can be seen quickly.

THINGS TO CONSIDER

Advanced access in a residency clinic

Advanced access can work in a residency clinic but with one caveat: Change the principle of a "physician/patient" relationship to a "care team/patient" relationship. Otherwise, full-time clinical faculty would find their schedules booked up. Meanwhile, residents who change rotations every few weeks and part-time faculty will be left with empty schedules. Establish a care team comprised of several faculty members and residents — at least one provider in the care team should be on site five days a week. Assign a nurse(s) to each care team. Name each team so that everyone, including patients, can readily identify the team. Using colors (e.g., red, blue, green) or other themes (e.g., river, mountain, desert) offers instant remembrance, and enables the practice to develop visual recognition, if needed, as well.

Next, apply the principles of advanced access to the care team. Schedule patients' acute requests with a care team using "care team blue" — versus specific physician — slots so that any team member who is available can perform the encounter while the team nurse(s) provides day-to-day continuity for the team.

Give each member of a care team a "business card" that prominently lists the contact information for the team members, including the assigned nurse(s). This will help the team build a relationship with patients and perhaps improve patient compliance with the physicians' medical plans.

WORDS OF WISDOM

Words of wisdom about follow-ups

Never schedule follow-up visits on Mondays unless the patient specifically requests it. Patients demand acute appointments after the weekend; be prepared for them.

The benefits of advanced access

Medical practices large and small that successfully implement advanced access reveal its benefits:

- ➤ Increase patient satisfaction;
- ➤ Enhance physician efficiency and satisfaction;
- ➤ Allow swifter service to meet our instant-access culture's demands;
- ➤ Fulfill patients' needs today;
- ➤ Decrease appointment no-show rates;
- ➤ Improve practice performance ratings by insurance companies that set access standards;
- ➤ Enhance coordination of care because patients see their own physicians;
- ➤ Enhance the practice's market position as access attracts new patients who could not get timely appointments with competitors;
- ➤ Improve providers' relationships with referring physicians;
- ➤ Reduce resources spent to create barriers to access the practice;
- ➤ Reduce malpractice risks because the practice isn't deflecting its patients' clinical problems;
- ➤ Reduce the time spent explaining poor access;

➤ Increase the level of work per visit (i.e., more relative value units (RVUs)); and

➤ Improve physician satisfaction because physicians see their own patients.

KEY CONCEPTS

Advanced access boosts RVUs

Advanced access helps physicians increase their production of RVUs because:

➤ More work is done during each visit;

➤ No-show rates decrease;

➤ More patients are seen – both new and established – because the practice is more efficient (e.g., nurses are nurses instead of deciding whether to schedule an appointment); and

➤ More surgeries and procedures are performed because there are more new patients, therefore, gross charges, collections, and income are higher.

Advanced access requires flexibility and preparation. Rigid scheduling templates aren't allowed and appointments scheduled today cannot become a crisis. Further, it will fail if your practice never gets through its appointment backlog.

Advanced access offers a useful solution to a problem that is growing worse throughout our nation's health care system. Implementation of advanced access is not effortless, but remaining focused on what your patients value will make the transition easier.

If implemented and managed properly, advanced access scheduling will boost your practice's operational performance, reduce risk, increase profitability, and keep patients coming back.

WORDS OF WISDOM

Words of wisdom about primary care panels and advanced access

For primary care practices, between 0.75 and 1 percent of your patients will seek care each day. If offered a same-day appointment, 75 percent of adults and 80 percent of children would accept it.

For a panel of 2,500 active patients, this means that 20 to 25 patients will seek care each day, whether on their own initiative or because you've scheduled a follow-up visit for them. Of course, this can fluctuate based on the severity of your patient panel, your follow-up protocols, and seasonal issues (flu season, school physicals, etc.).

Source: Mary Murray, MD

Monitoring advanced access

Monitor your access performance indicators closely. (For details on the indicators, see Chapter 5, "Patient Access.") If you have trouble accommodating patients' requests for appointments, check the following areas:

Follow-up visit protocols. Are physicians bringing patients back in out of habit? Can the nurse check on patients by telephone or via secure e-mail? Can patients be referred to a group visit instead of an individual appointment? Can the physicians do work today instead of three weeks from now? If so, they can likely bill for a higher-level visit *and* allow that future appointment slot to be taken by a new patient. For a specialist, can you establish protocols to offer appointments to patients you can treat? Or, offer a more detailed plan of care when transferring the patient back to a primary care physician?

(See the section on pre-appointment screening in Chapter 5, "Patient Access," for more information.)

Operational efficiency. Are you operating as efficiently as possible? Do you have supportive staff and facilities? Is everyone doing the right work the right way? Is your staff preparing for patients adequately so they don't waste precious time looking for the necessary supplies and equipment after the patient arrives? Often, a simple review of the next day's, or even the next morning's, appointments can reduce time wasted scrambling around at the last minute to find a special supply while a patient and physician wait in an exam room.

Nonphysician provider and physician capacity. If the practice has maxed out its efficiency, maybe it's time to add another provider. (See the Recruiting section in Chapter 5, "Patient Access" for more information on determining when it's time to recruit another provider.)

Insurance companies. Before you add another provider, look at the profile of your patients' insurance companies. Although not recommended in most cases, your practice could close to new patients. An alternate tact would be to target which part of the panel to close. Do this by performing a cost/benefit analysis of each insurance company when its contract comes up for renewal. Consider not renewing contracts with insurance companies that reimburse your practice below cost or below your market's average.

If advanced access is too radical for your practice, review the following tips designed to make scheduling easier – and your practice more productive.

Scheduling staff

Make the scheduling process run faster and smoother is by reducing the number of times a patient is transferred or put on hold. Allow the staff members who already handle telephone duties to also schedule appointments. Or, accept appointment requests via your Web portal. Allow direct scheduling into your system, or train the same telephone-based scheduling staff to accept the request and communicate with the patient to schedule a mutually convenient time.

Spreading the scheduling duties out and delegating them downward to less-skilled staff works fine until a patient asks an unusual question or seems to have a more urgent medical need. When that happens, the patient is transferred from the scheduling area to someone who has more medical training. Then, to make things more inconvenient and inefficient, the patient is transferred back to the scheduler because the clinical person cannot – or is not allowed to – make an appointment for the patient.

Here's a way to reduce the handoffs and transfers and make the scheduling process run smoother: delegate the scheduling responsibilities up, not just down and out.

Insist that all staff, to include clinical assistants, are trained to schedule appointments. Nurses and medical assistants with additional training can put their skills to work triaging patients, giving basic facts, and judging the potential level of visit a patient may require. It will save the practice time and effort – and offer a better service to your patients – to train these clinical staff members to schedule appointments for the patients being triaged.

Doctor, may I schedule this patient?

One of the most inefficient scheduling practices routinely used by practices is to force anyone scheduling a patient to request verbal permission to do so. Some practices force scheduling staff to jump through hoops for patients with certain diagnoses, those who need certain services, or for same-day appointments.

This scheduling practice keeps an already distressed patient on hold while the scheduler tracks down a physician to review the case. When a physician demands that all new patients be pre-qualified before getting appointments by him or her personally, appointment schedulers must leave their workstations, wait for the physician to come out of an exam room, and ask for permission to schedule the new patient. While this is going on, the physician is interrupted from working with another patient, and the patient making the scheduling request waits on hold. Telephone lines are tied up and other patients cannot schedule their appointments. It's a no-win situation.

Solution? First, consider whether your screening process really adds value. What exactly are you screening for? It makes good sense for a specialist to determine if apatient can be helped clinically before scheduling an appointment. Instead of forcing staff to verbally review the patient's case and ask the physician for permission to schedule, train staff on the screening protocols the physicians use. Give schedulers basic guidelines including prescribed questions and information needed about the patient's condition and, once they are trained, learn to trust their judgment.

See Chapter 5, "Patient Access," for advice about appropriate screening for specialty practices.

Free your template hostages

When new physicians are hired by a practice, they often spend the first few days developing the ideal scheduling template. After years of dealing with whoever walked in the door of their residency program's clinic, new physicians are eager to see the patients they want to see. So, many spend hours setting up schedules to reflect their ideal number of consults, acute visits, new patients, and procedures.

This personalization can often result in the new physician's schedule never being full. Although practices realistically take time to mature, a lower-than-expected volume could be the fault of the scheduling template. Physicians – particularly new ones who are not familiar with the patient population – tend to develop templates that meet *their* needs but not those of their patients. Rigid scheduling templates can hold patients – and physician productivity – hostage.

When physicians are recruited to join your practice, ask them to share their scheduling preferences. Don't let those preferences become barriers to productivity or patient access. Help newly recruited physicians build templates that reflect their needs as well as the needs and expectations of their new population of patients.

Empower schedulers to make decisions when a physician's supply of open appointments appears mismatched with patient demand. For example, let the scheduler set up an office consultation in an acute-care slot if it appears that slot will go unfilled (or the opposite). When that happens, remind the physician to praise the scheduler's quick thinking instead of criticizing himor her for not following directions.

Meet with new physicians monthly. Ask them what's working and what's not with their schedule. Get another physician involved in these meetings to assure new physicians that their flexibility is critical to the practice's success.

Consider establishing the templates for all new physicians to your practice. Your practice knows best when it comes to the needs of your patients.

Remember, the ultimate goal of good scheduling is to deliver value to your patients, not to cling to a perfect-looking template that doesn't work.

Emergency calls

While I argue for spreading out scheduling duties, don't overlook the need to train staff. Suppose a 50-year-old patient calls your practice and asks for an appointment because he or she suddenly feels short of breath and has a sharp pain, first in the jaw and now in the upper back, but hasn't had any dental work recently and hasn't lifted anything heavy.

How would your scheduling staff respond? Would they take a message and tell the patient that the physician will call back? Or would they tell the patient to go to an emergency room because the patient is exhibiting signs of a heart attack?

It is critical to establish emergency protocols and to keep re-examining and updating them. Teach every member of your staff who answers telephones when to tell a patient to go directly to an emergency room or dial 911.

Scheduling gaps should spur staff shifts

Gaps in schedules can cause problems, too. If fewer patients are scheduled on Wednesday afternoons, the front office and clinical staff may welcome the time to return telephone calls and catch up on the work from the previous week. It's nice to have a little breathing room to catch up on paperwork, but it doesn't bring in any revenue to the practice.

Maybe there's a way to shift some of those staff members whose compensation and benefits are a big part of the practice's fixed costs to a busier part of the week. If so, they'd be in a better position to assist patient flow and help boost the physician's productivity.

Few practices do enough to adjust staffing to actual workflow. Although staffing might be worth a whole chapter on its own – if not an entire field of study – getting a little creative about your workforce can smooth out the rough edges in patient scheduling.

How do you know which days are busier than others and, thus, need additional staffing to help solve patient flow problems? Staff may know intuitively which days are busier. Usually, Monday mornings are busiest. But you can do better than rely on intuition. Here's how.

Examine the weekly schedule for all of your physicians. Next, make a grid for an average week. Let's say your physicians have six hours set aside each day for direct patient contact – three hours in the morning and three hours in the afternoon. For example, 9:00 a.m. to noon and 1:00 to 4:00 p.m.

YOU KNOW...

...your practice has the "Monday mentality" syndrome when one of your staff tells an outsider:

"If you'd only been here on a Monday, you would have seen how hard we really work."

If the practice is open five days a week with morning and afternoon sessions each day, your chart will have five vertical columns (days of week) with six boxes (hours of the day) stacked under each column. Put a check mark into each box for each patient scheduled during that hour block. Then, add up all the check marks for each hour and for each morning and afternoon session. Next, calculate the average patient volume associated with each morning and afternoon session for each day. That is, determine the number of patients seen. Make sure that you use actual volume, which will account for cancellations and no-shows.

In addition to patient volume, another excellent determinant of staff work is telephone calls. Measure patient and call volumes by day of the week, at minimum, and perhaps by month. (See Chapter 3, "Telephones" for tracking and responding to call volume.)

Look for fluctuations that repeat themselves. That is, do you experience 20 percent more work on Mondays? Does that happen every Monday? If so, you are a candidate for flexing your workforce.

Now, look at the work schedules for all nonphysician staff on both the clinical and non-clinical sides of the practice. Apply those staffing ratios to each morning and afternoon session. If your practice is like most, the pattern you'll see emerge is that staffing numbers remain constant while the actual workload fluctuates from mornings to afternoons or from day to day.

Fluctuations in patient volume can be particularly profound in surgical practices where the outpatient practice is scheduled around operating room availability. Let's look at an example of a general and vascular surgery practice shown in Exhibit 4.3.

 STAFF BENCHMARKS

Scheduling

Function	Workload range
Appointment scheduling without registration	75-125 calls per day
Appointment scheduling with full registration	50-75 calls per day
Surgery scheduling	25-30 surgeries per day

Forget trying to staff appointment scheduling based on the number of physicians in your practice. The number you need depends on how many appointments need to be scheduled.

The workload range depends on patient population, information system, level of automation, and work processes utilized at the practice. The more information you gather and/or deliver during the scheduling call (thus, the higher the transaction time), the lower the productivity you should expect.

Given the multitude of variables, measure the time it takes your staff to schedule an appointment, and apply that transaction time to reach your practice's ideal workload range.

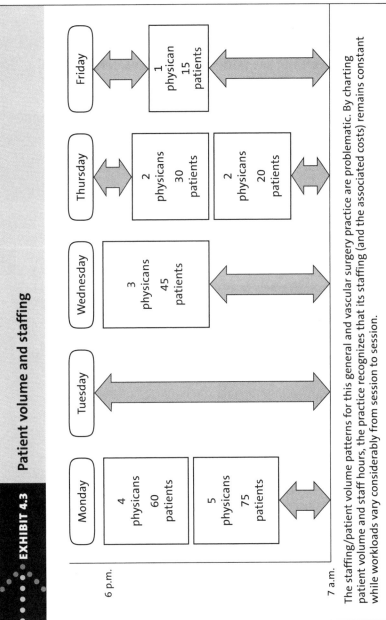

EXHIBIT 4.3 Patient volume and staffing

The staffing/patient volume patterns for this general and vascular surgery practice are problematic. By charting patient volume and staff hours, the practice recognizes that its staffing (and the associated costs) remains constant while workloads vary considerably from session to session.

Blocks of idle time exist throughout the week. Although some idle time is necessary for any practice, staff must be productive at all times. By making a few scheduling shifts at this general and vascular surgery practice, the result will be reduced idle, non-productive time for staff and a lower overhead.

Improve staff scheduling

Use the data you gather about your practice to help set up more effi-cient staff schedules. That is, let the work, not tradition, dictate how you staff.

In surgical or procedural specialty practices, consider covering the office with a skeleton staff of one person per function – one person for the front office and telephones, and one for clinical assistance – on days that physicians are out of the office. Some specialty prac-tices have shifted office staff to four- or five-hour workdays with no reduction in revenue performance.

Alternately, implement the skeleton staff when you know volume will be light, such as some practices experience on Friday afternoons. To keep staff engaged, rotate these duties. Putting staff on a slightly reduced workweek, perhaps of 36 hours, means slightly less pay for them, but they may welcome having most Friday afternoons off.

Another strategy to better match staff to the actual workload is by hiring part-timers to work only on the busiest day(s) or hectic morn-ings or afternoons. You may just attract intelligent, motivated stay-at-home mothers who want to reenter the work force but wish to limit work hours with their children's schedules. Depending on the complexity of the duties, you might also be able to tap into the tal-ent pool of students who are looking for internship opportunities.

Sometimes fluctuations in the schedule are hard to predict. For help handling those unanticipated needs, develop a per-diem corps. Keep in contact with good employees who leave your practice (and thus, are trained in your processes and systems), particularly those who are taking time off for education or other reasons. This infor-mal cadre of staff can be called upon to help out in both administra-tive and clinical duties on a per diem basis during a busy day, a week, or for longer periods to cover an employee who is on extended temporary leave.

Scheduling for seasonality

If your practice is like most, it seems like everyday is the busy season, but a closer look at past schedules might find some times of the year really are busier. Most primary care practices expect the annual flu season and the wave of back-to-school physicals to bring increased volume during certain months. Other specialists will notice trends, too. That's why it may be worth the time it takes to plot out patient appointment data for the previous 12 months.

It's simple: just take your schedule for the past year. Record how many patients were seen each week of the year. Maintain the graph with current scheduling data, relying on patients seen versus patients scheduled. Watch for predictable patterns of utilization, which can provide guidance to staffing your practice. (See Exhibit 4.4.)

There are ways to influence how patients use your schedule. Considering the cost and difficulty of finding and retaining talented staff, it may be worth taking some of the following steps to gain control of seasonal scheduling demands:

Carve out time for same-day access. If April blooms in your region routinely bring in more rhinitis or asthma patients with acute needs to your primary care practice, prepare your scheduling template accordingly. Leave open an extra appointment slot or two each day during your specialty's busy seasons.

Be flexible. Adding some flexibility to the schedule – perhaps working late one day a week or starting 30 minutes earlier three days a week – during the busiest few weeks, might improve accessibility for your patients. The short-term adjustment may also reduce some of the stress on you and your staff because you'll know what's coming. And, likely, you will end up working those hours anyway unless other factors (a change in payers, a mild winter, etc.) changes that demand.

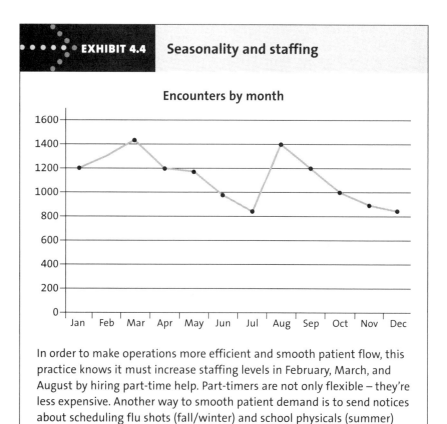

●●●●●● **EXHIBIT 4.4**   **Seasonality and staffing**

Encounters by month

In order to make operations more efficient and smooth patient flow, this practice knows it must increase staffing levels in February, March, and August by hiring part-time help. Part-timers are not only flexible – they're less expensive. Another way to smooth patient demand is to send notices about scheduling flu shots (fall/winter) and school physicals (summer) well in advance – or schedule special hours or days to take care of this extra demand.

Hire help. Consider hiring a nurse to help with the extra patient flow, or hire an extra receptionist to work on busy days or as a temporary worker just during the busy season. Don't forget that seeing more patients also means more claims to process, so make sure that you allocate enough resources to the business office so cash flow doesn't suffer.

Evaluate follow-up protocols. Adjusting policies and medical decisions as clinically appropriate can help juggle patient demand. For example, look for other ways to accommodate follow-up visits during busy seasons. Could certain follow up visits during the busy season be handled via a telephone call from your nurse? During the month before the expected busy season, could physicians instruct some patients to return in six weeks instead of four?

Evaluate demands on the physician's time. Physicians should plan to wind down or put some of their other obligations on hiatus during the busy weeks. Perhaps committee memberships, specialty society activities, alumni group activities, and other non-clinical professional work could be put on hold for a few weeks. Consider opting out of e-mail forums and other non-essential activities for a few weeks. (See Chapter 2, "The Physician's Time," for more time-management tips.)

Stop scheduling routine follow-up visits on Mondays. Unless patients demand otherwise, steer non-acute visits to other days of the week to lessen the stress of hectic Mondays.

Predict the times of heavy demand. Don't let the stress of seasonal workloads become a distraction, or a surprise. Most practices intuitively know when patient demand rises during the year. If you can predict it, you can manage it. Staff up instead of just letting frustration rise.

Use better scheduling to contain facility cost

Removing scheduling gaps doesn't just reduce staffing costs; it also helps hold down facility and real estate expenses.

Practices often look for new space thinking that they have grown out of their existing space without really looking at the capacity. A simple exercise known as a *facility capacity analysis* might reveal that the problem is not square footage but rather inefficient scheduling. The clinical areas of a supposedly full facility are often in use less than 25 percent of the time.

Utilize the same analysis that you developed to evaluate staffing – but this time, look at space. Take your patient encounters per hour and divide them by the patient encounters that your facility can handle. So, if you have the exam rooms to handle six patients per hour and see five patients per hour, your space utilization would be 83 percent (5 divided by 6).

The first hour of the morning and afternoon clinics offer the most opportunity. As a result of our pre-encounter processes, exam room usage lags 20 to 30 minutes behind the "start" of the clinic. Plot your space utilization by hour of the day in a chart to understand your daily facility capacity – and the opportunities to improve it (see Exhibit 4.5).

Your historical scheduling template may reveal that your practice has more untapped space capacity than you realized. Maybe better scheduling can allow you to put off an expensive facility expansion or a move to a larger office.

Most physicians spend between 5 percent and 10 percent of their revenue stream on real estate. That's considerably higher than what most practices spend on information technology and telecommunications. But what most practices forget is that their building investment offers capacity 24 hours a day, seven days a week. Of course, you won't get many patients to schedule their appointments at 2:00 a.m., but here are some ways to get more out of your facility:

Examine a typical week to find the busy days. Maybe you're stuck with too much facility downtime on certain days. Monday's are booked solid but your practice, like many, has a light schedule on Friday afternoons. Everyone wants to wind down before the weekend but you're paying extra overhead – and opportunity cost – for that desired downtime.

Review surgery schedules. Keeping your facility at optimal capacity may also be a function of scheduling the physician's time at the

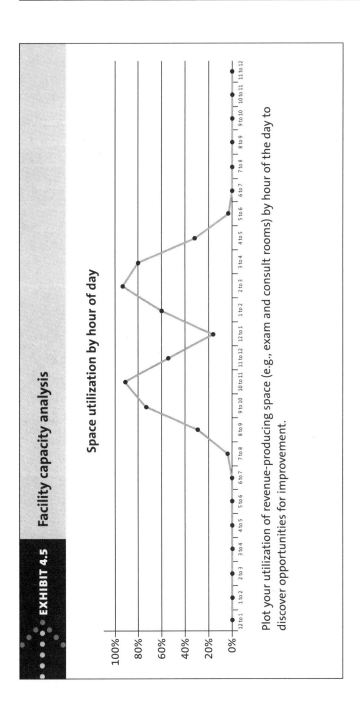

EXHIBIT 4.5

Facility capacity analysis

Space utilization by hour of day

Plot your utilization of revenue-producing space (e.g., exam and consult rooms) by hour of the day to discover opportunities for improvement.

hospital or surgery center. Work with your hospitals to gain the operating room time you need. Consider Saturday mornings as an alternative to weekday surgeries; patients have reported high satisfaction with this option, and your office can be used all week. If office hours become secondary to operating room time, then physicians are left holding the bag for expensive office space that isn't being used.

Use an alternative – the patient's home. Practices that draw from a limited geographical area may want to revive on old idea: home visits. There is no building overhead, no-shows are nearly wiped out, and patients absolutely love being seen in the comfort of their own homes.

Analyze how your office is really used. Yes, you have office hours posted, but is your facility really in full use during those hours? Most practices don't start seeing patients for 20 to 30 minutes after the office doors open. Often, just one or two patients are seen during the last quarter hour of the day. Your practice might be jammed from 9:00 to 11:00 a.m., slow during midday, and hopping again from 1:30 to 3:30 p.m. Are you really out of space when most of your exam rooms sit empty for two or more hours during your posted hours? Try starting at 7:00 a.m., which is a growing trend for practices particularly in urban areas because it makes for shorter commute times for patients – and staff.

Use your facility capacity analysis to make a difference. For example, try alternating lunch schedules among physicians so that your revenue-producing space – your exam rooms – always remain in use. Schedule the day's first appointments to start 15 to 30 minutes before the physician's posted hours. A clinical assistant can greet and process the day's first patients so that they are waiting in the exam room when the physician walks in to the office. Consider extended hours; a growing trend is for medical practices to stay open from 7:00 a.m. to 7:00 p.m. two to four days a week. An extended schedule can transform six to eight hours of a day's worth of capacity into 10 to 12 hours – and it doesn't cost you any more rent.

All of these solutions can have a positive impact on revenue, staffing costs, and patient service. As you can see, scheduling ties into many other corners of the practice, including the very building itself. Before you consider any facility expansions or relocate to gain more clinical space, make sure you're getting full use out of your current facility.

Give the patient a heads-up

Another way to make a schedule run on time is to train schedulers to tell patients exactly what they should bring to their appointment (e.g., payment, radiology films, forms, etc.).

The scheduler also should give patients a best estimate of how long to expect their appointment to take on average. That is, "physicals for your age group take an hour on average in our practice." Repeat this information during the appointment reminder call, if one is made, but make sure it's the same information. Many automated reminder systems can be customized. Reducing the surprise factor will create a more informed patient. Don't, however, make time estimates if you aren't sure that you can meet – and then try to beat them.

Smoother communication smoothes schedule delays

Take a lesson from the airlines: keeping customers in the dark when there are delays just makes them madder.

Medical emergencies can cause a physician's scheduled patients to wait longer. But there are good and bad ways to deliver this news. When an emergency arises and a physician can't see scheduled patients on time, take these steps:

➤ Ask physicians to notify the office immediately. Make sure the news gets passed on. Too often, the clinical support staff hear about a physician's delay but forget – or not think – to let the

front office know. Front office staff bear the brunt of patients'
frustrations, so keep them in the loop about delays.

➤ Require that a member of the clinical support team, whenever
possible, deliver the news to waiting patients. Patients may
perceive the nurse as the physician's spokesperson, but see the
receptionist as only a gatekeeper.

➤ Immediately give delayed patients the choice of rescheduling
or waiting. People tend to feel less put-upon when they have
a choice. If necessary, bring extra staff to the front office to
help with rescheduling.

➤ Ask the receptionist to telephone scheduled patients who may
be affected by the delay. Give patients who have not yet
arrived the opportunity to reschedule if it appears the delay
may be lengthy.

➤ Delayed physicians should deliver the news, too. Ask delayed
physicians to step into the reception area when they arrive to
apologize for the delay, thank the patients for waiting and
indicate that they will be with them as soon as possible.

You can never tell when a medical emergency will happen but you
can try to alleviate patients' frustrations over these inevitable delays.

THINGS TO CONSIDER

Handling delays

I once observed a physician handle an emergency-related delay
with great skill. He went into the waiting room to apologize and
explained to patients that a medical emergency caused the delay.
His staff had made the announcement earlier but the 60 seconds
it took for the physician to tell his patients personally had a great
calming effect on the entire reception area – even for his partners' patients. Handled differently, the same situation could have
created an uproar, rather than a roomful of loyal patients.

When patients create delays

Your practice is a service business – not a factory – so you should expect that some patients will show up late for appointments. Instead of dancing to the tardy patient's tune, attack the problem head on.

Create a window. Most practices consider the patient late once 15 minutes has passed. If parking is scarce or traffic is heavy around your practice, give patients some grace time. Inadequate parking or congested roadways may be the facts of life for your practice, so don't take it out on patients.

Offer options. Consider offering patients who show up more than 15 minutes after their appointment times the opportunity to reschedule or wait to be seen when the physician finds time, which could be an hour or two. Regardless of whether patients opt to reschedule or wait to be worked in, they will walk away feeling accommodated – and you will have prevented them from inconveniencing other patients.

Prevent late arrivals. Set expectations about promptness when patients make appointments. Warn them of road construction near your practice that may cause delays. Advise them if parking is a problem at certain times of the day.

Fix internal problems. You won't convince patients that promptness matters if *you* routinely run late. When physicians consistently run late, the percentage of late arriving patients accelerates. Besides, if you always run 30 minutes behind, it's difficult to justify turning away someone who is just 15 minutes late. Make sure your house is in order before you set up a policy to discipline late patients. Physicians who run on time rarely, if ever, complain about patients who are late.

Target the worst offenders. Some patients always show up late. Identify these patients in your practice management system by entering "CLA" for "chronic late arriver" or some other code in the system's account alert notes. Avoid scheduling these patients for the first appointment of the day or late in the afternoon. If setting expectations, issuing warnings, rescheduling, or treating these as walk-ins don't produce any effect on the patient's behavior – and you don't want to dismiss the patient – then at least keep that habitual late arriver from forcing everyone to stay late or start the day off on a bad note.

Don't fine late arrivers. Can you charge late patients? And if you can, should you? Some practices treat late-arriving patients as though they missed their appointments and may want to levy a small charge to discourage that behavior. Beware: those charges are costly and difficult to collect, and some payers don't allow them. The charges will likely incite the anger of patients who were late because they were caught in traffic or faced other delays they felt they could not control.

No-shows happen for a reason

No-shows are the bane of smooth scheduling. They are one of the frustrations cited most frequently by physicians, and with good reason. Not only do no-shows put a crimp in the daily flow of patients, they are money losers. No one reimburses you for a no-show, yet the overhead related to that missed appointment – staffing, leases, insurance, utilities, and so on – remains on the books. But there will always be no-shows. Three questions to answer about no-shows are:

➤ How many can you expect?

➤ How can you prevent them from disrupting your day?

➤ How can you reduce their frequency?

What is the average no-show rate for medical practices? It can range from as low as zero percent to as high as 60 percent of all appointments. Most practices experience an average of 5 to 7 percent. What makes the difference in handling no-shows is your understanding of them and how your practice deals with them.

Here are some things that may cause your no-show rates to be higher than expected:

The patient–physician relationship. Practices in which physicians routinely rotate, including residency clinics and those which employ locum tenens, tend to have higher no-show rates. So do practices in which physicians rotate between different sites through-out the week. Patients may get confused about which site to visit. The less loyalty patients have to the practice, the more likely they will be no-shows.

Payer mix and your hours. Some patients may not have reliable transportation, dependable childcare or enough flexibility at their workplace to schedule appointments during your practice's regular hours.

The amount of time to next appointment. Practices that schedule appointments too far in advance may find that patients make alter-nate plans. Patients given appointments well into the future may locate other physicians who can get them in sooner, start to feel bet-ter, or simply forget.

Specialty of physician. Psychiatry and certain other specialties may experience higher no-show rates. Some patients may perceive that there is a stigma in having to seek help from certain types of specialists.

 WORDS OF WISDOM

The emotional side of no-shows

No-shows aren't just an administrative problem. Their causes may be deeply rooted in emotions and attitudes about your practice. Consider these comments and what's really behind the emotion expressed:

➤ "You're so busy, you won't miss me." Warn practice staff not to express relief at a no-show or cancellation, even on the busiest day. Patients will get the message that their absence is actually welcomed.

➤ "I hope I can remember this appointment." Patients tend to lose those little appointment reminder cards. If your patients are forgetting about their appointments, don't schedule them more than three months in advance. Instead, call the patient six weeks ahead of time to schedule.

➤ "I feel wonderful; is there any reason for me to come in to be seen?" Remind patients, especially those with chronic illnesses, that routine preventive visits are important to their care, even when there are no symptoms to report.

➤ "I'll just hear bad news." Handle the emotional side of medical care by addressing patients' fears head on. For patients you're concerned about or for the services most patients find fearful, ask a nurse to make contact two or three days before the appointment to give last-minute support.

➤ "I tried to cancel, but I couldn't get through." Set up 24-hour/seven day-a-week cancellation voice mail and e-mail address so patients can cancel or ask for schedule changes at any time. Make sure someone is held accountable to monitor all such messages and to contact patients to reschedule within one working day of their communication.

➤ "You're the ones who moved my appointment." Avoid cancelling clinics without ample notice, and offer alternative access to patients whose appointments have to be moved. (See the section of this chapter on bumping patients).

➤ "I just don't like you." Well, that's a reality. Some patients just don't like some physicians. Offer avenues for physicians and staff to exchange constructive, non-threatening criticism about each others' people skills. Consider sending exit interview forms to patients who leave – you may learn some powerful lessons.

Being knowledgeable about the emotional side of no-shows will help prevent at least some of them – and improve the care delivered to your patients.

Managing no-shows

I worked with one physician who had his staff schedule chronic no-shows during his lunch hour. If patients didn't show up, he had the full hour for lunch. If they did, his lunch was a little shorter but he made a little more money that day. While this tactic may work great for managing the chronic no-shows that you aren't ready to cut loose from your practice, it doesn't get to the heart of the problem, which is to prevent no-shows from happening in the first place.

Good data can help a practice manage no-shows instead of letting them manage (and disrupt) the practice. If you figure that your practice's no-show rate is 10 percent and your physician has slots to see, say, 20 patients per day, then expand your scheduling template to 22 slots. If your data are reliable, you can expect that, on the average day, two patients won't show up. Commonly known as overbooking, this practice is widespread but don't let it prevent you from trying to become more efficient. That is, don't rely on over-booking as the only way to increase the practice's productivity.

While you can't eliminate no-shows altogether, you can reduce their frequency.

Here are some steps you can take to reduce the frequency of no-shows in your practice:

Improve your relationship with patients. A strong relationship with patients strengthens the commitment they feel toward your practice. One way to build this bond is to send birthday cards to patients (use the date of birth from your registration database) or greeting cards at the holidays.

Create stronger nurse-patient relationships. Assign nurses to patients, especially those who have chronic conditions and who make many return visits to the practice. It may also help increase patient compliance. Print business cards for nurses to distribute to patients.

Maintain timely patient access. The longer a patient has to wait to be seen, the more likely that he orshe will find care from another source – mostly likely another physician. Or the patient may start feeling better. In either case, the patient will rarely call you to cancel the appointment. How do you create more timely appointment access when you already work a full schedule? Strategies may include using nonphysician providers and other clinical staff to help handle more appointments daily – seeing just one more patient a day can produce big results over the course of a year. In some cases, it may make sense to stop participating with a payer that may be sending you lots of patients but not much income.

Stop creating no-shows. Do you or other physicians in the practice often cancel clinics? More than once a month is too much. Cancelling or bumping clinics accelerates the no-show problem because:

> ➤ You lose revenue but not any overhead;

> ➤ Rescheduling takes a lot of staff time;

> ➤ Patients get frustrated with your staff and, eventually, you; and

➤ Patients stop taking your appointment scheduling needs seriously.

Identify offenders. Detect your no-show problems early. Use your practice management system to track no-shows. Identify patients who chronically miss appointments. Place an alert note or another simple identifier, such as "CNS" for chronic no-show, in a part of the patient record that is accessible to schedulers during the scheduling process. Instruct staff who schedule appointments to give those patients less desirable appointment times, such as at the end of a clinic or whenever else a no-show will not disrupt patient flow.

WORDS OF WISDOM

What to do *after* a patient fails to show

From a compliance perspective, it's important to identify and review the records of a patient who fails to show. Determine who is accountable for deciding on the action to be taken. If a preventive visit was missed, a reminder call to reschedule should be placed; if news of a malignant tumor was forgotten, tracking down the patient becomes more urgent. Remember, it's your responsibility to care for your patients even if they sometimes miss appointments. Work with your malpractice carrier to determine the best possible route to follow up with patients if this is a problem for your practice. Document your efforts in the patient's record, to include method of communication, timing, and responsible staff.

Handle chronic offenders. Patients who habitually fail to show up for appointments are more than nuisances – they are risk management issues. Make a policy on when to dismiss a patient from your practice and whether it is three, five, or some other number of missed appointments, be consistent. State your missed-appointment policy in the practice's new patient literature, and ask new patients to review and acknowledge by signature. (Don't develop a new form for patients to sign, but include acknowledging your chronic no-show policy in the registration process.) Inform current patients, too. At the same time, make sure to carefully review with your malpractice carrier any planned dismissals of patients for whom you have ongoing management of care.

Manage to it. Track no-shows to find patterns. You may find that your highest no-show rate is between 3:00 p.m. and 5:00 p.m. on Fridays. You may see them peak during summer months. Discovering when no-shows are most likely to occur gives you more options to manage the problem. For example, it might be safe to book more patients than you normally would during the heaviest no-show periods because you can reasonably expect that one or more will not show up. Or, save on staffing costs by shutting down the practice on Friday afternoons during the summer.

Set up a virtual "no-show doctor." Assign a "no-show doctor" template for staff to schedule patients who are chronic no-shows. When and if patients show, they can be moved to a physician's schedule on a rotating basis – or to the physician who has time to see them. Or, perform the same process by slotting patients into "stand-by appointments" for their requested physician. Inform the patient that the slots are just that – stand-by – as a result of their history of no-shows. This system will prevent these patients from blocking appointment slots for other patients, and staff from possibly wasting time to prepare for their appointments in advance.

Remind patients. Assign staff to remind patients 48 hours in advance of their appointments. Use automated telephony solutions if you're concerned that your workforce does not have the capacity to remind all of your patients. For those with capacity, or patients who may need an extra reminder, a live human voice is preferable.

It creates a more compelling reason for the patient to show up. This doesn't have to be an expensive option. Try hiring college students or retirees to make reminder calls at night (it vastly increases the chances of reaching patients instead of their answering machines or voice mail). And people with caller identification do tend to pick up the phone when they see that it's their doctor calling. Telephone reminders also can play a role in your practice's health care mission. Nurses or medical assistants who make reminder calls can emphasize that showing up for the appointment is part of the continuity of care process.

Know when to require confirmations. For procedures and other encounters that consume a lot of your time, ask the patient to call back to confirm no later than 24 hours in advance of the appointment. If the patient doesn't call back, shift that appointment to a patient on your waiting list. Be sure you tell patients about this policy in writing. You don't want to create a bevy of incoming telephone calls for every appointment. Getting confirmation for lengthy visits and procedures will make sure your time and overhead are not wasted.

Personally remind patients. Oftentimes patients are surprised to learn at check out that their physician wants them back in a few weeks. Close each encounter with a review of your follow-up plan. If it includes a follow-up appointment, then say so. Emphasize how important it is to stay on the treatment plan, which includes showing up for the next appointment.

Don't schedule too far in advance. A scheduling template that extends many months into the future can increase no-show rates because patients will likely forget about a routine follow-up appointment that is scheduled 12 months in advance. The patient may have made other plans by the time he or she receives your appointment reminder call or postcard. To reduce no-shows and cancellations when visits must be scheduled several months out, put those appointments into a manual or automatic queue. The queue can trigger a printed or telephonic reminder notice to the patient six to eight weeks before the scheduled appointment.

Regardless of why the patient failed to show, mark the fact in your practice management system. No-shows have an impact on billing and collections because you must be sure to bill all of the patients who present at the practice. Without knowing who did not show up for an appointment, you cannot track the patients who did indeed come.

If you've done your tracking well, you will notice certain patterns emerge in your no-show rate. You may need a month of data or more. You may need to track over several months to see if, as some practices have noticed, seasonal differences in no-show rates relate to holidays and summer vacation times.

There's no simple solution to preventing no-shows. Maybe a more realistic goal is to reduce the overall rate to a relatively low level so they don't ruin your day and erode physician productivity.

Should you charge for no-shows?

No-shows cost your practice money through lost opportunity. For years, practice management experts have debated whether it was worth it to charge patients who missed scheduled appointments. With practice overhead costs rising every year, your practice may soon join the growing number of practices that do charge for no-shows.

What should you charge? Typical no-show charges range from $15 to $25. You may end up waiving many of these charges – patients may have legitimate transportation or childcare problems that occur at the last minute. Counsel them on what to do the next time it happens. Billing patients for not showing up for appointments does get their attention but capturing these nominal charges is not the primary goal; it's reducing the rate of no-shows.

Is it your fault? If you do decide to charge for no-shows, do your homework. Have you addressed your own access issues? Make sure your house is in order before you start penalizing patients. You may face some bad publicity and bad feelings if you make patients wait six months for appointments, then charge $25 if they happen to forget the appointment – or saw one of your competitors in the meantime.

Will payers allow you to charge a no-show? First, determine if your payers allow you to charge their beneficiaries for missed appointments. Most insurance companies, including Medicare, will not pay for no-show charges, although some insurance companies may allow you to charge the patients (their beneficiaries) directly. Check with the insurance companies to ensure that your no-show strategy is in compliance with their rules. And, consider that if some payers allow these charges but others don't, can your office processes track who can be charged and who cannot? Will it work? You know your patient population. Will the chronic no-shows just pay up but keep not showing up? Will they ignore attempts to charge them? Can some of them really afford it?

Is it worth it? You might spend more money charging and trying to collect no-show charges than you'll ever realistically collect. Billing statements for missed appointments cost money in supplies and stamps. It also can divert your business office staff from more important tasks, such as working outstanding accounts, following up on claims denials, and so on.

How will patients react? Follow up on recent chart transfers to make sure no-show charges are not driving away patients. I worked with one practice that realized many of the patients they were charging for missed appointments also brought in the best reimbursement. By comparing chart transfer requests and no-show charges, the practice soon realized that a significant minority of these more lucrative patients transferred their care after receiving a billing statement that contained a no-show charge.

If you charge for no-shows, communicate the new policy in advance to all patients. Send them a letter, post signs in the office, and ask schedulers to remind patients of the policy when they make appointments.

WORDS OF WISDOM

Look for definition of covered services

Look to see how you your participating payers' contracts define "covered services" to see if you can charge for no-shows. Negotiate for a definition that supports your ability to charge their beneficiaries no-show fees. For "non-covered services," the decision to charge is yours. No-show charges, and other fees like interest on overdue accounts, as well as cosmetic services, would fall under non-covered services.

THINGS TO CONSIDER

Reminders

➤ Keep the appointment fresh – don't make calls more than 72 hours in advance of the appointment.

➤ Do not leave a voice mail or answering machine message that mentions the nature of the patient's visit.

➤ Ask new patients if you can leave future appointment reminders on their answering machines, voice mail or with others who might answer the telephone for them, or via e-mail. Make sure their consent is in writing and included with appropriate HIPAA documentation.

➤ Use the 15-minute rule when you can't confirm every appointment. Identify which patients may need longer (than 15 minutes) or more complicated visits; make sure to send them reminders and seek confirmations.

➤ Automate the appointment reminder process to ensure that all patients are reminded – and to redirect your staff effort to greeting, answering phones, and other important front-desk functions.

THINGS TO CONSIDER

You can't bill them if you can't find them

Don't even try to charge for no-shows if your practice serves an indigent population or other hard-to-reach populations. You'll spend more on mailing bills for the $15 no-show charge to wrong addresses than you could possibly hope to collect.

Don't ignore cancellations

Cancellations come in two forms – the ones given with several days of advance notice and the ones given with very little notice. The difference between cancellations and no-shows is that the patient is at least attempting to be considerate. The two are similar in that they both can affect practice income and both may be warning signs of other problems.

Let's take a closer look at the impact of appointment cancellations that are made with little notice to see why tracking and analyzing them is every bit as important as tracking and analyzing no-show rates.

Understand the impact. Your staff will not have time to schedule another patient when a cancellation is made on short notice. The time they have spent preparing for the patient to present – pulling and previewing the chart, and perhaps stocking special supplies – is now wasted.

Establish policies. Inform patients that cancellations must be made no less than 24 hours in advance (or an alternative period of time you set) so you have time to schedule another patient in that slot. Be sure to announce the policy in advance of enforcing it. Handle a last-minute cancellation as you would a no-show with the same penalties. These could include offering less favorable scheduling for repeat offenders, a nominal charge in some cases, or – for the worst offenders – dismissal from the practice.

Be nice. Every once in a while patients have legitimate emergencies that require them to cancel appointments on short notice. You don't want to alienate patients who are trying to be considerate, so require that any decisions about penalties for short-notice cancellations are made by a supervisor, not the front-line staff.

Emphasize performance. Make sure your staff knows that cancellations must be converted into appointments whenever possible. Instruct them to remind patients of the practice's cancellation policy whenever appointments are scheduled, appointment reminders are sent, or cancellations are requested on short notice.

Keep a waiting list. If you keep a list of patients who have asked for earlier appointments, then you are better equipped to deal with cancellations, as well as no-shows. The waiting list can be kept in a spreadsheet file and should include patient's names, contact information, and account numbers. Include the date the patient is placed on the list and when the appointment is scheduled so you can purge the list weekly. Highlight the names of all patients who are accommodated and be sure staff closes the loop by releasing those patients' originally scheduled appointments. In addition to providing an easy way to convert cancelled appointments into revenue-producing visits, the very fact that you keep a waiting list may get a positive reaction from patients.

Recognize warning signs. Patients who cancel are sometimes making their last call to your practice. They cancel out of respect for your time but do not intend to return. They may be frustrated with your practice or have found another physician. Instruct your staff to follow up within five working days with any patients who cancel but do not reschedule. You can retain patients by encouraging them to schedule another appointment or gather feedback about their dissatisfaction. Either way, it's a call worth making.

Remove obstacles. Make it easy for patients to cancel. Don't make them wade through a complex telephone system and speak to several staff just to get the opportunity to tell you they want to cancel. Putting the phones on hold at lunch makes this process even more frustrating to patients. Making it hard for patients to cancel effectively increases your no-show rate. Offer a cancellation voice mail box as well as an e-mail address. Be sure a member of your staff is accountable for checking the voice mail and e-mail boxes several times a day and responding within one working day to reschedule the appointment.

Analyze trends. Produce a daily report to monitor your appointment fill rate. (For more information on your fill rate, see Chapter 5, "Patient Access.") This will tell you how well your cancellation policy works and how well your staff manages the cancellation conversion process. Compare the number of patients each provider is expected to see per day with how many patients were seen. For example, if your practice had the capacity to see 60 patients last Wednesday but physicians and other clinical staff only saw 52, then your fill rate was 87 percent. Ideally, your fill rate should be at or close to 100 percent. Anything less is excess capacity and likely caused by no-shows or cancellations that were not converted into appointments. Focusing on your fill rate helps you and your staff spot opportunities to improve your income.

Physicians can cancel, too

Patients aren't the only no-shows who disrupt the practice's business. Sometimes, physicians cancel appointments because they want leisure time or want to attend other functions at the last minute. We tend to use code words like "bumping" the appointments, but whatever term you choose to use, this behavior is hazardous to practice productivity and customer service.

I worked with one practice that did not realize how big a problem it was until a patient called to complain about being rescheduled three times. It may seem like the physician bumping a clinic is sufficiently penalized by not receiving the revenue (thus compensation) related to those missed visits. But, in a group practice, all of the partners may bear the overhead related to the cancelled clinical sessions. Three little words – "cancel my clinic" – do more than send shudders up a scheduler's spine, they also cost your practice a lot of money. The rescheduling process, as well as the under-utilization of staff, equipment and facility, are the true costs of rescheduling. See Exhibit 4.6 to develop a better understanding of the costs of bumps.

Physician bumps are worse than no-shows and cancellations because they cost staff time to reschedule patients. More importantly, bumps can destroy the loyalty and satisfaction of patients and referring physicians. Bumping patients also does nothing to improve patient care.

An increase in the rate of bumps can indicate problems with how you are scheduling the physician's work, how patient flow is being handled or, possibly, a problem with the physician's attitude or personal life.

Approach the problem of physician bumping by measuring it, sharing it, exploring its causes, and managing it.

| EXHIBIT 4.6 | Calculating the cost of a bumped patient |

Tasks	Time per task (mins)	Cost
Review bump request	2	
Locate and review chart for relative urgency and clinical issues (e.g., medication renewals)	3 to 15 (EHR vs. paper)	
Review future appointment availability to accommodate relative urgency	5 to 10	
Pull contact information	2 to 5	
Make phone call(s) until bumped patient reached	2 to 15	
Explain situation and reschedule patient on the phone	5 to 10	
Compose and send letter to patient if he or she could not be reached	10	
Reschedule patient when he or she calls	(included above)	
Document the situation in bumped patient's chart	2	
Handle outstanding clinical issues (e.g., converse with physician, call pharmacy, etc.)	0 to 15	
Total administrative and clinical staff	31 to 84 minutes	$10.33 to $28.00[1]
Unused office overhead	n/a	$59.61[2]
Total cost of a bumped patient	n/a	$69.94 to $87.61

[1]Calculated at $20 per hour, which includes compensation and benefits; assumes clinical assistant is involved in steps related to patient's clinical needs.

[2]$290,541 of overhead allocated to 4,874 encounters; source: MGMA Cost Survey for Multispecialty Practices, 2006 Report based on 2005 Data. $378,254 reduced by $87,713, which account for variable costs (e.g., administrative supplies, drug supplies, etc.).

n/a = not applicable

I estimate that bumps, on average, cost medical practices $69.94 to $87.61 per bumped patient. Note that the cost rises significantly (from just the staff time to include staff and overhead) when one accounts for the unused overhead. If another physician can hold clinic during that time period, the cost associated with the fixed overhead ($59.61 per encounter) is eliminated but, even without that cost, there remains a $28 price tag. Of course, these costs do not include the lost revenue associated with the bumped appointment. In summary, bumps are quite costly to your practice.

Measure bumps

Over several months, track the number of patients whose appointments are cancelled and rescheduled at the provider's request. Be sure to track all physicians so the outliers will see how much they deviate from the norm. Track these occurrences by time of day, day of week, and type of appointment so you can spot potential causes.

Ask your scheduler to log the number of attempts made to reschedule each bumped appointment during the tracking period. It's a bit of work but developing a picture of how much additional time is spent rescheduling a bumped appointment helps you come up with a staffing cost. Do a quick calculation of the dollar amount that each rescheduled appointment typically consumes, and then add in the lost reimbursement as a negative amount. Create your own version of Exhibit 4.6 to document each process.

Add in the lost reimbursement as a negative amount (unless, of course, the encounter is unbillable, such as a post-operative visit. The results will depend on your specialty, ancillaries, and payer mix. While these may seem like small dollars at first, the cost – and the lost revenue – adds up quickly.

Also ask your scheduler to jot down comments heard from the bumped patients or staff at the patients' referring physicians' practices. Be sure to note if the appointment is never rescheduled.

The goal is to track the cost of the rescheduling, as well as to record customer dissatisfaction.

Share information about bumps

Put the data, costs, and comments into a report. Present it at the next physicians' meeting or to physician leaders who are most attuned to the problem's impact. Some physicians will change behavior after seeing how they compare with the rest of the group. Make it clear in your report that the *entire* practice bears the cost for physicians who bump patients.

Explore what causes bumps

Maybe the root cause of the bumps is not a lazy physician or a burning desire to play a round of golf on a nice afternoon. Ask your physicians' help to determine the root cause of the bumps. It could be that an obstetrician routinely bumps office patients to handle deliveries. If so, then maybe there should be a different arrangement between physicians to share these duties. Perhaps, the bumps always seem to occur the morning after the gastroenterologist's busy day at the surgery center or on the Monday after the pulmonologist has been on call all weekend. Maybe, you should not let the provider schedule early morning office appointments the following morning.

Manage physician bumps

Managing starts with tackling any issues related to individual physicians who are cancelling their clinics. It also helps to set broader practice policies. Many practices now require physicians to announce their continuing medical education (CME) and vacation schedules at least eight weeks in advance. If physicians demand more flexibility, then set a time limit of, say, six weeks for cancelling appointments unless there is an emergency. With a policy or without, introduce a form to capture information staff need to process the requests. See Exhibit 4.7 for an example and follow the script or letter in the "Words of Wisdom" box to best manage the bumped patient.

If one physician keeps bumping appointments anyway, consider asking the physician to reschedule those appointments personally. The physician will soon realize how much time it takes and hear patients' frustrations firsthand. If all else fails, levy a fine in the amount of the administrative burden of the bumps. Don't forget that while a fine may cover the rescheduling cost and missed opportunity, it cannot resolve the image of providing poor service.

How you handle bumps, or if they are even a problem, depends quite a bit on your practice's culture. Some practices never bump appointments. Others – perhaps yours – have a significant or developing problem with the issue.

Set a goal of no physician bumps. A cancelled appointment can disrupt a patient's life in many ways: a patient will have to re-arrange time off work and potentially cause disruption to co-workers. The patient may also have day care, family activities, and any number of other obligations to rearrange.

Bumps are more costly than patient no-shows, and, over time, they can degrade your practice's reputation with patients and referring physicians. If your practice has a problem with bumps, it's time to start working on it.

EXHIBIT 4.7 Appointment bump rescheduling form

Bump details

Physician:_____

Date: _____ Time: _____

Total number of patients impacted: _____

Date bump approved: _____

Date schedule blocked: _____

Physician must complete requested action:

☐ Physician (or nonphysician provider) _____ will see my patients. Notify the patients of the change of physicians.

☐ Add a clinic to my schedule on _____ (date) from _____ to _____. If patients cannot be seen on that date, the following accommodations can be made:_____

_____

_____

☐ Reschedule patients for next available appointment. The urgency of the appointment time is marked below next to each patient's name.

Staff member assigned to
communicate with patients: _____ Date: _____

Patient name	Phone	Address	Chief complaint	Urgency (by phys)	Action (by staff)

(NOTE: a print-out of the schedule can be used to capture and record this information. If so, it must be attached to this form.)

1.

2.

3.

4.

5.

6.

7.

8.

Date completed: _____

Staff signature: _____

Practice manager signature: _____

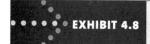

EXHIBIT 4.8   Appointment bump rescheduling letter

(ON PRACTICE LETTERHEAD)

NOTE: *Do not fill in blanks. Type a letter to every patient affected by the bump using a macro for the body of the letter.*

March 1, 2009

Ms. Janet Wood
123 Anytown Drive
Atlanta, GA 30307

Ms. Wood:

Dr. Robert Jones requested that I contact you personally. Regrettably, your appointment with Dr. Jones on Tuesday, May 15, 2009, must be rescheduled.

We attempted to contact you by telephone at the number which you provided to us upon registering at our practice. We are very sorry that we were not able to reach you.

Dr. Jones has alternative appointment dates and times available.

Please contact our office at 222-222-2222 at your earliest convenience so that we may schedule another appointment.

We apologize for any inconvenience that we have caused.

Thank you for choosing Medical Associates for your care.

Sincerely,

Merrilyn Burke
Practice Manager
Medical Associates

WORDS OF WISDOM

Script the rescheduling call

Develop a script for staff to follow to handle a patient who must be bumped. Managing the rescheduling process is critical to maintain customer service.

"Ms. Smith, this is Gloria from Neurology Consultants. Dr. Jones asked me to contact you personally. There has been a change in his schedule which will impact your appointment. He asked me to personally contact you to tell you that..."

...(go to option A or B):

Option A: "...one of Dr. Jones' partners, _____, will be seeing you on your appointment date. Dr. Jones wanted me to reassure you that he will review your care with _____ following his return. Do you have any questions about this change?"

(Respond to the patient's questions. If the patient has no questions, thank the patient for choosing Neurology Consultants and conclude the conversation.)

Option B: "...your appointment with him will need to be rescheduled. Do you have your calendar available? (Pause for the patient's response.) Thank you. The dates that Dr. Jones has available are ... Dr. Jones is very sorry that he inconvenienced you."

(Once the patient is scheduled, thank the patient for choosing Neurology Consultants and conclude the conversation.)

If the patient cannot be reached by telephone, send the patient a letter (see Exhibit 4.8) to inform him or her of the bump.

CASE STUDY

Southeast Surgical Partners cuts "bumps"

There were so many cancelled clinics at Southeast Surgical Partners that it took almost 40 hours a week in combined staff time just to manage all the tasks involved in contacting patients to reschedule clinics that physicians had cancelled. The administrator calculated that the cost of physicians cancelling appointments for non-emergency reasons was almost $30,000 a year. Once alerted to how much Southeast Surgical Partners was spending to reschedule clinics, the physician leaders introduced administrative policies similar to those described in the "Physicians can be no-shows, too" section. Since then, the "bump" rate at Southeast Surgical Partners has been cut by 80 percent. The reduction in staff time dedicated to this rescheduling function was worth $24,000.

Surgery scheduling

For practices with physicians who perform surgeries or procedures, the scheduling of these out-of-office services is a critical component of practice operations. All of the scheduling techniques described thus far have related to office appointments; I'll now spend some time on out-of-office surgery and procedure scheduling.

Scheduling a surgery or procedure is an essential process that must be conducted in a timely manner to ensure that both the patient's and the physician's time are respected. It is important for the individual scheduling the appointment to know the physician's individual scheduling preferences (based on the duration of the surgery, lead times to gather necessary test results, order instrumentation, if necessary, and so forth).

Once the service is identified, the scheduler should meet with the patient. Ideally, the meeting will take place near the end of the patient's encounter in the office. Contacting the patient later is batching work. Pull in the work; the patient is right there.

The pre-authorization or pre-certification process, as well as the arrangement of the patient's financial responsibility is typically coordinated with the scheduling of a surgery or procedure. Although the specifics of the process depend on the medical specialty, state law (in the case of consents) and the insurance companies involved, some processes are standard. They include:

➤ **Consent to treat.** The patient must consent in writing to have the surgery or procedure performed based on the state's required consent. Typically, the physician presents the consent form for signature in the exam room. However, the scheduler must always check that this important form has been completed and is attached to the patient's file. Consent forms are regulated by each state, so be sure to check with your state medical society to make sure that you're using the right one.

➤ **Schedule.** The time and date of the surgery or procedure are determined based on the physician's calendar. Then the hospital or ambulatory surgery facility is contacted to put the patient on the schedule. Any required pre- or post-operative arrangements should be made at this time.

➤ **Pre-admission.** The scheduler must ensure that the hospital or ambulatory surgery center has all of the appropriate diagnostic test results, a clearance physical and/or any other clinical and administrative requirements required by the patient's clinical needs and/or the facility.

➤ **Pre-authorization/certification.** If required, the insurance company must be contacted on the telephone or online to request authorization to perform the surgery or procedure. The scheduler usually makes this contact, although sometimes a nurse or the business office may be responsible for this component. Typically, the insurance company will request some background information about the diagnosis and treatment, so the staff member handling the details of this step should have clinical training or a solid clinical knowledge base. Whether you need a pre-authorization or certification will be dictated by the insurance company and the services your physician intends to perform. Maintain a detailed list by service and by insurance company so that you know when to call. If you don't get the appropriate authorization, your physicians won't get paid.

➤ **Financial responsibility.** Practices attuned to patient collections take the opportunity to introduce a patient's financial responsibility during the scheduling process. During the contact with the insurance company about the pre-authorization, the scheduler asks for details of the patient's financial responsibility to include the deductible (what, if any, is remaining), coinsurance and any other responsibility. A worksheet is developed for the patient that outlines his or her responsibility. Many practices also ask for some – if not all – of the patient's portion of the payment before the surgery or procedure.

At all stages in communicating with others (primary care physician, hospital, and insurance company), it is important for the physician's staff to record the date, time, and the person(s) with whom they speak. If problems arise, this information can be invaluable in determining who said what, when, and to whom.

Keep track of surgery scheduling

Develop a single template to track all information involved in scheduling surgeries or procedures. Maintain the template electronically, with the ability to print and scan when necessary.

If one person is assigned to conduct the process for the practice and has a particular method, it is essential that someone else be cross-trained in how to schedule these services. You don't want the process to be put on hold or fall apart if the individual who normally handles the task goes on vacation, takes sick leave, or resigns. Problems that occur at this stage, such as a missing authorization or consent form, can come back to haunt the practice.

A single form (see the sample template in Exhibit 4.9) containing all of the required information and communication regarding the surgery or procedure can help this function move smoothly, efficiently, and accurately.

For the purposes of tracking, record the surgery or procedure in your main scheduling system, in addition to a personal calendar that the physician may hold. A record of the service in your scheduling system will allow your business office staff to make sure that they have charges for every service performed.

THINGS TO CONSIDER

Operating room (OR) scheduling

For surgery practices that can never seem to get enough OR time, ask your hospital(s) if "block scheduling" in the OR is offered. In this arrangement, the hospital provides a guarantee for your surgeons to have full use of its OR for a specific block of time (for example, 7:00 a.m. to 5:00 p.m. every Tuesday). The advantage is that instead of managing your surgery day around the hospital's schedule, your physicians get full use of a dedicated time block. This allows your practice to manage its time better and create a schedule that maximizes the surgeon's time.

EXHIBIT 4.9 — **Surgery scheduling template**

Date:	Initials:
Patient's name:	DOB
SS#	Phone (h) (w)
Address:	
City/State/ZIP:	
Referring MD:	Phone: Notified? / /
Will they do H&P? Y / N	Will they schedule H&P? Y / N
PCP:	Phone:
Diagnosis?	Procedure(s)?
Scheduled for: Date: / /	Time: Hospital:
Scheduled by: (hospital)	(office)
Anesthesia:	
Pre-Op:	
Patient instructions:	
Patient notified? Y / N	/ / (date)
Insurance:	
Policy No.	Group No.
Patient financial responsibility:	
Deductible met? Y / N	If not, what amount remains?
Coinsurance? Y / N	
Total balance:	
Amount collected from patient?	Amount on payment plan?
Pre-certification needed? Y / N	
Obtained by: (office)	(insurance co.) / / (date)

Pre-Certification No.

Notes:

Appointment recalls

Appointment recall systems prove valuable in assuring timely and appropriate care management. Appointment recalls are the practice's method of tracking the next visit(s) that the physician has recommended. For example, if a patient receives a well-woman checkup in November and a follow-up visit for a small mole is recommended in March, the practice should record, track, and communicate with the patient in February to remind her of the follow-up appointment needed in March.

Recalls can also be an effective alternative to giving patients appointments in the distant future. When the physician asks a patient to return in 12 months, don't make an appointment; instead, record the request in your recall system. Proactively reach out to the patient in 10 months to schedule the appointment. Use your patient population and history of cancellations and no-shows to determine when to start recalling. If your patients tend to forget – or cancel or don't show – for appointments made three or more months in advance, set the recall process to cover three months and out. This will be necessary, of course, if you don't have your templates set beyond three months.

Regardless of the nature of the recommended return visit, don't leave the recall solely up to the patient. Inform him or her of the physician's recommendations, ask if the patient wants to schedule an appointment (unless you don't have the ability to schedule it that far in advance), and if not, place the patient on a recall list.

Most practice management systems and electronic health records systems can conduct the recall process by automatically sending appointment notices telephonically or in writing to patients. Alternatively, a recall list can be generated to prompt a physician to review a patient's medical records to decide if a recall is appropriate. Or, develop manual recall logs, in which staff record all appointments or other reminders in date order to prompt the recall.

Scheduling is the key to managing patient flow. Combining the physician's work style with processes around that physician will leave your practice – and your patients – satisfied.

CHAPTER 5

Patient Access

Key Chapter Lessons

➤ Calculate your fill rate – and why it's critical to access

➤ Identify barriers to access – and how to overcome them

➤ Understand the essential balance between physician supply and patient demand

➤ Discover alternatives to rebalance supply and demand

➤ Examine your contracting strategy to improve patient access

➤ Develop a pre-appointment screening process that works for you, patients, and your referring physicians

➤ Identify the benefits of creating a medical home for patients

➤ Set the stage for a new physician joining your practice

Initiating patient access

Once you successfully field a call or electronic request from a patient desiring to be seen, you must find a place for that patient in the schedule. Creating this access for patients effectively initiates the patient flow process.

It's important to remember that patient access is the strategy underlying the scheduling process. Without actively managing patient access, patient demand can overwhelm the number of scheduling slots. When that happens, the scheduling process is doomed to fail and none of the tips described in Chapter 4, "Scheduling" will succeed. Instead, appointment backlogs will commence, and your staff will spend more time deflecting demand than accommodating patients.

Patients don't want a backlog and they don't want to be deflected. They derive value from appointment availability – and consider the lack of it frustrating and even detrimental to their care. Moreover, patients won't value the scheduling processes your staff use to try and deflect their demand. Value, from the patients' perspective, centers on getting access to your physicians' time. By allowing patients to pull the value of access management, practice operations can only benefit.

Managing patient access demands good planning, good data, good information systems, and good staff. Too often, this final key element – good staff – is overlooked. Workers must be trained, committed, and empowered to provide top-notch customer service, which includes striving towards minimizing patients' waiting time for appointments – and the time they wait in the practice.

If your practice is one of those where patients are easily accommodated because physicians have lots of extra time during the day, then patient access is simple: schedule patients when they want to be seen and move on to the next request. (Of course, the problem with too little patient demand is that you won't have sufficient revenue after expenses to keep the practice running for very long, so it's important to focus on marketing; see this chapter's "Words of Wisdom" on tips to fill your schedule.)

Problems arise when there is no room in the daily schedule to work in the patient who has an acute but non-life-threatening medical issue. Or, it may be several months before any appointment slots for new patients are available.

If either these scenarios ring true – no way to work in acute patients or long waits for new patients – the root of your access problem may be poor scheduling processes. Perhaps your operator has trouble transferring telephone calls to the scheduler, or the scheduler doesn't understand how to schedule patients. In contrast to patient access, the scheduling process is just that – a *process*. It's comparatively easy to solve a process by using the ideas explained in Chapter 4, "Scheduling."

If the problem is that physicians don't have enough time in the day to see all of the patients asking to be seen, then you have a bigger problem – your strategy for patient access if faulty. No amount of tinkering with the details of the scheduling process will get you back on track. Don't apply a micro solution to a macro problem.

GETTING STARTED

Access performance dashboard

Measure these key access indicators each quarter so you can identify and evaluate changes over time.

➤ **Time to Next Available Established/New Patient Appointment**
Number of days to next available appointment slot that can accommodate an established/new patient

➤ **Appointment No-Show Rate**
Percent of appointments that patients do not keep; that is, the appointment is scheduled but the patient doesn't show up

➤ **Appointment "Bump" Rate**
Percent of appointments that the physician cancels in which patients must be "bumped"

➤ **New Patient Appointments as a Percent of Total Appointment**
Percent of new patient appointment slots as a percent of total appointment slots

➤ **Cancellation Conversion Rate**
Percent of cancelled appointments that are converted to an

appointment in which another patient is seen — often, through a waiting list or accommodating a patient who calls in the meantime

➤ **Fill Rate**
Percent of patients actually seen divided by the capacity as defined by appointment slots available

WORDS OF WISDOM

Tips to fill your schedule

If patient demand is lacking, it's important to market your practice. Try these tips to fill your schedule:

Pull several charts a day and review them for services that it would be appropriate to recommend. For example, if you last saw a 50-year-old female two years ago, contact her to suggest a physical. For a practice with 1,000 charts, you can get through the entire pile in a year by reviewing just four or five charts a day.

Query your registration database for ZIP codes. Look for underrepresented ZIP codes, and target those communities for marketing.

Target established patients who have not been seen within a year. Send them a postcard with your contact information and consider following up with a courtesy call.

Contact schools, senior citizens centers, religious institutions, childcare centers, and other potential sources of new patients with a request to speak at an upcoming function. Or, offer to perform free screenings on site and make appropriate recommendations about follow-up care with you.

Volunteer for community activities. Not only is volunteering good for your community, it gets your name out there and allows you to meet others.

Get to know the members of your community who routinely meet new arrivals; employer benefits officers and real estate agents are two places to start.

Thank established patients, referring physicians, and staff who refer patients to you. Avoid giving them lavish gifts, which can be construed as paying for referrals, but be sure to acknowledge the referral by sending a note.

Hone your customer service. Patients who are impressed by your service will spread the word.

Don't ignore the traditional marketing avenues, such as having a Web site and listing your phone number in the Yellow Pages and local physician referral listings. However, the most effective marketing may be right under your nose: it's the service you give and the reputation you build in the community.

. . . .

Waiting for appointments

Access correlates with patient satisfaction. One measure of access, and one that is important from the patient's perspective, is how long patients must wait for appointments. What is the ideal time-to-next-appointment for your practice? Let your patients' needs determine it.

The ability to offer timely appointment availability to patients is a key characteristic of a successful medical practice. In addition to requests for appointments from patients and the referring physicians managing their care, it is important to recognize that your physicians also prompt the need for access in the form of follow-up appointments. In any case, if patients cannot be seen when requested, both service and care will be compromised.

Access does more than support good customer service and quality care. It also can have an impact on your practice's financial health. Your practice's growth depends on accommodating new patients. In the first two to three years of a practice, physicians may see 25 patients a day. During the next three years, those 25 patients will produce less revenue than they did at first. Why? Well for one, the physicians may have helped them to get better and they don't need to come in as often. But even if they are returning for chronic conditions that require careful monitoring, established patients generate significantly less revenue per visit than new patients. Moreover, in a specialty practice that doesn't have a large panel of chronically ill patients, new patients equate to future procedures and surgeries. Regardless of the specialty, poor patient access also puts a drain on practice resources as staff must dedicate themselves to managing and deflecting demand. Phone-based care skyrockets, and the scheduling process increases in complexity. The additional overhead provides little value to the practice, and only increases the waste perceived by the patient.

Determining the root cause of the problem

The first step in sorting out patient access is to determine if there's really a problem. Patient access stems from a mismatch between supply and demand.

Within a medical practice, "supply" can be defined as physician capacity. There are two important measurements: the number of hours a physician is willing to dedicate to patient care and the patients a physician can see during that time. The time providers dedicate to patient care may range significantly, from 30 hours per week per provider to more than 60. Because this book is focused on patient flow in the practice setting, let's identify the supply of time in the office. (Notably, if there isn't enough time for office consultations, for example, surgeons won't have the surgeries needed to fill their operating room schedule, thus patient access in the office is even critical to surgeons.)

In addition to the varying hours physicians commit to the office, some physicians work faster than others, perform more procedures, or see more patients per hour.

For our purposes, the critical measurement of supply is how many hours a physician is willing to provide and the number of patients a physician can see during that time.

This measurement can lead us to determine the physician's capacity – how many patients the physician can realistically see each day. For many practices, this indeed is what the schedule is based on; for a minority, the schedule is only a basis for staff to overbook to what they perceive the physician's true capacity to be. If your schedule doesn't match your capacity, you'll need to determine what it really is before you can take a bite out of your access problems.

 THINGS TO CONSIDER

Although improving the scheduling process won't offer a permanent solution to an access problem, don't rule out how scheduling strategies can help achieve your access goals. As discussed in detail in Chapter 4, "Scheduling," these scheduling techniques complement patient access improvement initiatives. They include:

➤ Simplifying appointment types;

➤ Reducing handoffs in the scheduling process;

➤ Implementing modified wave scheduling;

- Clustering appointment types;
- Offering group visits;
- Performing online consultations;
- Extending office hours;
- Rolling out advanced access;
- Preventing appointment bumps;
- Managing patient cancellations and no-shows;
- Executing pre-appointment screening;
- Reminding patients of their appointments;
- Handling appointment recalls; and
- Improving provider efficiency.

There's no single solution to perfecting patient access; use all of the tools at your disposal to achieve your goal.

How supply overwhelms demand

Let's say there is a solo allergist who spends 40 hours in the office. During those 40 hours, the allergist can see 160 patients (based on the average per-encounter time of 15 minutes spent with each patient, or four per hour). The allergist supplies 40 hours, which creates a capacity of 160 patients per week or 32 patients per day.

In total, 20 patients per day request appointments. In addition, the physician, on average, schedules another 10 patients per day to follow-up from previous visits. The demand is 30 patients, on average.

The allergist has enough supply to meet current demand.

The allergist also practices in a community geographically separated from other towns. In addition to this practice, one other allergist practices in the same town. If the only other allergist in town closed, and the population of patients seen at that practice was similar to his, it is likely that patient demand would rapidly overwhelm supply. The allergist could not handle another 32 patients a day.

Bottom line, patient access is a strategic issue, and not one that a tweak to the schedule can solve.

Your fill rate

Most practices choose to solve problematic patient access by either increasing supply (hiring more providers or making process changes to use existing ones more efficiently) or reducing demand by closing the practice to new patients.

Before you add more physicians or, even worse, put the brakes on accepting new patients, measure your fill rate to make sure that you don't have a false sense of overwhelming demand.

Although your average time to next-available appointment may extend weeks or even months into the future, get a reality check by looking at yesterday's schedule. Look at how many slots you had yesterday – your capacity – and how many of those slots were actually filled by patients. Divide the latter into the former to calculate your fill rate. For example, if patients were seen in 23 of the day's 25 appointment slots (perhaps two patients failed to show up), then your practice's fill rate is 92 percent (23 ÷ 25 = 0.92). Measure this rate over time. If your schedule represents your capacity and your fill rate is consistently less than 100 percent, on average, demand is actually *not* exceeding supply.

Note that you don't want to be operating at 100 percent, on average, over time. That would mean that you are consistently exceeding your capacity, which creates frustration (if your capacity was indeed realistic and desirable), generates staff overtime, and leads you down a path to push work into the future in order to protect yourself from this excess demand. In fact, you want to be operating right at or slightly less than 100 percent in order to accommodate same-day requests from patients and referring physicians. (Later, you will see how to use a contracting strategy to benefit from a 100 percent fill rate.)

Accurate measurements

For some physicians, the schedule doesn't define true capacity. Notably, you may always be running at 110 percent of your schedule as a result of overbooking (e.g., you squeeze patients in), but it begs the question of what is the *real* capacity? If you routinely overbook patients, wouldn't it be better to add in the capacity in a proactive, defined way instead of randomly overbooking?

Contrary to our perception, the schedule most certainly doesn't define patient demand. Remember, it's very difficult for us to truly understand demand in our industry. The schedule only defines the patients who were successful at (1) reaching you; (2) being serviced by one of your schedulers; *and* (3) making it through your schedule process to be keyed into the scheduling module of your practice management system. Consider that your real demand may be totally different than what your scheduling system reports to you. You may have patients who never get through to your practice (e.g., they call and get the answering service), as well as patients who abandon the call because they don't want to hold for the next-available staff member. Further, there are those patients who do get a hold of a scheduler but don't show up as a "demand" because they hang up or say they will call back but don't when the practice cannot offer their desired appointment time.

Although it may be impossible to identify exactly what your capacity is (based on arguments over "ideal" and "realistic" capacity), and even more difficult to estimate patient demand, the achievement of the balance of these factors equates to good patient flow. Although admittedly imperfect, looking at your fill rate over time is an excellent measure of whether your time-to-next-available appointment truly reflects the balance of supply and demand at your practice.

KEY CONCEPTS

Access Performance Dashboard

Maintaining the balance between supply and demand is critical for medical practice operations. Use these key access indicators to develop an access dashboard to keep your practice on track.

Time to Next Available Established/New Patient Appointment.
This metric tells you if your practice is providing your existing patient base with timely access to physician's and provider's services, not just to your phone nurse(s). To uncover this metric, ask your appointment scheduler for data from your practice management system regarding the average time to next available appointment for both established and new patients. Some practices choose to look at data per physician, but obtaining a practice-wide average will likely be sufficient to see how well you are doing. With data from your practice, you can start to keep a pulse on your competition by figuring out their wait times as well. How? Just call them and ask. Don't let telephone triage take over (see Chapter 3, "Telephones" for more information). Unless your payment is based on capitation, your receptionists' first question to patients who call asking to speak to you or your nurse should be, "Ms. Jones, would you like to be seen?" Ideally, you would like to reallocate resources, such as staff, into helping your providers see more patients in person, rather than trying to handle their needs over the telephone.

Appointment No-Show Rate. It's important to monitor the percent of appointments that patients fail to keep; that is, they don't show up for scheduled appointments and don't bother to call to cancel. No-shows directly impact access. A high rate of no-shows can be an indication that the time-to-next-appointment metric is too large and your patients might be seeking care from other practices. Another reason this metric is important is that physician's time is precious. A last-minute cancellation or no-show fails to allow you the opportunity to schedule another appointment in that slot.

Appointment "Bump" Rate. The percent of appointments that physicians cancel (in which patients must be "bumped" to other appointment slots) is the tip of an iceberg that negatively affect patient access – and frustration. Below the water-level lurk many other hazards: multiple phone calls and letters between the practice and the patient to reschedule; additional phone calls from patients and with pharmacies regarding prescription renewals or other medication questions; and the negative impact on patient care for those patients who are not seen within an appropriate timeframe.

New Patient Appointments as a Percent of Total Appointment. Your rate of new patients as a percent of total should be steady or growing, unless the physician closes to new patients or prepares for retirement. Because new patients equate to a higher reimbursement (consider your payment for a 99204 versus a 99214), the rate correlates to financial performance. While important for all medical practices, this indicator is especially vital for surgery practices. New patients are candidates for the procedures and surgeries from which a surgeon derives the majority of the practice's revenue.

Cancellation Conversion Rate. Knowing the percent of cancelled appointments that are converted to appointments in which another patient is seen tells you how well internal coping mechanisms, such as waiting lists or walk-in appointment strategies, work.

Fill Rate. Evaluate the number of patients you saw in the past month compared with the number of patients for which you had the capacity to see during that period. Ideally, your fill rate should be close to or at 100 percent. Falling short of that represents unused, thus unprofitable, capacity. This may be because a patient failed to show, there was a last-minute cancellation, a patient was bumped by a physician, or an appointment slot just wasn't filled. Knowing your fill rate can help you evaluate which of the various operational strategies explained elsewhere in this chapter would be helpful in reducing rates of no-shows, last-minute cancellations, and bumps. It might also help you refine a marketing strategy to attract new patients. If your fill rate is consistently above 100 percent, then make sure that you are not also using resources to deflect excess demand. The more time the staff spends to protect the physician, the less time they have to help the physician see patients. With a 100 percent fill rate, you'll know that future growth of any significance can only occur if you hire another provider or physician, or perhaps you'll seek a slower growth strategy by dropping participation with a low-paying insurance company.

Addressing truly poor access

If your fill rate analysis confirms your patient access problem, don't look for a single or easy solution. You'll want to carefully evaluate your options to rebalance supply and demand. Look carefully at both sides of the equation – patient demand and provider supply.

Determine your goal

Before you begin your journey of improvement, set the goal you wish to achieve. Try setting a series of goals to gradually improve on your current time-to-next- appointment instead of trying to resolve this issue in one large gulp. Managing patient access is challenging. It's not a process that can be solved by acquiring a piece of technology or assigning a staff member to handle. Access problems are sticky issues because they can be caused by waste, poor design, or sloppy execution in many other processes.

Most physicians find that patients demand same-day access to primary care and two-day access to acute specialty care but consider a time period of two weeks adequate for non-acute specialty care. Although some experts recommend specific access measurements, the most important consideration is what your customers want and need. Gather feedback from your patients and referring physicians, and discuss your own expectations for patient access based on clinical guidelines.

As you consider your patient access goals, develop an awareness of the time-to-next-available for appointments with competitors in your market.(Notably, the concept of 'market' depends on your specialty; an internist may pull from a 10-mile radius, while a pediatric neurointerventionalist may pull from a multi-state area.) If your practice can only offer appointments three months into the future, and your competition is scheduling the same service next week, you may be losing patients to them.

After gathering information from patients, referring physicians, competitors, as well as your own expectations for providing quality care, set a goal for patient access.

Decreasing demand

Most practices rely on increasing supply – or capacity – to solve patient access challenges, but the demand side may offer more fruitful opportunities.

Decreasing demand can be as simple as closing your practice to new patients but this is a drastic and typically unwise decision.

Closing to new patients will quickly cause a drop in your revenue, considering that most insurance companies pay as much as 35 percent more for the same level of new patient evaluation and management as they do for an established patient. In addition to a reduced per-unit reimbursement, you'll lose your ability to alter your payer mix if your practice closes to new patients.

If you don't want to expand your practice, another (and arguably better) way to reduce demand is to review your contracts with payers with an eye to eliminating contracts that aren't worth the trouble. Perhaps a certain insurance company pays you less than your costs and still denies every claim. Consider re-negotiating or dropping that contract when it comes up for renewal. Some payers will immediately come back with better terms, paying you a higher rate per encounter.

Dropping participation doesn't necessarily mean that you'll eliminate all demand from that payer. What it does mean is that you'll need to collect directly from the patients (or reap the benefit of higher out-of-network rates), and let the patients deal with their insurance company directly. Alternatively, you may find that the payer returns to the negotiating table with higher rates. It's not uncommon for practices to come out on top under this scenario.

In light of the focus on lean thinking, I recognize that actions like dropping payers are not valued by patients. Unfortunately, the responsibility of handling the balance of supply and demand has been placed squarely on the shoulders of physicians. Even as demand has increased, and the supply has decreased, the per-unit reimbursement for physician services has plummeted – and the cost to collect the declining reimbursement has skyrocketed. It's time for physicians to recognize that participation with an insurance company is just that: *participation*. And, participation requires a relationship between two parties. Physicians can no longer be unwilling, unassuming price-takers. It's time to bring the insurance companies into the challenges associated with managing patient demand.

Using supply and demand to make strategic decisions will ultimately provide value to the patient. Without recognizing and addressing the underlying strategic matter of the role of insurance companies, physicians will soon be forced to shut off their supply to *all* patients. Before your practice is forced into this position, analyze your relationships with payers.

In fact, some practices aim to operate at or slightly above capacity so they can be in a better position to make strategic decisions about payers with which to participate – and those not to. These practices argue that strategic payer selection is a more successful financial approach than expanding supply because the practice can effectively increase its per-unit reimbursement over time. When combined with strategic contracting, managing at capacity to optimize reimbursement can be very financially rewarding.

 BEST PRACTICES

Increase profitability without working harder or hiring more providers

Managed care expert Randy Cook, MHA, senior medical practice consultant, State Volunteer Mutual Insurance Company of Brentwood, Tenn., reveals the science of using a contracting strategy to determine ways to reduce demand that also can boost profits.

"Once a practice is at or near capacity, the amount of reimbursement per unit becomes the most important element of measure to consider. A practice that has reached capacity cannot provide more services in order to increase revenue or profits. The only route to increased profits for this practice is to increase its average per-unit reimbursement. Although pursuing the highest rate payers would seem logical, the fact is, this practice is at, or perhaps over, full capacity. Therefore, the first step in raising its average per-unit reimbursement is selling *fewer* units (coded services, procedures, etc.) to its lowest-rate payers. This requires the practice to understand its reimbursement per payer, and ideally, its per-unit cost to render each service. If these factors are understood, the practice can target the least profitable payers with which it does not want to continue contracting to drop participation. As long as demand exceeds capacity, volume is a secondary consideration to reimbursement."

Create your own chart of reimbursement and volume, and add your cost for comparison, similar to Exhibit 5.1. Use the chart to evaluate the appropriateness of each payer's rate and to consider how to increase that rate.

Reducing patient demand by discontinuing participation with an insurance company requires careful thought. If competition abounds, your payer may gladly shift its business to another practice. Some payers that are barely profitable to you might also provide a large number of patients, some of whom may be candidates for your more profitable procedures, such as ancillary services.

Regardless of the tact you take, scrutinizing payers closely may help your practice solve two problems – end money-losing relationships and reduce excess demand on your schedule – without closing the doors to all new patients.

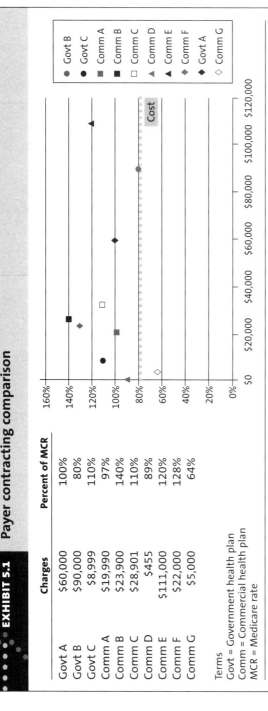

EXHIBIT 5.1   Payer contracting comparison

	Charges	Percent of MCR
Govt A	$60,000	100%
Govt B	$90,000	80%
Govt C	$8,999	110%
Comm A	$19,990	97%
Comm B	$23,900	140%
Comm C	$28,901	110%
Comm D	$455	89%
Comm E	$111,000	120%
Comm F	$22,000	128%
Comm G	$5,000	64%

Terms
Govt = Government health plan
Comm = Commercial health plan
MCR = Medicare rate

Use this chart to focus your payer contracting efforts. The payers that are plotted above cost and close to, or above the rate/volume line are worth keeping. Seek to increase the volume of business you do with these payers. Payers that fall below the rate/volume line have a payment rate that is too low given the volume of services purchased. Further, if a payer's rate is below cost, they are not paying enough to cover the total cost of the services to their beneficiaries.

Find the lowest-rate payer and consider the implications of terminating this payer. If your practice is at capacity and has plenty of demand, then dropping this lowest-rate payer will give you room to see more patients from the payers that have higher rates. As you see more of these patients, the average rate for the practice will increase but – most importantly – the practice's costs will not increase. In order to improve profitability, the physicians will not have to increase the total number of patients they have to see each day or the volume of services provided per patient.

WORDS OF WISDOM

"Quantifying the relationship between reimbursement and volume is helping us deliver more timely and efficient care to our patients because we now have the ability to negotiate from a point of strength. We have data to determine if a payer's reimbursement is sufficient to cover costs as well as data to measure each payer's relationship to one another. We can decide whether to eliminate the below-cost payers from our practice or negotiate for higher reimbursement rates. This strategy has increased our practice's per-patient receipts. The best outcome has been that we have a better way to determine if we should hire another provider to accommodate the increased volume of patients covered by the appropriately paid contracts."

Kathy Rice, CMPE, administrator, The Plastic Surgery Group and Hayes Hand Center P.C., Chattanooga, Tenn.

Pre-appointment screening

If your specialty practice focuses on a narrow field of clinical care or your specialists receive too many referrals for patients whose diagnoses lie outside their area of expertise, you can consider reducing demand by screening appointment requests.

Pre-appointment screening is the process of carefully evaluating patients' or referring physicians' requests for appointments before scheduling appointments. The goal is to determine whether these patients really are appropriate for your practice. For example, if your otolaryngology practice focuses only on neurotology, then a patient calling about a sinus problem should not be given an appointment. Instead, the patient should be referred to another otolaryngologist or sent back to the referring physician for advice.

Specialists can also screen patient appointments by educating refer-ring physicians. Talk to your primary referral sources. Tell them what your group of specialists handles best, what they can't or don't want to handle, what kind of access to expect for referred patients, and where to refer patients who don't fit your practice's areas of expertise. Describe your physicians' areas of expertise in written materials and on your practice's Web site. A careful approach to your education efforts can avoid annoying or confusing referring physicians.

For patients who self-refer or want a second opinion, outline con-crete instructions about what information to submit and to whom. Be clear about what tests, notes, physical characteristics, and other information you will need to make a decision.

The entire appointment process – information gathering, review, and setting or denying the appointment – should be handled in a short, defined period of time. Empower one or two individuals on your staff, typically nurses or nonphysician providers, to make those decisions. Don't route patients or referring physicians through an extensive and frustrating maze of gatekeepers and processes.

Provide a scheduling flow chart, automate a scheduling algorithm to the staff member responsible for screening appointments, or automate the process through a Web portal that referring physicians can access directly. Include key questions to ask persons requesting appointments, as well as a list of any test results, imaging or other documentation your physicians want to review in advance of the appointment.

Pre-appointment screening can backfire if your process of informa-tion gathering, clinical review, and communication about the appointment is too cumbersome and time-consuming. That's why you must monitor this process carefully.

If managed effectively, pre-appointment screening can help specialists who do not wish to handle all of the general issues their specialty's name implies. It also can mean getting the right care to the patient more efficiently.

CASE STUDY

Dermatology department clears backlog

The ambulatory clinic of the University of Michigan Department of Dermatology was plagued with appointment backlogs that frustrated patients and referring physicians alike. In late 2001, appointment availability exceeded six months despite several major customer service initiatives targeted at internal and external customers. As the access problem expanded and overbooked clinics and patient no-shows blossomed, requests for more faculty, space, and triage nurses flooded in. Department leadership, recognizing that these tactics would only be a temporary solution, established an Access Work Group in December 2001 to address the strategic issues that were creating the problem.

After determining that the department's goal was to be the "tertiary referral center for dermatological problems" the department gathered data regarding access, schedules, and capacity. The Access Work Group identified three key findings:

1. Faculty were seeing all types of skin problems and providing primary care for many common skin conditions;

2. The scheduling template had too-few new patient slots; and

3. Faculty requested patients to return to clinic when conditions did not warrant a return visit.

By identifying key areas to address, the Access Work Group accomplished the following in its shift to become a tertiary referral center for dermatology:

➤ Reached desired rate of new patients to returning patients – 25 percent of the schedule is available for returning patients (the target was set for the general dermatology clinic; subspecialty clinics (melanoma, surgery, and cosmetic) had other targets).

➤ Developed and distributed the "Handbook for the Non-Dermatologist – Seven Skin Conditions" for primary care physicians with patients in ongoing management and discovered that primary care physicians were eager to coordinate care when specialist communication was clear and contained specific management recommendations.

➤ Required patients to see their primary care physician before being referred to the dermatology department.

➤ Initiated a standard dermatology consultation request form.

➤ Controlled faculty patients' return visits by scheduling return visits only when clinically appropriate, and extending the intervals for return appointments when appropriate.

Within two years, the department reduced its average appointment wait time to 10 days. Satisfaction ratings soared, as did the department's bottom line. To date, new patients are seen within 15 days, and the department opened the "Today Clinic" for same-day appointment requests with its additional capacity.

Sources: Benjie Johnson, Annemarie C. Lucas, MHSA, Philippe Sammour, CPA, MBA, MSA, Faculty Group Practice, University of Michigan, Ann Arbor.

CASE STUDY

Electronic pre-appointment triage system improves access at neurosurgery practice

Michael Gilligan, FACHE, president and CEO of Cincinnati-based Mayfield Clinic, knew that patient access needed to be addressed – and soon. Established patients were waiting three weeks on average for appointments with the clinic's neurosurgeons. The wait for new patients had stretched to eight weeks. In 2001, the neurosciences practice launched a pre-appointment screening system by creating a collaborative database. Designed to facilitate triage, the results were almost immediate.

Under the new system, calls for appointments are handled by intake specialists (appointment schedulers who had trained in the new system). Using guidelines, the electronic triage system gathers information about the patient's condition, including the type, intensity, and duration of symptoms, as well as any prior testing and treatment received. Based on clinical algorithms authored by Mayfield neurosurgeons, the intake specialists use the system to ask and record additional information about patients as well as coordinate the receipt of all diagnostic images.

Within two days of the receipt of all information, a neurosurgeon is able to review a patient's case to determine the recommended next steps. These steps may include a surgical consultation, an appointment with a physiatrist, therapy, or other treatments. Because the system is able to complete a patient's case, it now takes just five to seven minutes for neurosurgeons to review each case.

Based on the surgeon's recommendation, the intake specialist can make an appointment with a Mayfield neurosurgeon, physiatrist, or therapist. A registered nurse care coordinator then contacts the patient to discuss the surgeon's recommendations, offer education, and coordinate any additional therapy and diagnostic imaging. The care coordinator maintains communication with the patient and follows up with the patient at the end of the treatment period. The follow-up includes discussion of next steps and may include a surgical consult.

The results are impressive: patients can get appointments with neurosurgeons consistently within 20 days. In the first year of the program, the rate of surgery per new spine patient doubled from 22 percent to 41 percent. Gilligan reports, "The neurosurgeons used the talents of other professionals to improve productivity and efficiency while ensuring the highest quality of care."

Mayfield Clinic is so passionate about its electronic pre-appointment triage system that it is now marketing its database to others.

Sources: Michael Gilligan, FACHE, Mayfield Clinic, Cincinnati, Ohio, and www.priorityconsult.com

. . . .

Medical home

Peeling the layers of the onion may reveal another problem with access – patients need coordination and advocacy, as much as they need access to medical care. Instead of deflecting the demand of these patients, consider embracing the concept of a medical home to proactively manage the demand of a subset – or all – of your patients.

The complexity of the health system can be overwhelming to many patients, particularly those with significant medical issues. At times, these patients may even be considered "nuisances" as they communicate their needs. Often, what appears to be an inappropriately demanding patient is one who is ignorant or just overwhelmed. Embracing the medical home concept allows your practice to support the medically needy patient – and get them the best medical care.

As far back as the 1960s, physicians have espoused the value of providing a "medical home" to patients. Advocates of the medical home, the American Academy of Pediatrics, offer the definition:

> "A medical home is not a building, house, or hospital, but rather an approach to providing comprehensive primary care. A medical home is defined as primary care that is accessible, continuous, comprehensive, family centered, coordinated, compassionate, and culturally effective.
>
> In a medical home, a pediatric clinician works in partnership with the family/patient to assure that all of the medical and non-medical needs of the patient are met. Through this partnership, the pediatric clinician can help the family/patient access and coordinate specialty care, educational services, out-of-home care, family support, and other public and private community services that are important to the overall health of the child/youth and family."

Other specialty societies have praised the model and extended the concept into specialty care. Patients suffering from chronic conditions such as malignancies, asthmas, diabetes, and cardiovascular disease naturally look for a home in the specialty field dedicated to managing their condition, but our practices are often not structured to provide all that these patients need.

In contrast to a gatekeeper of the HMO era, a physician providing a medical home to a patient coordinates all aspects of the patient's care. This includes providing advocacy and guidance to patients and their families in all aspects of their care. A practice providing a medical home creates:

1. An integrated, comprehensive, coherent plan of care.
2. A structure to provide enhanced communication and a true partnership with all providers of care to the patient, to include physicians, nonphysician providers, and community agencies.

3. An infrastructure to identify and measure key quality indicators related to the patient's care (see Chapter 12, "Technology," for information on the related topic of pay-for-performance).

4. A means for the patient (and/or family) to effectively capture, maintain, and organize information related to the patient's care.

5. A sensitivity to, respect for, and incorporation of the cultural and emotional needs of the patient, family, and support team.

6. A structure to support the emotional and social needs of the patient and his or her family.

7. Guidance in maintaining, organizing, and optimizing communication with medical providers.

To accomplish these goals, many practices that embrace the medical home concept use an EHR. This technology is especially supportive of the medical home concept because it allows multiple care providers to access the patient's record, ideally regardless of the site of service. The electronic record can then seamlessly track encounters, test results, consultations, etc., thus enabling all providers to gain the information they need to provide better quality and better coordinated care.

A Web portal can extend the information to the patient through a personal health record, and provide a platform for referral management (see Chapter 12, "Technology", for more information on Web portals). The practice may have designated care coordinators on staff, or train clinical assistants.

Regardless of the specialty, a significant part of the success of a medical home is engaging the patient. Resources for medical homes abound. Consider providing patients with care notebooks. Many practices find these essential tools for patients to document, store, and organize all information about their medical care, including their social and developmental issues (see Exhibit 5.2).

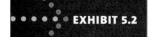

EXHIBIT 5.2   **Care notebook, apppointment information**

Use this form to keep track of your loved one's medical appointments.

Appointment date/time:

With:

Where:

Phone:

Reason for appointment:

Insurance coverage:

> Changes in condition? Treatment progress?
>
>
> Procedures/Tests performed? Results? New tests scheduled? Time, date, location of these tests?
>
>
> Outcomes from current medication? New medication? Reason for prescription? Side effects?
>
>
> Support services recommended? Name, address, phone?
>
>
> Next appointment:
>
>
> Follow up:
>
>
> Notes:

Source: Huntington's Disease Support Information

The medical home truly provides the value that patients with significant health care issues want and need. A significant number of practices have identified state or private grants to cover the expenses associated with offering a medical home. You'll also find that by putting some of the power of tracking into the patient's hands, the medical home can reduce the demands of your most demanding patients, or at least help them to focus their requests better so you can help them faster.

Increasing supply

You have two options to increase supply (and therefore, capacity): do it yourself or hire help. To decide if you can do it yourself, look at your practice's efficiency. How do you compare to industry benchmarks for patient encounters? If each of your physicians sees 45 patients in eight hours, you've probably reached capacity. If you think you can boost physician productivity, decide how much of an increase is possible. Remember, there are lots of ways to improve efficiency without speeding up visits. Before you draw conclusions, carefully assess whether the resources around you are being used efficiently.

You may be able to increase daily capacity in small ways by using tips found elsewhere in this book. Although it goes beyond the scope of this book, do not rule out facility redesign. You won't get the full value of recruiting another physician if that person is assigned an exam room so remote that he or she loses the equivalent of two or three patients a week in the time it takes to traverse to the room.

If you've met your capacity or are almost there, it's time to recruit. You can use a locum tenens physician for short-term supply but in the long-run, you'll want to have another provider join the practice permanently.

Analyze access and productivity

How do you know the right time to recruit another physician? Before you jump into the recruiting process – or worse, sit back and do nothing, a simple access and productivity analysis can make a difficult determination fairly easy.

Create a chart to measure access and productivity. Make the x-axis the number of days to your next available new patient appointment, and the y-axis physician work RVUs per day. Decide on your expectation for accommodating new patients based on the needs of your patients and referral sources, and obtain the industry benchmark for the productivity for your specialty or substitute the average of your physicians.

Feel free to choose your own definitions of "productivity" and "access." Instead of work RVUs, for example, you can choose total RVUs or patient encounters. Instead of measuring productivity on a daily basis, you can run the data on an annual, weekly, or per-session basis. The same theory holds with access; choose both new and established patient visits or choose business days instead of total days. The point is that there is no "right" way to define these variables, but once you make your choices, stick with them.

Plot the data for each physician in your practice, as well as the benchmarks. (Add each physician's fill rate to give you an additional analytical tool.) A sample chart (Exhibit 5.3) is presented for a urology practice with four physicians.

A productivity/access grid is a relatively simple way to get the answer to the very complex question of if and when to recruit.

Once you determine that you need help, consider whether a non-physician provider or a physician better suits the practice, then start the process. Don't delay. You won't find your dream partner in three weeks; it can take a good year to find someone who really fits.

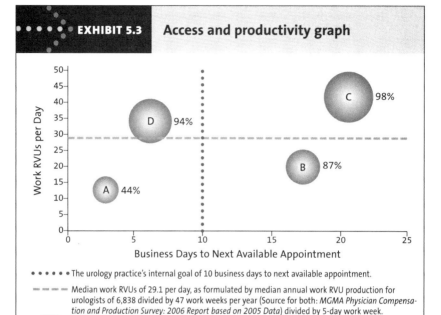

EXHIBIT 5.3 Access and productivity graph

• • • • • • The urology practice's internal goal of 10 business days to next available appointment.

– – – – Median work RVUs of 29.1 per day, as formulated by median annual work RVU production for urologists of 6,838 divided by 47 work weeks per year (Source for both: *MGMA Physician Compensation and Production Survey: 2006 Report based on 2005 Data*) divided by 5-day work week.

The bubble represents the urologist's average daily fill rate (also known as percent of capacity filled).

The access and productivity comparisons are simple, but telling.

Physician A. If there is a physician in the lower left quadrant (like Physician A), you had better hope that it's a new physician. The combination of good access, poor productivity, and a relatively low fill rate are characteristics of a practice that has yet to mature. If the physician has been in the practice for many years, it's time to find out why he or she is unproductive and not in demand. If Physician A is not setting up a new practice, you may have a real problem on your hands that recruiting won't help at all.

Physician B. If some of your physicians are in the lower right quadrant (like Physician B), you have poor access and poor productivity. A fill rate of 87 percent demonstrates an even greater challenge. This is a problem, but not one that recruiting another physician can help with. Instead, find ways to make those particular physicians more efficient. Maybe they need more staff, smoother work habits, or a little motivation. If they are near retirement, displaying their data may be the impetus to exit.

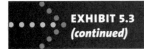

EXHIBIT 5.3 *(continued)*   **Access and productivity graph**

Physician C. If most physicians are in the upper right quadrant (like Physician C), you need to recruit or alter patient demand – soon. Quadrant C means your physicians are highly productive and optimizing their capacity, but patients have to wait to get in to see them. Since you've maximized supply, access will continue to be a problem. If you don't succeed in increasing supply or reducing demand, a backlog – and all of the inefficiencies that stem from it – will soon develop.

Physician D. If most of your physicians are in the upper left quadrant (like Physician D), you have good access and good productivity. "Good" is defined by exceeding industry norms for productivity and meeting patients' expectations for timely access. With a fill rate of 94 percent, there is some room for growth, but this is a physician who is operating very close to optimum levels.

Remember, it's a professional marriage. Assume that recruiting the right person will take 12 months, and be delighted if it turns out to be less.

New physicians

Has this ever happened in your practice? You hire a new physician but find months later that the new physician books just 10 patients a day – too few to cover his or her salary and overhead.

Try lending your new physicians a hand. Track performance monthly and look for ways to help them become successes in your practice. Here's how:

Check the new physician's schedule each month. Compare time-to-next-available-appointment averages for new and established physicians in your practice. Is the new physician's average time to next appointment much longer than established physicians' in the practice? Examine the new physician's fill rate – a retrospective view of the physician's schedule. Compared to how many slots are open, how many slots were filled? The new physician's scheduling template may be to blame. The template may have too many slots reserved for established patient slots that go unfilled. For the first two years at a minimum, ask new physicians to be very flexible with appointment types so they can build their active patient panel. See Chapter 4, "Scheduling" for additional discussion of scheduling templates.

Count the number of new patient appointments each month.
Compare new patient appointments to the total number of appointments scheduled. Plot this ratio on a graph, month after month, as shown in Exhibit 5.4. The number of new patient visits should stay steady or, better, it should grow each month.

If the average number of new patient appointments per month falls, it may be a sign that new patients – or the physicians who refer them – are not interested in the new physician. Or it might indicate a fault in the scheduling process, such as schedulers forgetting to send new patients to the new physician. It could even be caused by your practice's internal politics – a more established physician has told schedulers to keep sending new patients to him or her.

Promote the new physician. Hold an open house, a reception for referring physicians, and place an advertisement in the local paper to promote the new physician's arrival in the practice. If the new physician is replacing another physician, send an informational mailing to patients who might be reassigned to the new physician. And don't forget to include the new physician's name in your telephone directory ad and on your Web site. Make sure that the new physician is credentialed and signed up with all of your insurance plans as soon as possible; ask the physician to sign the paperwork the same day that he or she signs the employment contract.

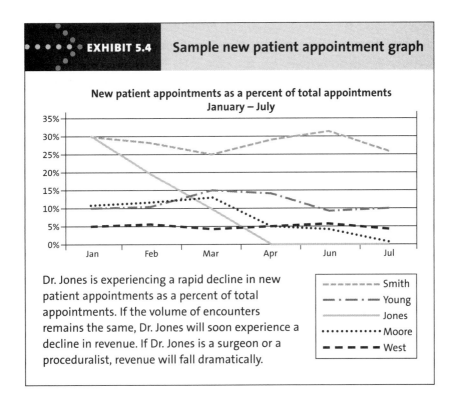

EXHIBIT 5.4   **Sample new patient appointment graph**

New patient appointments as a percent of total appointments
January – July

Dr. Jones is experiencing a rapid decline in new patient appointments as a percent of total appointments. If the volume of encounters remains the same, Dr. Jones will soon experience a decline in revenue. If Dr. Jones is a surgeon or a proceduralist, revenue will fall dramatically.

Smith
Young
Jones
Moore
West

Set expectations. A young physician might not know how many patients should be seen in a day. Set very clear goals and offer him real-world advice on how to meet them.

New physicians can help your practice tremendously. Monitoring their progress can help you and them.

If patient demand truly is overwhelming your supply of available appointments, your practice has a patient access problem. You'll need to manage the situation on a macro basis, that is, get a view of the bigger picture first. If you jump in and try to manage the problem on a day-to-day basis, you'll just create more operational efficiencies that will cause waste and unintended consequences elsewhere in this or even other processes. It pays to manage patient access before it becomes a problem. Proactively manage patient access, and you'll deliver value to your patients and your practice.

Once you've addressed the strategic challenges related to patient access, it's time to resume the focus on your operations, which will be addressed in the chapters that follow.

CHAPTER 6

Reception Services

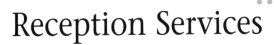

Key Chapter Lessons

➤ Identify the moment of truth

➤ Improve patients' impressions of your office

➤ Recognize the tools to create an effective reception services workstation

➤ Understand the value of registration in the revenue cycle

➤ Learn six ways to pre-register your patients

➤ Examine the process of insurance verification

➤ Learn the key components of site registration for new and established patients

➤ Familiarize yourself with check-in requirements

➤ Evaluate and find alternatives for the sign-in list

➤ Identify proven ways to enhance customer service at reception

➤ Develop a system to communicate the patient's arrival to the clinical team

➤ Evaluate your check-in process

Freshen up your office

What your office looks like can speak volumes about your practice, yet many medical practices give too little attention to making a credible and indelible first impression on patients.

Improvements don't have to cost a lot of money; in fact, the smallest things often make the biggest difference to patients. Do signs in your office contain spelling or grammar errors? If so, patients may wonder, "Are they smart enough to care for me if they can't spell?"

GETTING STARTED

The moment-of-truth checklist

"Any time a customer comes in contact with any part of your organization and uses that contact to judge the quality of the organization, this is a *Moment of Truth*."

— Scandinavian Airline System

☐ Is parking adequate?

☐ Are the grounds maintained and kept free of debris?

☐ Is the entrance accessible?

☐ Is the reception area clean, neat, and quiet?

☐ Is the receptionist welcoming? Does the receptionist make eye contact?

☐ Are patients greeted with enthusiasm, respect, and concern?

☐ Is printed information (forms, education, etc.) readable and concise? Is it explained to patients?

☐ Is there adequate space to wait?

You don't need to hire an interior design consultant, or even have a knack for design yourself. Instead, ask a few friends or neighbors to visit your office. Getting a few fresh observations from outsiders could point the way to needed improvements. You and your staff probably tune out that stain on the carpet or the dead plants on the front stoop. Your ad-hoc design team can quickly evaluate your office's appearance and, perhaps at a price of no more than a cup of coffee and light snack. Most people are just glad to be asked.

Ask your volunteer critics to not hold back on their opinions. Ask them to note everything about your office's appearance – good or bad.

The review should include:

➤ Grounds;

➤ Entry way;

➤ Reception area;

➤ Bathrooms (in reception area and clinic);

➤ Front desk;

➤ Hallways;

➤ Signage;

➤ Exam rooms;

➤ Check-out desk; and

➤ Any other areas that patients typically see, even through a doorway in passing (e.g., your staff lounge, nurse's station, etc.).

Ask your reviewer to make brief comments about the impressions of each area's:

➤ Cleanliness;

➤ Appearance include color, décor, and layout;

➤ Odors;

➤ Lighting;

➤ General impression; and

➤ Clarity (for signage).

If you are renting space, some issues that your team uncovers may require action by the landlord. If those impressions are strongly negative and the landlord won't budge on such issues as replacing worn-looking carpet, removing dead foliage from the exterior grounds, etc, then you may need to consider relocating. A bad impression is just another handicap that you don't need in today's era of tight revenue, high costs and increasing competition.

Remember, your office's appearance is a reflection of you and your practice. It's worth your time to try and improve it.

WORDS OF WISDOM

Big improvements that cost little

Refurbishing an office doesn't require a ton of money. You've probably seen television shows, magazines, and Web sites that show you how to "design on the cheap." It's possible for a medical practice, too. If an office cabinet or bookshelf is falling apart, browse an antique market to find an interesting replacement that can be painted. Get rid of artwork that is outdated by framing your child's school project, holding a photography contest that your staff (or even patients) can enter, or hiring art students from a local college to paint a mural in your hallway.

"The patient has arrived! Now what?"

After scheduling and reminding a patient when to come and what to bring, your next contact is when the patient arrives. As with telephones and scheduling, this function offers many opportunities to make your practice more efficient.

The pre-encounter process should be quick, efficient, and painless for both the patient and the practice. Attention to detail at this early point in the patient flow process will save your staff and physicians considerable work down the line. Attention to courtesy will keep "patients patient" if physicians are running late. Most importantly, courtesy will keep patients satisfied and willing to come back to your practice instead of another one. If you deliver service that wows your patients, you'll find that they not only come back, but they also spread the good word about the great experience they had at your practice.

This chapter will examine ways to streamline the functions within the check-in process, including pre-registration, registration, and sign in.

Don't make registration a source of pain

Does your receptionist greet patients by avoiding eye contact, pointing to a clipboard and mumbling, "Sign in"? Or, does the receptionist simply open the glass partition at the reception desk and stare at patients, waiting for them to respond? If so, your practice is saying, in effect, that it takes patients for granted. Remember, patients' loyalties to their physicians are growing thinner than ever thanks to retail-based quick access clinics and frequent changes in insurance plans. They don't need any help from your staff!

Unfriendly and inefficient check-in processes will irritate patients before they've even taken a seat in your waiting area. They also will raise staff stress, and even increase claims denials.

I know a practice manager whose reception services employees averaged just 28 registrations each per day. That's approximately one patient registered every 15 minutes –more time than most of the patients spent with their physicians. This practice needed a shakedown of its registration and check-in process to see what was making it run so slowly. But even if your practice's registration function gets patients in faster than four-per-hour per employee, it never hurts to measure for improvement. Remember, our patients don't want a lengthy registration process – they want to see their doctor.

Take the perspective of your patient, and start improving your registration process by answering the following questions:

➤ How long does it take to register a new patient versus an established patient?

➤ What's the ratio of new to established patients?

➤ What are the required tasks of registration staff? How long does it take them to complete each task?

➤ How much time must registration staff spend on other tasks, such as answering telephones, acting as the "information desk" for other staff (or other practices if you're at the front of the building), handling patients who walk in to pick up prescriptions and forms, greeting and routing pharmaceutical representatives, and so on?

➤ Does registration staff seem to sit and wait for the practice management system to accept information and move from screen to screen?

➤ Are extenuating circumstances – language barriers or poor location of copiers and other machinery – slowing down registration?

Most importantly, ask your registration staff what suggestions and ideas they have for improvement. Perhaps a computer with higher processing speed, a scanner placed at the front desk, and a pre-registration initiative for new patients are in order. As you gather information about how this critical position functions, and seek feedback from the people who perform it every day, you'll recognize that there are opportunities to improve.

Every medical practice is different but oftentimes reception services average between five and eight minutes to register patients of all types: two minutes or less for established patients with no changes to their demographic or insurance information, and up to 14 minutes for new patients. At that rate, between 60 and 80 patients can registered per day, including all necessary insurance verifications, registration updates, new patient registrations, collection of copayments, and greeting patients. If insurance verification has already been performed, the volume of patients who can be registered per staff member soars to 100 to 130 patients per day.

STAFF BENCHMARKS

Reception services

Practice operations task	Workload range
Pre- or site registration with insurance verification	60-80 patients per day
Check-in with registration verification only	100-130 patients per day
Site check-in with registration verification and cashiering only	75-100 patients per day

Forget trying to staff reception services based on how many physicians are in your practice. The number you need depends on how many patients need to be received.

The workload range depends on the number of new patients, the extent of cashiering responsibility, as well as the patient population, information system, level of automation, and other work processes used at the practice. The more information you gather and/or deliver during reception services (thus, the higher the transaction time), the lower the productivity you should expect.

Given the multitude of variables, measure the time it takes your staff to register a patient, and apply that transaction time to reach your practice's ideal workload range.

Speed up your front desk

Often, it is processes, training, and equipment – not slow employees – that slow down patient registration. Try some of these ideas:

Pre-register. Ask staff to try and pre-register new patients, either over the telephone when they schedule appointments, by mail when appointment reminders are sent or via downloadable registration forms or an interface with your practice management system on your practice's Web site. Or, provide patients with the opportunity to pre-register via a kiosk interfaced with your information systems as soon as they walk through your door.

Streamline paperwork. Ask patients to mail or fax in their paperwork before they come in. Better yet, have them complete it on your Web portal, or direct them to an on-site kiosk or tablet PC that interfaces with your practice management system. In addition to facilitating the capture of information, look at your forms: What signatures do you really need? Are you making them sign every time? Are you covering all of the issues in a succinct format, or is the patient faced with reams of paper to review?

Huddle. Anticipate problems by holding a mandatory five-minute "huddle" before office hours commence to give everyone a rundown of what's going to happen that session or day. Involve the reception services staff in the huddle, or provide a quick summary of the important issues that will impact them, such as an appointment cancellation because the patient was admitted to the hospital during the night. Involving your front office staff will help them anticipate problems – and keep the flow from getting bogged down by crises. (More on huddles in Chapter 8, "The Patient Encounter.")

Prepare. Create a preview checklist of the administrative issues related to each visit. Review patients' accounts the day before the visit and record the information on the printed schedule, the encounter form or better yet, electronic notes attached to patients' accounts. The preview will remind staff of what information to capture during the visit (e.g., copayments, account balances, and copies of insurance cards).

Speeding up check-in is not a matter of telling everyone to work faster; it's about improving efficiency. That not only delivers value to patients, it benefits your practice's bottom line.

WORDS OF WISDOM

Why you should try to "wow" patients

Seeing the MD or DO after the names on the placard at your door, most patients expect to receive quality health care in a safe environment. Although patients are more attentive to prices, cost remains a secondary decision-making factor for most patients when choosing a practice (as a result of our insurance system). What they really want is to be treated well. You may have the world's best reputation, snazziest facilities, and most advanced computer systems, but it's your people who will make a difference. The Ritz Carlton® hotel chain reports that 50 percent of lost customers are a result of poor quality staff. Technical reasons (e.g., access and facility) rank at 15 percent, price at 15 percent, and inattention at 20 percent.

Remember that you can teach employees to schedule appointments, but you can't train them to smile. Hire right, and retain the good ones.

GETTING STARTED

Reception services workstation requirements

➤ Computer with practice management system

➤ All necessary forms

➤ Telephone

> ➤ Desktop scanner or photocopier
>
> ➤ Daily schedule (manual or automated)
>
> ➤ Office supplies
>
> ➤ Communication tool for patient arrival

Does reception services staff handwrite patient information changes for someone else to enter into the practice management system database later on? If so, you are just piling more work on your business office. In doing so, you are slowing cash flow by delaying charge entry and claims submission tasks. Real-time work processing is more efficient than batching work.

Now let's look at the various processes within the check-in function and see how each one works to support the entire function.

Does your front office staff have to walk more than 10 feet to get to the nearest printer, photocopier, or scanner? If so, the few extra seconds those additional footsteps take can add up to hours over the course of the year – time that would be better spent gathering and updating patient information, greeting incoming patients and seeing to other critical reception services tasks. Make sure your workstation is just that, a workstation with all of the resources needed by the front office staff.

YOU KNOW...

...check-in procedures need improvement when you see...

➤ Reception services employees leaving the reception area for several minutes at a time to go into a separate room to photocopy insurance cards and do other registration tasks

➤ Employees sitting at the front desk eating snacks while on break

> A "take-a-number" system for registration

> The sign-in sheet is on a ledge outside a closed sliding window with a sign on the window saying, "Knock/ring bell if you need help"

> The triage nurse at the front desk talking to a patient on the telephone about a medical problem within earshot of the patients

> Completed forms or other paperwork from patients lying on top of the reception services edge

> Urine samples sitting on the front office ledge for pickup

The list of poor check-in practices witnessed in medical practices, large and small, new and established, could go on for many pages. Let's just say there is room for improvement in all practices.

Find the stars in your reception services

Your reception services employees are critical to both patient service and collections. If you want to create an outstanding front office you may need to reconsider your view of the front office.

Front-office employees are by far the most undervalued and under-appreciated in the practice. High-performing front office staff must be extraordinary multi-taskers: capable of greeting patients, checking them in, collecting their money, answering the phone and giving a message to a clinical assistant – all at the same time and all with a smile. They need intimate knowledge of the practice management and EHR systems, as well as the telephone, e-mail, and insurance company eligibility systems. Spend a day working the front office, and you'll respect what they do. Employees who are appreciated deliver better performance because they know their work is valued, so it's worth your time to understand the value of your front office staff.

Many employees are hired into front office positions as receptionists. Make it clear that you require them to also be partners with the
business office. Explain the check-in process and incorporate the
billing-related responsibilities (e.g., registration) into job placement
ads and job descriptions for your front office staff. Set expectations
during the hiring process – and continue to do so periodically
throughout the employee's tenure.

Evaluate your wage scale to determine if you are paying competitive
wages. Don't be bound to medical practice survey data, as most
practices pay too little to get the quality staff they need. Your investment will pay off quickly. Quality employees in the front office can
free up the business office staff to concentrate on productive work
processes instead of spending time fixing mistakes.

Hire enough staff so the front office can manage its daily workflow
in a timely and accurate manner. If patients and other staff complain about the front office and you see errors in their work but you
know you have good employees, re-engineer work processes to redis-
tribute responsibilities or hire additional staff.

In addition to regular personnel training and orientation, provide
front office staff with training on specific issues, such as how to
handle difficult patients, patient flow delays, and patients who resist
paying copayments.

Train front office staff in payment posting and train payment
posters to work in the front office. Cross-training will help front
office staff see how much work their errors can cause. Payment
posters will see the chaos that often resides in the front office. If
employees in both areas gain a better understanding of each other's
work processes, they may be more apt to do their jobs correctly or,
at the very least, stop spending so much energy complaining about
each other.

Give front office employees daily reports on registration errors (as a
percentage of total registrations) and time of service collections (as a

percentage of total *potential* time of service collections). Break out the numbers by employee and ask them to fix their own errors. Seek feedback on the tools and resources they need to perform better.

In addition to sharing data about registration errors and time of service collection, offer feedback from patients, other staff, and physicians. Set employees' expectations about what needs to be improved and when you want to see results. When applicable, offer a "thank you," some hours off, or possibly a bonus to employees who make performance improvements.

Focus time and energy on creating a good staff, and you and your patients will reap the rewards.

BEST PRACTICES

Look for talent

Advertisements for support staff positions at medical practices seem always to contain "experience required." Standard hiring practices in our industry place more weight on experience than personality. Although experience is a plus, high-performing prac-tices are placing equal if not more emphasis on fit. Savvy prac-tices recognize that it's much easier to teach someone to check-in a patient, but you can't teach them to handle challeng-ing situations under pressure, work as a team member, multi-task, or for that matter, to smile.

Take another view of registration

One hundred percent accuracy in registration and pre-registration will save you much time and effort later on. But, no matter how you design your registration process, it must be patient-friendly. Too many medical practices have designed processes that may be practice-friendly or physician-friendly, but are definitely not patient-friendly. To achieve your goal, the patient-centered registration process should include:

Seeking pre-arrival completion of paperwork. Handing a stack of papers to complete in the reception area confirms to patients that they will be waiting. Plus, patients may not have brought the necessary items to complete the paperwork, such as an insurance card. Finally, patients will rush through the forms to try to gain faster access to the provider. Directing patients to a Web portal where they can download or directly transmit the necessary paperwork allows patients to complete the process before arriving and feel more relaxed about the wait. Or, provide a kiosk for on-site, electronic registration. The corollary benefits for you are more accurate information and a less anxious patient.

Greeting the patient. Mostt receptionists claim to greet patients, however, not all are pleasant interactions. Train receptionists to:

➤ Greet arriving patients – don't just check them in like a package the delivery service just dropped off;

➤ Use their name and make eye contact – every time; and

➤ Be upfront and keep patients informed about delays.

Confirming coverage. Developing a process so that each patient will give correct insurance information helps assure that your business office can send an accurate claim to the patient's insurance company and a correct bill to the patient for any uncovered amounts. In addition to verifying coverage, your practice may want to go two steps further: confirm benefits eligibility and query about unmet deductibles.

WORDS OF WISDOM

Problems with claim rejections and denials in your business office?

➤ Study your front office processes and procedures. One internal medicine practice discovered that 10 percent of its claim rejections were direct results of registration problems based on patients seen in the office – from ineligibility to incorrect policy numbers. In order to understand your registration errors, your business office staff must monitor rejections and post denials according to specific adjustment codes that can be reported on a summary basis. If you can't get information from your practice management system, take a sample of 500 claims and count the number of rejections (claim pre-adjudication) and denials (claim post-adjudication) by category versus the total number of claims submitted. "Hire" a community college intern to do the job if you're too busy.

➤ A multi-site primary care practice found that reporting "the error rates" (the percent of claims rejected due to registration errors) to each of their 15 registration desks (one per site) on a weekly basis brought the point home ... and the errors down. As your error rate decreases, the cost of billing declines, cash flow increases, and your staff work on the rejections generated by the insurance company, not their fellow staff members.

Pre-registration

Pre-registration is a process primarily used for new patients. However, some steps in the process are useful for gathering information from returning patients who may have changed insurance companies, addresses, telephone numbers, employers, or may have other important information changes. Any of these changes may affect what your staff must do to handle that patient's records, billing, financial responsibility, referral(s), prescription(s), and so forth.

Unless they have just walked in off the street unannounced, new patients will already have been in contact with someone on your staff, often through a telephone call to schedule the first appointment or a request made online. If it is a referred patient, the initial contact to schedule the first appointment may have been with another physician's practice. Make the best of these contacts, however brief. They are your chance to gather some necessary information before the patient shows up for the appointment.

How much information is reasonable to gather from a referring practice when it makes an appointment for a new patient? Generally, you should be able to obtain the patient's name, home and work (and possibly cell) telephone numbers, the chief complaint and/or diagnosis (the latter particularly important for imaging services), the insurance company and a referral number if the insurance company requires it. Or better yet, provide access to a referral management function in your Web portal so that the referring practice can refer patients directly. At the very least, make it possible for the referring practice to transmit the patient's data to you electronically through a secure connection or fax a registration form or face sheet for that patient.

Register patients when they request appointments

Now let's look at the various processes within the check-in function and see how each one works to support the entire function.

The person who schedules appointments can either conduct a "mini registration" (gathering critical demographic and insurance information) or a "full registration" (all information needed for registration) at the same time the appointment is made. This allows you to gather data in a timely manner. But some patients may not have all the information you need handy when they request appointments. For telephone requests, your scheduling staff will spend more time on the telephone with each patient if you register patients, especially new ones.

If resources are constrained – you don't have enough people to schedule and register at the same time – ask patients if they wish to make their scheduling request on-line. You can ask patients to submit the information needed for the registration process through a Web portal, or they can be asked to have it ready for when they call to schedule.

Some practices allow patients to directly book open appointments online, but if this process seems to create no-shows, or you just want the flexibility to arrange patient appointments based on the most efficient use of a physician's workday and/or the patient's complaint, then continue to take online requests for appointments. However, call the patient back to complete the appointment booking. As you learned in Chapter 3, "Telephones," an outbound call is always more efficient than an inbound call because you can handle it on your schedule.

There's one important exception to combining scheduling and registration in tandem and in real time, and that is when the environment of your practice doesn't support accuracy. This could be because the skill level or performance of your current staff is inadequate. Or it could be an outdated computer system. Ultimately, accuracy in registration is more important than pure speed – accuracy means your practice will get paid; inaccuracy means it will not. If you must, handle scheduling the patient and registration as two separate processes then try to complete as much of the registration portion before the patient arrives.

GETTING STARTED

Six ways to pre-register a patient

Register patients at the time they call for an appointment.

Patients expect one-call service

Information is obtained in real time, thus eliminating the need for any transfers

Patients may not have all needed information handy

Staff spends more time on the telephone and is unavailable for other duties

Transfer patients to a "pre-registration unit" immediately after they schedule.

Makes the pre-registration process more efficient

The practice must have sufficient staff and telephone system

Patients will hang up if forced to wait on hold for a long time and, if so, less information is gathered

Call patients back.

Allows the practice to control the workflow of callbacks

Staff can perform callbacks when inbound flow of work is down

May be difficult to track down patients

Patients may view callbacks as inconvenient

Register patients through a Web portal or interactive voice response (IVR) system.

Convenient for patients and practice

Allows the practice to reduce staff or reallocate resources if information obtained can be scrubbed, verified, and interfaced electronically

Patients may not complete all the necessary information

Not accessible to all patients

Technical glitches can happen

May raise security of information and privacy concerns you'll want to address

Register patients at a "pre-registration" station at your practice.

Keeps registration separate from the "check-in" desk so fewer employees need to be specially trained and accountable for registration duties

Patients often arrive at the clinical area and must be directed back to the "pre-registration unit." In a larger facility, that unit might even be on another floor. Unless you are mindful to request early arrival, new patients will arrive at their appointment time, not realizing that the "pre-registration unit" might consume up to 20 minutes and delay their actual appointment – and the productivity of your physicians.

Register patients via a kiosk at your practice.

Keeps registration separate from the arrival process

Welcomed by technologically-savvy patients who dread standing in lines

Won't totally replace employees because some patients will have questions and a smaller subset of patients will refuse to use a kiosk

Patients who want personal interaction will consider this option uncaring

Patients may not always key in correct information

Registering patients AFTER scheduling the appointments

Although registering patients at the time they are scheduled is ideal, there are essentially three ways to register a patient after the appointment is scheduled:

Transfer patients to a "pre-registration unit." Immediately after the appointment is scheduled – but before patients hang up – transfer them to a specially staffed "pre-registration unit." Staff dedicated to this function can efficiently complete a mini- or full registration over the telephone. This can make the entire pre-registration process much more efficient but you must have enough staff to pull it off. Call volumes can be unpredictable, which makes these units difficult to staff in order to maintain optimal levels of patient service.

Don't get caught putting patients on hold for more than 15 seconds while they are transferred to your pre-registration unit. Patients who wait on hold will feel inconvenienced and may hang up before your pre-registration information is gathered. Customer service should be an important consideration before embarking on this path, as your customers in the pre-registration process are mostly new patients. Their first impression is an important one, and you don't want it to be that dealing with this practice always means an indefinite wait on hold.

Call patients back to complete pre-registration over the telephone. If the "pre-registration unit" is unavailable at the time the appointment is scheduled or your practice cannot dedicate sufficient staff to this function, the scheduler can gather quick necessary information (insurance coverage and patient demographics). Then, the designated pre-registration employee can call the patient back later to do a full registration over the telephone. The same process holds for patients who request an appointment online.

Be prepared to play a little telephone tag if you go this route – many patients won't be available when you attempt your call. Or they may be on a cell phone in a public location where they should not be asked to go into great detail about their medical issues. Moreover, patients may find it intrusive if you call them back in the evening, even though that's when you have a better chance of contacting them.

Use better technology to pre-register patients. Develop a system for patients to register online, ideally through a Web portal with an interface into your practice management system. Look for a system that can perform automated scrubs (searches for possibly incorrect or mistaken information). If your automated system of scrubbing pre-registration information can't be integrated, or you don't trust the software, be sure to keep your staff involved so not to sacrifice accuracy.

Insurance verification can ensure payment

Many insurance companies will give you access to their database of enrollees to help you verify that their beneficiary – and your patient – is actually covered by the insurance company.

Gathering insurance information from your patients is important, but it cannot guarantee accuracy. Insurance cards are rarely stamped with the eligibility expiration dates, and patients may abuse this fact or mistakenly provide you with inaccurate information. Insurance verification from the insurance company itself ensures that the patient is covered. (Although insurance companies update their systems often, please note that there may be terminations that have not yet been updated on their verification system because of the delays inherent in the employer communicating to the insurance company, and the latter updating their database. Although verification isn't a guarantee that the claim will be paid by the insurance company, it's the best tool that exists.)

Online insurance verification can be done directly with the insurer or through a third-party vendor. Ideally, an interface is created to download information directly from the scheduling system to the applicable payers via a batch transmission, with no manual intervention. Online verification should occur one to three days prior to the date of the appointment. This helps avoid the cost of dedicating more staff resources to calling insurers (and spending lots of time on hold). It also helps prevent claim denials that occur because the patient provided inaccurate coverage information or was not actually covered for the service your physicians provided.

If online access is unavailable or not comprehensive enough (i.e., you can verify coverage, but not benefits), then the telephone is your next best option. Even though telephone verification may be more time-consuming for staff, the cost of denied or delayed claims is a much greater expense to the practice in the long run.

Don't limit your activities to verifying insurance coverage. For many specialties, determining the patient's eligibility for benefits is equally important. That is, if you are proceeding with fertility services on a patient covered by ABC Insurance, you'll want to make sure that the patient's contract with ABC Insurance covers fertility services. Determining benefits eligibility is particularly important for services that are not routinely covered by all insurance companies. Often, these are expensive services. Many insurance companies will provide the details of the patient's plan, including covered benefits, through online verification.

While you're at it, gather information about payments, including unmet deductibles, copayments, and coinsurance. Since these amounts can change often, patients are sometimes unaware of the most current obligations of their own insurance.

Finally, find out about covered laboratory and imaging facilities, referral, and authorization requirements, as well as any other information that you can learn about the patient's plan that would help your practice.

Many practices have developed insurance verification and benefits eligibility forms that are completed and maintained manually or electronically for every patient.

The more data that you have prior to the time the patient arrives for the appointment, the better you can serve the patient and support the physician – and the greater the chances are that you will be paid appropriately for the services.

If you have limited resources for verification, consider limiting your verification activities to new patients, patients covered by insurances other than Medicare (because Medicare is so ubiquitous among seniors, coverage is rarely declined), patients who are scheduled for procedures, surgeries or any other services that have fees in excess of $200 (or, a value that you set to represent a level above your average per-encounter revenue), and patients presenting to receive services that insurance companies may not cover (e.g., immunizations.).

For surgery practices, this verification process should automatically be conducted for any patients scheduled for surgery at the time you call the insurance company for pre-authorization. The insurance company will inform you at that time if the patient is not on its roster. Thus, if resources are constrained, you could limit insurance verification activities to just those insurers that do not require pre-authorizations.

THINGS TO CONSIDER

Registering patients via the Web

Patients and staff alike will find registration through a Web portal extremely convenient. Here are some tips to follow when giving your patients options to pre-register or update their information over the Internet.

➤ Develop electronic forms that are simple to complete and easy to submit. Patients accessing your Internet must be able to quickly find the forms on your portal;

➤ Ensure that everything works – no missing links, dead ends, etc.

➤ Use an experienced Internet service provider.

➤ Make sure information can be easily loaded into your practice management information system; re-keying is a waste of time.

➤ Send patients a confirmation notification that their information was received.

➤ Maintain a "print the form" option for those patients who are more comfortable completing forms by hand and bringing them to the practice.

➤ Security and patient privacy are paramount. Discuss encryption and security options with your Internet provider. Make sure that your portal meets HIPAA guidelines.

➤ If real-time data interchange is not available, ensure that patients are informed about when they should register prior to their appointments.

➤ Make sure that your online registration process works flawlessly with all of the most popular Web browsers currently in use, including older versions.

➤ Try to make your online registration process as simple and straightforward as the ordering forms used on any major retailer's Web site; otherwise your attempts to increase convenience will be seen as incompetent.

For more information on Web portals, see Chapter 12, "Technology."

Don't make the pre-registration process unbearable to patients. If you decide to transfer callers to a pre-registration unit, the best way to create a dissatisfied patient is to put them on hold! Whatever method you choose for registration, make sure it provides top-notch customer service. Get rid of the waste by focusing on the needs of your customers. Let patients pull the value they want from the registration process.

Although the pre-registration process itself is optional, collecting the information is not. Doing as much of it as possible before patients walk in the door will make their flow through the practice smoother and reduce administrative burdens on front and back office staff.

Registration

Some parts of the check-in and registration processes cannot be done over the Internet, telephone, by mail, e-mail or otherwise. You may need patients present to sign certain forms, to confirm key information, such as current insurance company, address and telephone number(s), and to provide time-of-service payment. Face-to-face is also the best time to make sure that the patient has read and understands your practice's financial policy.

When "how" is as important as "what"

Medical practices across the country are working hard to improve patient service and get higher patient satisfaction scores. But all that preparation you put into what staff should say to patients will be wasted if your staff doesn't know how to talk to patients.

In his groundbreaking book, *Silent Messages,* University of California Los Angeles Professor Emeritus Albert Mehrabian[1] concluded that 93 percent of a customer's perception in sales situations is formulated based on the seller's body language, gesture, and tone of voice. Non-verbal qualities also represent the controlling factor in consumer perception in situations that are not face-to-face, constituting 82 percent of perception (see Exhibit 6.1).

Based on the teachings of Mehrabian and ample research by others, here are some tips for staff and physicians to keep in mind when speaking to patients:

→ **Watch your tone.** Train staff to understand how the tone of voice conveys feeling. In a medical practice, the tone should be soothing and caring. Use an appropriate rate and volume when speaking but be prepared to slow down when speaking to patients who do not hear well or who do not speak English well.

→ **Be positive.** Teach staff to give positive-toned replies. Instead of saying, "I don't know" and moving onto the next task, tell the patient, "That's a great question. I'll find the answer for you."

→ **Watch body language**. Your body language conveys as much as your words. Patients appreciate it when staff make eye contact, smile, and lean slightly toward them when assisting.

→ **Be professional.** Appropriate personal appearance creates a strong positive impression without words. If your practice has not already done so, develop a policy about personal appearance standards for inclusion in your personnel handbook.

EXHIBIT 6.1 **Verbal vs. visual cues in communication**

Face-to-face communication	Percent that accounts for the meaning of the message
Body language	55%
Tone of voice	38%
Words used	7%

Telephone communication	Percent that accounts for the meaning of the message
Tone of voice	82%
Words used	18%

Source: Albert Mehrabian, 1981

Non-verbal cues represent a majority of what the patient takes away in person — and over the phone.

Face-to-face communication

Words used 7%
38% Tone of voice
55% Body Language

Telephone communication

18% Words used
82% Tone of voice

→ **Stay calm.** Train your staff to say, "I'm sorry we didn't meet your expectations" when patients complain. By acknowledging that you didn't meet a patient's expectations, you satisfy the need to have someone recognize the concern. Teach staff to diffuse the situation as quickly as possible by their words, accompanied by an understanding tone and body language.

→ **Use the "mother test."** Ask staff to ensure that all patient interactions – verbal and non-verbal – pass the "mother test," that is, they should always ask themselves: "Would I want my mother to be treated this way?"

Train your employees what to say and how to say it, and you'll be well on the road to improving your patients' satisfaction with your services.

Frustrated patients? Use prevention and remediation to control unpleasant situations

Patients may already be sick or worried when they come to your office and, thus, more likely to get frustrated at small inconveniences. Sometimes you can control the causes of patient frustration by reducing wait times or improving the telephone system. This frustration may also be fueled by a force out of your control, such as patients' increased financial responsibility for health care or unrealistic expectations. Regardless of the cause, your staff must be prepared to prevent small incidents from escalating into serious problems.

Here are some ways that you and your staff can keep difficult situations under control.

Acknowledge the patient. People who are frustrated want to be acknowledged. Listen carefully. Use eye contact when speaking to them in person. Use the patient's name to indicate you are attentive. Defer to formality, using "Mr. Smith" or "Ms. Jones." State the problem by saying, "You say you are frustrated with all the forms we are asking you to fill out." This shows the patient that you are listening.

Respond with caution. When a patient expresses frustration, don't say, "relax" or "calm down." That may only escalate the situation. So, too, will expressing frustration through your tone of voice or body language. Instead, remain calm. Respond by saying, "I'm sorry we haven't met your expectations." Apologizing immediately usually diffuses the situation. Toning things down early can prevent the situation from deteriorating into anger, which is harder to manage. Anger is another step closer to the disruptive or possibly violent behavior that you want to avoid altogether.

Seek solutions. Determine what you can do to help the patient. If the patient is frustrated by a lengthy wait, offer to reschedule the appointment. Stock a supply of inexpensive gift certificates for a nearby coffee shop or restaurant so the patient can use the certificate and return at a later time. Better yet, get the patient's cell phone number and call when the clinical team is nearly ready. Even if you can't offer the exact solution the patient seeks, your attempt to assist will show that you sympathize with and respect the patient's time.

Control the damage. Recognize when you're creating the frustration. Medical practices with inefficient operations undoubtedly have more numbers of frustrated and dissatisfied patients. Patient dissatisfaction can be the result of poor staff morale, but it also can contribute to poor morale – who wants to work around angry and frustrated people all day? It also may contribute to more patient unhappiness because the time you and your staff spend dealing with and resolving one patient's frustration is precious time taken away from other patients. Unhappy patients can turn into bad publicity machines – customer service experts say an unhappy customer will tell 10 other people on average about the bad experience.

Have a back-up plan. Despite your best efforts, frustration and anger can escalate into violence. Make sure you have a plan of action. Train your staff to recognize when a situation is getting out of control, and to call 911 if they feel threatened. If you are in a building with security personnel on campus, consider installing a panic button at the front desk.

Frustrated patients are a reality. Look closely what role, if any, you and your practice play in creating their frustration. Talk with colleagues and staff about the best ways to handle frustrated patients. Encourage staff to consider how they would want to be treated on the job. Use staff meeting time to discuss the issues, do role-playing and establish protocols regarding potentially violent patients. This is one of those situations in the workplace where you have to be both proactive and reactive. Like so many other areas of the practice, keep your patient at the center of good planning and execution.

Greeting the patient

Do whatever you must in arranging workspace and job assignments but make sure that somebody actually greets patients as they enter the practice. Even if you do not make any of the egregious oversights of common sense and courtesy already listed in this chapter, you are still dropping the ball if your reception services staff must:

➤ Answer the bulk of incoming telephone calls while trying to deal face to face with patients;

➤ Wear telephone headsets but make no effort to let patients know if they are talking to them or to someone on the telephone;

➤ Get up frequently to copy or scan documents, or search for forms and patient records; and/or

➤ Work without all the information they need to accurately answer patients' most common questions such as about their bills or whether the physician is running on schedule.

YOU KNOW...

...your registration process isn't working when you see staff walking around.

Do a mini time/motion study of the check-in process. How often does your front office staff have to get up and walk to a scanner, printer, copier or computer terminal? Multiply those extra seconds by the number of patients you register during a typical month. Now imagine what other tasks could have been attended to in that time.

Making staff walk just an extra 10 feet for each patient lengthens processing time, removes the employee from the greeting position, and tires the employee unnecessarily. Give your receptionists the tools needed to do the job at their workstations.

On-site registration of new patients

As with pre-registration, the on-site registration of new patients and established patients will require different administrative steps, information and time on your part.

If the patient has been pre-registered in one of the ways we've discussed, your practice should still verify that the information gathered so far is correct.

For new patients who have not pre-registered, your front office employees should have on hand a registration form that requests the patient's demographic and insurance information. The form should also include the information presented under the section below on "necessary signatures," which will need to be presented to all new patients, regardless of whether they have been pre-registered.

Finally, collect the new patient's insurance card and a form of identification, such as a driver's license. Ask, "May we make a copy of your driver's license?" (Make sure staff know that patients can legally refuse to allow scans or photocopies of their drivers' licenses.) Copy the cards on the photocopier or scan them on the scanner you have conveniently placed in the check-in area.

For optimum efficiency, set up the registration desk so staff can enter patient information directly into the practice's information system as soon as it is gathered from the patient. If, however, this direct keying cannot be done with accuracy, then simply gather the information and deliver it to a person(s) who can concentrate and key the information without error.

Deploying technology to take over the on-site registration confirmation process can serve your practice and your patients well. Consider setting up a kiosk in the reception area where a patient can opt to complete many registration functions, including the collection of information, verification of eligibility, and capturing of time-of-service payments. If you've been to an airport, grocery store, or library lately, you'll see that self-service is not only possible, it's being embraced by people who would much rather not stand in line.

BEST PRACTICES

Call them by name

Staff at high-performing practices use the patient's name as often as they can.

If you know or are expecting the patient, greet him or her by name. Be sure to use the patient's name during conversations both in person and over the phone. Using a person's name demonstrates that you're tuned into his or her needs. In addition to showing that you're listening, addressing a person by name in a formal way sends a message of respect.

On-site registration of established patients

Be sure to ask established patients at registration if any of their key information has changed since they were last in. Do not assume that asking, "Has any information changed?" will bring the required response. Instead, ask a few specific questions, such as:

➤ "Are you still located at 123 Anywhere Drive in Anyplace?"

➤ "Do you still hold Anybody's Insurance?"

➤ "Is your home telephone number still 555-1212?"

Alternatively, ask the patient to provide the information via another registration option – on your practice's secure Web site or at a self-service kiosk in your office.

It used to be acceptable to collect and scan patients' insurance cards only once a year, but the labor market often dictates multiple employment changes, even within the year. It's time-consuming, but making a record of the card upon each visit improves your practice's odds of getting paid.

As with new patients, strive for optimum efficiency by recording any changes into your system on the spot. Real-time work processing is more efficient than batching work.

THINGS TO CONSIDER

Cluttered signage

I recently visited a practice where the reception room looked like a used car lot. Signs covered every spare ledge and nearly obscured the view into the registration area. The practice had posted notices about everything from its privacy policy to its expectations for time-of-service collections. The sheer volume of signage was bad enough, but the wording – the technical and legal jargon – on the signs was even worse.

Registration forms

Registration forms can be overwhelming to patients. It's easy to forget that most patients don't understand our insider abbreviations and regulatory lingo.

For all new patients and often for many of your established patients, you distribute manually or electronically a packet of information upon registration that includes all of the forms, policies, procedures, and so forth. Although each practice will have its own set of forms, it's important for the information to be communicated clearly.

Here are some ways to make sure you communicate more effectively:

Keep the message simple. According to the Association of Medical Directors of Information Systems, "To communicate effectively with a general audience in the U.S., we need to write at a 6th to 8th grade reading level." Look for complex words in your registration packet – "deductible," "nonparticipating," "compliant," and "assignment of benefits." Is there a simpler word or phrase that you could substitute? Is there a simple explanation that you could give of the term?

Watch the abbreviations and acronyms. ABN, EOB, CMS – these mean nothing to many people. Take "HIPAA," for example. Do you know what the acronym stands for? Even many health industry gurus get confused about it. Your patients will, too, if you hand them a complex Notice of Privacy Practices form and simply say, "HIPAA requires it." If you use the terms, explain them.

Take your registration packet home. Ask your spouse, neighbor, or even your 12-year-old to look at it. If they can't understand it (assuming they don't work in health care), your patients won't either.

Understand regulatory requirements; don't just pass them along. For example, the "Notice for Privacy Practices" is required by HIPAA.

Some practices use a complex template that was drafted by a lawyer and is more than seven pages long. Some legal language is required, of course, but take time to understand what HIPAA requires you to include in the privacy notice and figure out how to say it simply. For example: "We will call you to remind you about appointments" makes much more sense than "Expect telephonic, minimum-necessary communication concerning upcoming opportunities for regulatory compliance."

Provide scripts and educate your reception services staff. It is much more efficient for staff at the front desk to answer patients' questions about ABNs, HIPAA, time-of-service payments, medical records releases, and so forth. Teach your staff what the various forms are used for and provide them with lists of frequently asked questions and the appropriate answers.

Simplicity is key when communicating to patients about regulations, policies, money owed or, really, anything else. Patients aren't stupid; they just don't live and breathe our health care jargon.

 WORDS OF WISDOM

Make your staff part of continuous registration improvement

➤ Consider the registration process an integral function of your revenue cycle.

➤ Involve registration staff in business office meetings and written communications about revenue cycle practices.

➤ Base part of employee performance measurements on registration error rates because accurate registration information will have a positive effect on your practice's cash flow. Obtain this information from pre-claim rejections outlined in reports from your electronic claims transmission and/or the denials you receive from insurance companies.

➤ Make sure staff training for registration personnel includes a two to three week rotation in the business office so new staff can understand their integral role in the revenue cycle.

➤ Create a registration "certification" process. Require all staff who register patients to pass a proficiency test to ensure they are qualified. Don't limit this process to new employees; test or assess annually to ensure the proficiency of all staff who register patients.

➤ Count over a 30-day period the number of claims that come back and need rework because a piece of patient information was not gathered or updated at registration. You may be amazed. Share this information with staff.

Necessary signatures

In order to seek payment from insurance companies on behalf of your patients for services rendered, there are several agreements to which patients must attest. They do this by reading and indicating by signature that they understand those agreements. Many of these agreements are signed one time only when they register as new patients. Others must be renewed at each visit.

The most common agreements for which you seek the patient's signature are:

Assignment of Benefits (see Exhibit 6.3): The patient agrees to assign insurance benefits to the practice so the practice may bill and receive payment on his or her behalf. The form should be signed by every new patient and upon change of insurance.

Medical Records Release (see Exhibit 6.4): The patient agrees to permit the practice to release medical records on his or her behalf to third parties. This includes medical documentation requested by insurance companies when a claim is disputed. The form should be signed by new patients and upon change of insurance.

Waiver Form: The patient agrees to be responsible for service(s) that the practice recognizes the insurance company will not pay. One form – Insurance Coverage Waiver (see Exhibit 6.5) – should be used for patients for whom insurance coverage cannot be verified. Another form – Non-Covered Services (see Exhibit 6.6) – should be used for specific services that an insurance company will not cover. These waiver forms should be signed only when circumstances dictate. The non-covered services form should be used only for services that the physician knows will not be covered by insurance. Some insurance companies maintain their own forms for this purpose. Having a signed form does **not** guarantee payment; it only sets expectations for the patient to pay. A waiver form should only be assigned if point-of-service collection efforts are exhausted.

Financial Policy: This optional, but highly recommended, form briefly states in non-legalese the practice's billing and payment

---

EXHIBIT 6.3   Assignment of benefits

I hereby assign to XYZ Practice any insurance or other third-party benefits available for health care services provided to me. I understand that XYZ Practice has the right to refuse or accept assignment of such benefits. If these benefits are not assigned to XYZ Practice, I agree to forward to XYZ Practice all health insurance and other third-party payments that I receive for services rendered to me immediately upon receipt.

_____

Signature of Patient/Legal Guardian   Date

SAMPLE ONLY

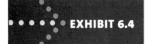

EXHIBIT 6.4   Authorization for release of information

I authorize XYZ Practice to release all medical information (including, but not limited to, information on psychiatric conditions, sickle cell anemia, alcohol and drug abuse, HIV, or communicable diseases) requested by my health insurance company, Medicare, or any other third-party payers. I authorize XYZ Practice to release all medical information to my referring physician and my primary (family) physician. I authorize XYZ Practice to contact my insurance company or health plan administrator and obtain all pertinent financial information concerning coverage and payments under my policy. I direct the insurance company or health plan administrator to release such information to XYZ Practice. I agree that these provisions will remain in effect until I provide written revocation to XYZ Practice.

_____

Signature of Patient/Legal Guardian   Date

SAMPLE ONLY

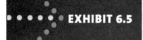

EXHIBIT 6.5   Insurance coverage waiver

I understand that my eligibility for coverage by (name of insurance company) cannot be confirmed at this time. I wish to receive medical service from (name of physician). If it is determined that I am not eligible for coverage, I understand that I will be responsible for payment of all services provided.

_____

Signature of Patient/Legal Guardian   Date

SAMPLE ONLY

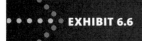

EXHIBIT 6.6 **Non-covered services**

Your insurance company will only pay for services that it determines to be medically necessary. If your insurance company determines that a particular service, although it would otherwise be covered, is not medically necessary, your insurance company will deny payment for that service. I believe that, in your case, your insurance company is likely to deny payment for one or more of the following reasons: [Statement regarding the service being provided and why the insurance company is likely to deny payment.]

I have been notified by my physician that he or she believes that, in my case, my insurance company is likely to deny payment for the service identified above, for the reasons stated. If my insurance company denies payment, I agree to be personally and fully responsible for payment.

_____

Signature of Patient/Legal Guardian   Date

SAMPLE ONLY

Please note that you'll need to make sure that the insurance company does not have a specific policy to which your practice agreed in contract that prohibits you from collecting payment from patients for non-covered services.

policies. The patient's signature indicates that he or she understands and agrees to the practice's financial policies. Signature is required according to a practice's policy; it should be signed by new patients and each time a patient changes insurance coverage.

Advance Beneficiary Notice (ABN): An ABN is a written notification made to a Medicare beneficiary before items or services are furnished for which the physician believes that Medicare will decline to reimburse. Although an ABN is addressed in this "Registration" section, it is likely that clinical staff, rather than reception services staff will use this form at the point of care when the service is provided. Find a detailed description of the ABN, when it is needed, and the required forms at www.cms.hhs.gov.

Notice of Privacy Release: The privacy regulations of the HIPAA require physicians who have a direct treatment relationship with an individual to post a notice of privacy practices in a "clear and permanent position" in the office. In addition to posting the notice, patients must acknowledge the notice by signing or initialing a copy. This is not a consent form, rather it is an acknowledgement.

STEPS TO GET YOU THERE

Follow the paperwork reduction plan

Many physicians ask new patients to bring in all of their medications for a thorough review. Why not conduct a similar review of your practice's paperwork? Gather up the forms you ask your patients to sign. Spread the forms out on a table. As you do, look for:

1. **Forms that can be put online.** Directing patients to complete or download, print and fill out your forms before they come in can save the patient time in the reception area and improve your patient flow.

2. **Forms you don't need.** One hospital-owned practice still used a form that the former chief financial officer had insisted on five years earlier. The form was no longer needed. Throwing it out cut 90 seconds off of each patient's registration. Ninety seconds per patient adds up to a lot of staff time by the end of the month. Another practice handed out a separate form describing its $25 charge for no-shows. Yet, the practice had never charged a no-show patient and had no intention of doing so. Solution? Toss the form.

3. **Forms that could be combined.** Administrative goals and clinical staff must find common ground. Gathering information in one thorough process instead of several different ones saves money and time.

4. **Forms that contain misinformation or mistakes.** Look for misspelled words and requirements that are no longer applicable.

5. **Forms that are ugly or illegible.** You can only photocopy a form so many times before it becomes difficult to read. Worse, it makes your practice look amateur, which is not a good way to build patients' confidence.

Be critical, but don't go overboard. If you eliminate essential forms, required information or forms that could save the physician time in the exam room, you'll soon be adding more forms.

The sign-in list

Think about it, a potential compromise to patient privacy and a leading source of discourtesy to patients is probably sitting almost right under your nose! It is the ubiquitous sign-in list. These lists compromise patient confidentiality because they display for all the world to see every preceding patient's name, appointment time, physician's name, and perhaps other information, such as their insurance company, home telephone number, and so on.

Once upon a time, the sign-in list was used primarily to gauge the patient's arrival time. It gave staff a way to manage the time it took to process patients who arrived at irregular and unpredictable times.

Unfortunately, in too many practices, this list has evolved to replace the function of greeting patients. How many times have I seen an employee seated at a registration desk tell a patient to "sign in" without even looking up and acknowledging the individual? More than I can count. Then, in all too many practices, the patient is ignored until called back up to the front desk to register. Even worse is posting a sign telling patients to sign in but then ignoring them for the next 15 minutes.

HIPAA does not require you to eliminate patient sign-in sheets. You can still use sign-in sheets and comply with HIPAA. That said, limit what you ask patients to write on this form to the minimum amount of information necessary to identify that the patient has arrived for the scheduled visit.

Do a better job of handling the sign-in part of the check-in function and your practice will go a long way toward improving patient relations and operating its patient flow more efficiently.

STEPS TO GET YOU THERE

Make the check-in process work in your favor

➤ Greet your patients. Say, "Hi, how are you doing today, Ms. Smith?" instead of immediately directing them to the sign-in list and barely acknowledging their presence.

➤ "Hire" a volunteer greeter. Call your local senior citizen's center and ask for volunteer greeters or pay a stipend to a former patient who is willing to serve as a greeter.

➤ Eliminate the sign-in list. Real-time registration is a much more efficient way to process patients.

➤ Use a sign-in "label" or "pad" system. Ask patients to write vital sign-in information on an individual piece of paper. Then, place the labels or notes in the order of arrival (or pre-printed with numbers) on a list kept at the front desk (but out of the patients' view).

➤ Purchase a kiosk to direct patients to self-service registration.

Communicating the patient's arrival

The patient has registered and signed in. Now, you have to let the clinical staff – who are often in another part of the office – know that the patient has arrived and is ready for the appointment. This internal communication need not require walking. And a few dollars spent on improving internal communications can save you time and money down the road.

Here are some of the most common methods of communicating the patient's arrival:

Line of sight: Once the patient is processed, place the chart where those at the nurses' station can see it. A chart rack can be placed on a ledge, counter, or wall. A strategically positioned mirror (convex or flat depending on the space) can create a line of sight if necessary at the turn of the hallway so nurses can see the chart rack and avoid many extra, unproductive steps. A small convex mirror with mounting hardware may cost as little as $25 or as much as $150, but it will be money well spent.

Lighting system: Lights can be used to indicate a patient's arrival. Someone at the reception desk can press a switch that turns on a lamp bulb at the nurses' station. Practices with more than one provider can use lights of different colors or flashing patterns. These systems are great for remote communication, especially in practices that are physically spread out, but they're not cheap. Think carefully about how much complexity you need in such a system; prices for simple systems are much lower. If all you need is to announce the patient's arrival, then drive over to your local technology store and ask for options. There are several simple lighting systems on the market, some of which are easily self-installed. This type of system may not work well in a practice where nurses or other back office staff are away from their stations frequently. For a large office, consider installing a lighting system outside and inside each exam room, as well as at the nurses' station.

Buzzers or chimes: A noise-making device can work through the telephone system or a separate low voltage system. Caution: buzzers or chimes that are too loud or have an irritating tone will quickly wear out their welcome with the people who have to listen to them day after day. These may not be useful if the clinical assistants are all in the exam rooms.

Charge ticket print out: Place a printer in (or adjacent to) the nurses' station. When a patient has arrived and is ready to be seen, the reception desk staff (or the kiosk) prints out the patient's charge ticket on that printer. This helps maintain the chart in the nurses' station, allowing the clinical team to review it prior to the patient's arrival. It also helps to ensure accuracy for staff who rely on the charge ticket's current registration information for making referrals, scheduling procedures and so on.

Pagers or radios: Give your clinical staff pagers or cell phones that can display text messages (e.g., the patient's last name, first initial). The cost of telecommunications has come down so significantly that you can outfit your entire staff with these devices for very little outlay. Registration staff can call or send a text-message when a patient is ready. In this arrangement, the clinical assistant who escorts the patient can easily retrieve paper charts, if applicable, from the front office. Alternately, paper charts can be kept in the nurses' station.

Wireless devices: Cordless devices with unattached ear buds that use wireless technology are readily available, and many retail at affordable price points. Cellular telephone vendors in your market may want to bid on supplying such devices or services. Your current Internet service provider also may provide wireless services for businesses, and may offer you a package of several telecommunications devices bundled with Internet service. The downside is that employees will have the devices, and may use them for personal calls or text messaging. If you go this route, implement a policy about personal use and a prohibition on long distance calls. Ask vendors what options they offer to restrict the unauthorized use of these devices.

Two-way radios: Another route is to use two-way radios, or personal paging systems. These systems use voice transactions instead of text messaging. Be aware that information broadcast on systems that use loudspeakers instead of ear buds might be audible to other staff and even patients. These systems are generally not designed to handle large volumes of voice traffic and are best used for quick notifications.

Messaging systems: As with pagers, messaging systems, such as secure and encrypted internal e-mail or instant messaging (IM) can be used to transmit the arrival information, but in more detail. IM is similar to email, but it's instantaneous. Your staff must still keep an eye on computer screens to tell when patients arrive, but the communication can be more complex than a simple lighting system would allow. For example, your staff could type in a patient's name along with a message, such as, "Mrs. Jones has arrived but she's completing her paperwork and will be ready in five minutes." Best of all, IM can be free from Web sites like MSN, AOL or Yahoo.com. The downside is security – most IM systems run via the Internet and are not secure. Talk to an information technology professional about security, including encryption and HIPAA compliance.

Information system: In many practice management systems – and most EHR and kiosk-based registration systems, an automatic alert is generated to indicate the patient's "arrival" once registration is completed. When the front office registers the patient – or confirms existing registration information – the system generates an arrival flag or some other notification. Once the patient's account is "arrived", clinical staff with access to the system will see the patient's name highlighted (or otherwise marked, according to the system's protocol) on a computer screen. The clinical staff must periodically check a computer screen or be alert for an audio cue, but it takes less time than walking down the hall and around the corner. If your practice management, EHR, or kiosk system offers this feature, place a terminal in the nurses' station or suspend the monitor from a wall or ceiling. Remember to keep the screen out of patients' sight for confidentiality reasons.

Although a messaging system can facilitate the communication of the patients' arrival, it shouldn't be the only bridge between the "front" and the "back." In order to work as a team, your practice needs these employees to be in constant communication.

STEPS TO GET YOU THERE

"Mr. Smith, front and center!"

Did you ever consider that a clinical assistant poking his head into the reception area and yelling out a name might not be the best way to retrieve patients? Instead, try one of these ideas to make this process friendlier:

1. Take a photograph of a new patient (with permission, of course), and attach the photo to the chart or store the digital image in the EHR to help staff find the patient in the reception area.

2. Photocopy the patient's driver's license (after asking for permission, of course) and secure or scan a copy on the chart to help staff identify the patient in the reception area.

3. Instruct the receptionist to write down a brief description of what the patient is wearing (but nothing that you would be embarrassed for the patient to see).

4. When new patients register, ask how they would like to be addressed. Note their response prominently in their charts so you can at least refer to patients in their preferred manner when you do have to call them.

Don't let registration and check-in snafus disrupt the patient flow process. You can handle the registration and check-in steps more efficiently and effectively with the right tools, right processes, and a well-trained staff.

References

1. Albert Mehrabian, *Silent Messages: Implicit Communication of Emotions and Attitudes,* 2nd ed. Wadsworth: Belmont, Calif., 1981.

CHAPTER 7

Waiting

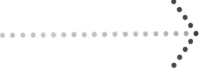

Key Chapter Lessons

- ➤ Analyze your waiting times
- ➤ Evaluate your cycle time
- ➤ Learn ways to improve the quality of patients' waiting times
- ➤ Identify options to reduce waiting times
- ➤ Recognize the value of communicating to your staff and your patients
- ➤ Calculate the impact of process time and staffing levels on wait time

The waiting process

We have built our medical practices around the concept that patients will wait for us. In fact, we even dare to call it a "waiting room"! With that mindset, it's no wonder that abuses abound at this step in the patient flow process. Improvements in communications and increasing expectations are making people less "patient" than ever. Lean thinking instructs us to design our processes around what creates value for our customers. Waiting is of little value to them, so our goal in lean thinking – and intuitively – is to make sure our customers wait as little as possible.

Do you know your practice's average wait time?

Most experts agree that patients will tolerate waits up to 20 minutes. But is "tolerate" what you're aiming for? Press Ganey Associates, a company specializing in measuring patient satisfaction, reports that patient loyalty is truly at risk when the wait exceeds 10 minutes. Based on more than a million patient surveys, the average patient satisfaction score drops from the 92.6 percentile for waits of less than five minutes, to 89.8 for waits of six to 10 minutes, and to the 84.3 percentile for more than 10 minutes.[1]

Before you can make any progress in improving waiting times for patients in your practice, you must understand how long they really wait. It might be longer than you think.

KEY CONCEPTS

Cycle Time

Cycle time is the measurement of time from the patient's entry to the patient's exit. The cycle time in a medical practice typically ranges from 30 to 90 minutes, with 60 minutes as the average. This period of time can be divided into two categories: customer value-added and non-value-added steps.

The concept is an important one for lean thinkers, as non-valued-added steps represent waste or "muda" and are targets for elimination or reduction.

THINGS TO CONSIDER

Patients can help you measure cycle time

If you don't have time to conduct your own timing survey to analyze wait time, let your patients do the study for you. Give every patient a clipboard (preferably with an integrated clock) with a survey instrument that highlights each point at which the patient should record the time (for example, reception, registration, escort to the clinical area, etc.). Provide a small token of appreciation for participants, such as a pen with your logo on it. Be forewarned that patients' perceptions will influence the survey, and do not try this if waiting is a significant problem in your practice. You may infuriate your patients by asking them to measure the waiting that they dread!

Cycle time

What is your practice's patient cycle time? In an efficient medical practice, patient cycle time – how long it takes a patient to get in and out of the door – averages 60 minutes. Of course, procedures, ancillary service, complicated office visits, and consultations will take longer.

Because the cycle time is dependent on the services you offer and may differ by patient, the key is not to aim for a particular *time*, but to provide defined *value* to patients in each step of the process. The goal is to streamline and optimize value-added steps, and to reduce and eliminate non-value-added steps. Undoubtedly, the easiest way to target non-value added steps is to identify and reduce waits and delays and improve the quality of waits and delays for the patient.

Here's how you can get started.

Measure cycle time. Start the clock when a patient enters your practice and stop the clock when the patient leaves. That's one cycle. Ask your reception services staff to note the exact time that each patient signs in, assuming that patients don't have to wait in line to sign in. The departure time can be noted at the conclusion of the practice services process.

Assess cycle time. Refine your cycle time assessment. Calculate the average cycle time for the patients whose visits make up 80 percent of your physicians' typical office visits.

Target one area for improvement. Eliminate a non-value added process – if you can – or reduce the transaction time. Measure reception time, for example. Can you make it go faster by reducing the amount of paperwork that patients must complete? Can you pre-register patients by phone, kiosk, or Web portal? Can you provide resources, such as a high-speed scanner, to your reception services staff so that they can reduce the time it takes to check in a patient? Can you also improve the quality of the transaction by enhancing customer service? Re-evaluate check-in time after making changes and assuring that the portions of the process you alter are running smoothly. It's important to recognize that workflow won't be perfected with a sweep of a wand or a couple of changes to a process. Mastering patient flow is a series of many, small changes that add up to optimized value for the patient.

Re-measure total cycle. After making changes in the area targeted for improvement, measure check-in time again, as well as the total cycle time for the average patient visit. Did cycle time go down, stay the same, or go up? Optimize the value-added steps, and decrease the non-value-added steps.

There is no "perfect" cycle time, but optimizing value-added time (the actual encounter between the patient and the physician) and minimizing non-value added time (asking patient's insurance information for the fifth time) creates a win/win situation for you and your patients.

Try to strike a healthy balance so patients and physicians spend more time together and both spend less time waiting for each other.

STEPS TO GET YOU THERE

Five ways to attack waiting time – and create value for the patient

1. **Eliminate check-in.** If your clinical intake process does not require a nurse, staff your front desk with care team associates who are trained to register and room patients, take vital signs, help patients fill out medical histories, and handle other duties.

2. **Eliminate the waiting room.** If your practice can verify insurance and benefits eligibility before the patient arrives, conduct the registration process in the exam room. Emergency rooms do something similar, known as "bedside registration."

3. **Eliminate checkout altogether.** Collect time-of-service payments upfront at check-in. Process any referrals, schedule tests, and arrange any follow-up appointments in the exam room. Stop giving the patients charge tickets to carry to another desk – just let them go after the exam.

4. **See patients in their homes.** While it was common for physicians to travel to their patients years ago, it's a rare occurrence today. But it's been a recent trend for physicians to truly optimize value to their patients by traveling to their homes. Home visits are on the rise, and patients are embracing the idea.

5. **Think out of the box.** Find a solution that works for your specialty and your practice. Imagine new possibilities, and you may surprise yourself – and your patients.

See Chapter 14, "The Patient-Centered Practice of the Future," for more information about eliminating the patient's waiting time.

WORDS OF WISDOM

Waiting affects patient satisfaction

The quality of the wait can influence the perceived value by the patient. Researchers measured patient satisfaction scores (see Exhibit 7.1) based on time (minutes in waiting room) and quality (comfort and pleasantness of waiting area), concluding that quality can improve satisfaction as waits get longer.

How to make the wait go faster

The nature of your practice's services, the fact that every patient is unique, and the reality that the exact arrival of your patients is unpredictable mean that you will never be able to achieve an

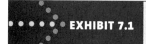

EXHIBIT 7.1   Ratings of waiting rooms

Minutes in waiting room	Comfort and pleasantness of waiting area					
	Very poor	Poor	Fair	Good	Very good	Total
0 to 5	41.3	64.2	75.3	82.4	96.3	90.6
6 to 10	44.0	62.3	66.9	74.7	90.9	82.9
11 to 19	41.1	54.9	57.6	68.5	84.8	74.9
20 +	15.0	23.6	34.2	49.0	66.1	51.1
Total	24.6	37.6	51.5	68.2	88.1	76.2

Source: K.M. Leddy et al. "Timeliness in Ambulatory Care Treatment: An Examination of Patient Satisfaction and Wait Times in Medical Practices and Outpatient Test and Treatment Facilitiies." *Journal of Ambulatory Care Management*, April/June 2003, Volume 26, Issue 2, 138-149.

Don't conclude your performance improvement initiatives without reducing wait times, but you can benefit from efforts to improving the *quality* of the wait.

average wait time of zero minutes in your practice. Spend time reviewing ideas provided in this book to reduce the time of the wait, but it's also important to note that you can easily add *value* to the waiting process.

Let's review ideas to improve the quality of the wait for your patients.

Change your "waiting room" to a "reception area." Changing what you call that area where patients wait before their appointment can help to create a new attitude for staff and patients. Support this by changing signage, as well as how your staff refers to the area. It won't cost you anything but will create a less negative impression on your patients. Instead of saying, "we expect you to wait," you'll be saying, "we're ready to receive you." Take it up a notch by calling it the "meditation area" or "relaxation room", but be sure to provide the atmosphere to support this new name, such as soft music and lighting.

Maintain the area. Children's toys should not be scattered about for someone to trip on. Torn or outdated magazines should be removed. Carpets should be clean. Any plants should appear healthy. The walls should not be dirty or have significant marks on them. Trash should be picked up nightly, or even twice a day. Someone should be designated for the responsibility to walk through the area before the doors open, and frequently throughout the day to tidy up.

Engage your patients. The self-serve salad bar is an example of how the restaurant industry tries to make the inevitable waiting for food more productive. You can try something similar in your practice by adding some value to the time your patients have to wait to see a physician. Offer them a blank form with the heading: "Things I wish to discuss with my doctor today." This allows patients to consider the information they want to convey to the physician so that the patient-physician interaction is more focused. Add another section, "Medications I would like to renew", so they won't forget to mention them during the encounter. Offer patient education materials for them to browse through via brochures or online by way of computers in the reception area.

Or, engage patients with a retail area. An ophthalmology practice can sell eyewear and an otolaryngology practice can sell hearing aids. Any practice can sell thumb drives on which the patient's record can be downloaded. Buy drives in the form of key chains and add your logo to the drive, and you have a marketing tool. In addition to adding value to the wait, this retail opportunity can increase your revenue stream.

Add amenities. Your reception area and exam rooms should provide entertainment or at least enough diversions to occupy your patients as they wait. Other ways to make the wait go faster for patients are by adding:

> ➤ Wireless network for patients to use their own laptops;

> ➤ Robes and slippers (particularly useful for replacing paper gowns used for patients in sub-waiting areas);

> ➤ Patient education materials;

> ➤ Computers loaded with materials relevant to the practice;

> ➤ Simple games on paper, such as Suduko, crossword puzzles, and word search puzzles will help pass the time. Create your own puzzles using Web sites for educators;

> ➤ Notepads for adults with your logo and coloring books for children;

> ➤ Jigsaw puzzles (but not if your practice serves small children who could choke on a small piece);

> ➤ A toy bin for children (but make sure toys are safe for all ages and are not left where other patients could stumble on them.) Be sure to clean toys after each child's play session to prevent spreading germs;

> ➤ A simple coffee bar, or ramp it up a notch with a machine that offers self serve specialty coffee drinks;

➤ A fish tank with colorful fish, or ramp it up a notch and stock turtles or other unusual aquatic animals;

➤ A working train on tracks suspended from the ceiling (for added affect, provide a "start" button on the wall for patients to push and decorate the train based on the seasons); and

➤ Recipe and coupon exchange boxes.

BEST PRACTICES

"Brand" your waiting areas

For large practices with multiple waiting areas, there's nothing more difficult to handle than a "lost" patient. To help patients get to where they need to be, high-performing practices develop and use a theme for each sub-specialty. Historically, practices have chosen themes based on specialty. Words like "rheumatology," "otolaryngology," and "gynecological oncology" are familiar to us who work in the health care industry; however, they may not be what engages the patient. The themes of the sub-practices can reflect the specialty, but also consider using area attractions (mountains, rivers, deserts, historical locations, etc.) as ways to identify these areas. They will offer more value to the patient. Employ similar colors, design, and signage for each theme so that each area is consistent with your practice's brand.

Review reading material. Get rid of tattered and out-of-date magazines. Stop using recycled magazines from you or your staff's home subscriptions – it makes your practice look like a cheapskate. Make sure reading material is up-to-date and relevant to patients by economic status, age, educational background, and native languages. Use a subscription service to ease the burden of managing several subscriptions and possibly get discounts. If money is tight, ask a local magazine vendor to provide you with reading materials that are being replaced with newer ones. And don't forget that your patients may bring spouses – men are frequent visitors to the reception areas of obstetrics practices, for example.

Hand out pagers. Allow patients to get up and walk around if there is an outdoor walking area adjacent to the practice. Pagers that combine simple video games will be appreciated (as long as the video game sound can be muted). Embed your pagers in a large (10" diameter) wooden holding device if theft is a possibility. Cut the wood into a shape to fit a theme, such as a fish.

Post a community board. Patients may want to peruse information about support groups, exercise activities, nutrition, etc.

Host an "art gallery." Ask local artists to display their work or perhaps some of your staff or patients are painters, photographers, quilters, etc. In addition to showcasing local talent, your reception area will be decorated for free.

Post pictures. Photographs of the physicians, staff and their families with some professional and personal information can help establish a "personal" relationship between patients and your practice. Try posting the baby pictures of your own staff and physicians; your patients will be delighted. If you have someone who specializes in scrapbooking on staff, pay them a nominal amount to set up your wall of photos.

Add history. Bring in historical photographs or other items from local yard sales or antique shops. One practice in a recently built-up suburb hung photographs of the area and memorabilia from the nineteenth century when it was still rural.

Entertain. Television can entertain but put some thought into what channels to show and at what volume. Take it up a notch by building a small movie "theater" into your reception area to play movies that you have screened for content and age level.

"Hire" a volunteer. A local retirement center may know someone who wants to volunteer as a greeter in your reception area – something hospitals have done successfully for years. Your volunteer could serve coffee, read to children, hold the door for the mother shepherding small children, or fetch a pen for someone filling out a form. Alternatively, ask or hire a former patient to perform the same duties.

Infuse pleasant smells. Use an air purifier to remove the "clinical" smell that pervades most practices. Or, take it up a notch by baking muffins and bread in your reception area. Offer the baked goods to patients. Not only will patients be delighted with the treat, the smell will provide a wonderful aroma.

Conduct patient satisfaction surveys. Take advantage of the patient's waiting time to ask just two questions: What do they think about the practice? Who referred them?

Staff. There's nothing that can demolish the atmosphere of a well-planned reception area faster than a staff member who turns patients off with his or her actions – or lack thereof. Hire pleasant staff and train them to be customer-oriented.

Test yourself. Consider asking a family member or friend to sit in your reception area for 30 minutes during a typical morning or afternoon. What ideas arise that could improve the wait. Find someone who does not normally visit the practice so you'll get an unbiased review. You might have grown accustomed to the shabby wallpaper, faded artwork, or dusty plants.

Improving the quality of the wait adds value for the patient. Be creative. Consider the population of patients you serve – and those new patients you want to attract, and integrate ideas that can improve the patient's wait. Improvements don't have to bust the budget because, often, just a few minor touches can improve the atmosphere of a room.

What patients value – or don't value – about waiting

David Maister, PhD, wrote these seven truisms about the psychology of waiting,[2] which I have translated into adding value for patients in medical practices.

1. Unoccupied time feels longer than occupied time.
    Entertain patients with reception-area amenities. See the section, "How to make the wait go faster" for lots of great ideas.

2. Anxiety makes waits seem longer.
    Keep patients informed about their wait. Even if long waits are inevitable in your practice, most of the customer service challenges can be stemmed by being proactive and open about the delay.

3. Pre-process waits are longer than in-process waits.
    People want to get started. Engage patients in the process by handing them a pad to write down their symptoms, questions, or medications that they wish renewed. Or, get them into the process faster by escorting them directly to the exam room. Finally, start the clinical process during intake by reviewing the medical history, current medications, etc.

4. Uncertain waits are longer than known, finite waits.
    Don't resort to the commonly used statement, "the doctor will be right with you." Train staff to estimate the wait time, and keep the patient informed every 15 minutes. Always overestimate the wait time by five minutes; your patients will be delighted that the wait was shorter than you had anticipated.

5. Unexplained waits are longer than explained waits.
    If the physician is running behind, proactively tell the patient that the wait will be longer. Explain why: "The doctor is delayed because of an emergency at the hospital"; estimate the time; and offer alternatives, "Would you like to wait? We'd be happy to reschedule."

6. Unfair waits are longer than equitable waits.
    If you're escorting patients back for lab work, for example, while those who are in process for the physician must wait, explain the

process upfront. "Ms. Jones, we did want to inform you that we have several clinics running today. Some patients may be served before you, but they are here for other services. I'm relaying your arrival to Dr. Smith's clinical team right now, and they will be with you in 20 minutes." Otherwise, your patients will just get increasingly angry as they watch patients who came in after them be served.

7. The more valuable the service, the longer you will be willing to wait.
There's that term again; it's all about value. If patients perceive value, the longer they'll wait.

Understand what's going through your patients' minds, and you can take steps to improve the perception, quality and hopefully, quantity, of their wait.

WORDS OF WISDOM

Learn to apologize

What's the most effective way to calm down a patient who is complaining? It is to simply say you are sorry. Unfortunately it's difficult for many employees to apologize when the problem is not their fault. Teach your staff that they don't have to embrace the blame, just say, "I'm sorry that we didn't meet your expectations." It's an apology that doesn't identify blame.

Pay attention to the signs around you

Take a close, critical look at the signage in your practice's reception area. At one practice, I counted 30 pieces of paper hung, taped, or tacked to the walls throughout the reception area. There were announcements of everything from charging for late payments to the appointment cancellation policy. Besides the visual overload, these signs often look unprofessional – containing spelling mistakes, smudges, and sometimes, they are unintelligible. Take a few minutes after hours to sit in your reception area and look around. What is the message you are getting from the signs on your walls? Is it "we don't do this," "we won't do that" or "we'll charge you extra for such and such?" Discard this negative messaging. Put those signs into a practice policy brochure or integrate the messages into your registration forms. Give those policies to patients in writing and post them on your Web site or portal, not all over your walls.

THINGS TO CONSIDER

Keep a pulse on your practice

Why wait for the results of your patient satisfaction survey? To keep a pulse on patient flow and the practice in general, the manager at an East Coast orthopedic practice walks through the reception area twice a day to talk to the patients. She says the 15 minutes spent over the course of the day doing the walk-throughs are the most valuable minutes of the day!

WORDS OF WISDOM

Pay attention to reception area furnishings

Cramped reception areas make waiting more stressful. I recommend having enough chairs to hold your expected number of patient visits per 90-minute period, plus an additional 1.5 chairs per patient for family members, friends, or guardians. If you expect to see six patients in 90 minutes, then you'll need 15 seats. It sounds like a lot but you'll want to account for the patients who arrive early for appointments, those who bring a spouse or child, and those waiting longer when their provider runs behind. Some patient populations may require an even higher number of seats. Pediatric practices and those serving certain cultural groups may find that patients arrive with a higher-than-average number of family members. Finally, make sure to provide individual seating; most patients don't want to share a sofa or loveseat in a physician's office with a complete stranger.

Can you eliminate waiting?

The short answer is "no" – no matter how adept you are at scheduling patients, your average waiting time will never be reduced to zero. Unlike the efficiency of a manufacturing operation, providing a service is susceptible to many factors, including variations in demand. For example, if every patient presented in 15-minute intervals (not even a minute off) and it took your office exactly 15 minutes to serve each one (again, not even a minute off), then you could create a no-waiting environment. But let's get real; we can neither expect every patient to present at exact intervals nor the service time to be exact. Don't forget that your service is perishable. That is, the "service" – your physicians' time – cannot be inventoried or stored until the patient arrives. So what can you do? You have three options:

1. Smooth demand through scheduling techniques. Encourage your patients to schedule their well-child checks before the flu season comes and avoid scheduling routine follow-up visits on your predictably busiest office days. Or, reduce your demand altogether by discontinuing your participation with one or more insurance companies (see Chapter 5, "Patient Access" for more tips on managing patient demand).

2. Adjust service capacity. Use part-time physicians, flexible work shifts (evening hours during flu season, for example), or schedule surgeries on Saturdays if operating room time and office space is at a premium. Study each physician's schedule to ensure they have the proper level of staff and space to match the demands created by their schedules. If every physician wants a Monday morning clinic, hire additional front office staff to serve patients on that morning. If you don't have enough space, start your clinic at 7:00 a.m. and run through lunch, to take advantage of previously unused space. Don't forget to use idle capacity to your advantage; give the task of opening mail to your telephone operators, for example.

3. Allow customers to wait. Knowing that your patients will have to wait, try to occupy their time to make the wait go faster. In other words, add value to the wait by using the suggestions described in this chapter.

Is it worth the effort to reduce waiting times even by a few minutes? Yes! Managing your wait times to minimize them is important to increasing patient satisfaction. Patient who wait four minutes to see the physician will be much happier than patients who wait 40 minutes, no matter how many jigsaw puzzles and magazines you place in front of them.

THINGS TO CONSIDER

When being extra nice to patients is fraud

Waiving the copayment for patients who have endured lengthy waits may sound like a good idea, but if you do so consistently, be advised that insurance companies will consider it fraud. Why? Because waiving a copayment interferes with the contractual relationship between the employer, insurer, and beneficiary. Waiving copayments on a routine basis is suspect on a number of grounds; routinely waiving copayments effectively reduces the practice's fee schedule. If you consistently reduce the patient's portion, insurance companies will expect the same courtesy; that is, they would expect to be given a discount as well. However, you can still try to mend fences with patients who have put up with long waits by offering them a coupon for a discounted beverage at a nearby café or cafeteria. Just make sure that whatever you offer is of nominal cash value.

BEST PRACTICES

End indifference

High-performing practices recognize that the key challenges of customer service relate to indifference. Most practice personnel do not overtly provide poor service. They don't shake their fingers and scream at patients, but they may be indifferent to patients' needs. It's easy to tell when a patient is lost, for example, but it's just as easy to avoid making eye contact, put your head down, and keep walking. That indeed is indifference, and it's poor service. High-performing practices recognize that customer service training starts with recognition about what service really is.

Other tips for the reception area

Communicate the wait time. When any staff member (nurse, medical assistant, receptionist, etc.) learns that a physician is unable to arrive on time or must cancel scheduled office hours, this information should be communicated immediately to all staff. Patients who are already waiting should be informed by the physician's clinical assistant and asked if they would prefer to wait (if it's an option) or be rescheduled. At the same time, the administrative staff (preferably an appointment scheduler) should contact the other patients adversely affected by the physician's delay and reschedule them.

When the physician gets more than 15 minutes behind schedule, tell newly arriving patients of the delay. Keep currently waiting patients informed and offer to reschedule their appointments if they so choose. Be sure to have a contingency plan that identifies who is accountable for what so that responsibilities for the tasks of communicating, rescheduling, and processing are clear.

Although communication should never take the place of striving to reduce your wait time, it's amazing how much impact proactively talking to the patient about the wait can have. It's not the actual words; it's the fact that you're demonstrating respect for the patient's time.

Be fair to your staff. Don't let the front office bear the brunt of patients' frustration over long waiting times. The idea of placing a sign in the reception area that says, "Please see the receptionist if you have been waiting longer than 20 minutes," can be unfair to staff when they must constantly apologize (and contend with angry patients) for a physician who consistently runs behind schedule. Not informing the front office about an emergency surgery that delays the physician leaves a receptionist vulnerable to angry patients who become even more agitated when the receptionist admits no knowledge of what's going on.

Your physicians may believe that their patients are "willing to wait" but that is not always the case. Many patients have other things on their schedule besides a doctor's appointment, and it's no secret that younger generations, who have grown used to instant access to information, are more intolerant of waits. Give patients and staff the information that they need to manage waits and delays.

Recognizing that waiting is inevitable should foster creative solutions to keep your patients informed, occupied and, possibly, entertained. Although waiting will occur, this fact is not an excuse to tolerate long waits in your practice; don't let an entertaining reception area lull your practice into accepting hour-long waits. Instead, measure and monitor wait times, using ideas that you learn in this book to reduce waiting during and between processes.

ANALYSIS

Calculating the impact of process and staff changes on wait times

If you were presented with evidence that a function provided by your practice results in long waiting times for your patients, how would you troubleshoot the problem? How would you estimate the impact of changing the process versus changing staffing to reduce long wait times? For example, can you determine how an increase in staff can reduce the wait time? A basic formula borrowed from industrial engineering (a field rich with methods for measuring and analyzing wait times in production and service processes) provides a quick, practical method. As demonstrated, this simple formula works to estimate average wait times and evaluate the relative impact of process versus staff changes.

Let's use the example of an in-house laboratory to demonstrate this concept:

1. Count the number of patient arrivals per hour (that is, how many patients seek out or are referred to the lab).

2. Determine the average lab processing time (that is, how long it takes on average for a technician to process a patient in the laboratory; include the time that the technician works with or on the patient and the test).

3. Count the number of technicians who staff the laboratory.

Here's the formula to calculate the relationship between staffing, process time, and waiting.

$$Wb = 1 \div (x - y)$$

x   = average service rate per lab technician
      (defined as the average rate of patients processed per hour per technician)

y   = patient arrivals per technician

Wb = waiting time

Your lab is staffed by three technicians who all handle the same services (i.e., there are not any tests that must be performed by any one technician; all are cross-trained). Twenty patients come to the lab each hour. The average processing time for each patient (preparation, drawing, and holding) is six minutes; that is, each technician has the capacity to handle 10 patients per hour. How long will each patient wait?

x   = 10 [average rate of 10 patients per hour per technician]

y   = 6.667 [20 arrivals per hour/3 technicians]

Wb = $1 \div (10\text{-}6.667)$

     = $1 \div 3.333$

     = 0.3 hours

     = 18 minutes [0.3 hours * 60 minutes]

As this formula shows, each patient will have to wait, on average, 18 minutes. If you assume that the volume of patients stays constant, and you want to bring the wait time down then either change the process (e.g., a five-minute processing time would reduce the patient wait time to 11.3 minutes) or change the staffing (e.g., four full-time equivalent employees would reduce the wait time to 12 minutes). Of course, we'd recommend changing the process if at all possible because increasing staff will definitely add expense while process re-engineering may not.

Next, try measuring your average wait time for your registration staff using the same formula.

Wb = $1 \div (x - y)$

x   = average service rate per registrar

y   = patient arrivals per registrar

Wb = waiting time

Now, we'll add a couple of steps for you to gather appropriate data.

a   = Number of registration desk staff (note: assume that all registrars are cross-trained and handle the functions)

b   = Number of patients who come to the registration desk each hour

c   = Average minutes to processing each patient registration

The formula then becomes

x   = 60 (minutes) $\div$ c

y   = b $\div$ a

Wb = 1 $\div$ (x $-$ y)

Don't forget to divide by 60 to convert your result to minutes. You can do this test for any other functions in your office in which the employees perform identical functions. This analysis would not work for nurses who perform different functions depending on the physician's request.

Note: This model assumes the demand for service times is constant. That is, during the morning session, service begins at 9:00 a.m. and finishes at 5:00 p.m. with a steady flow of patients seeking lab services. For further information on waiting times, please see E.J. Rising, et al, "A Systems Analysis of a University Health-Service Outpatient Clinic," *Operations Research*, vol. 21, no. 5 (Sept.-Oct. 1973); and J. Fitzsimmons and M. Fitzsimmons, *Service Management*, fourth edition (New York: Irwin/McGraw-Hill, March 2004.)

References

1. Press Ganey Associates Inc. *Press Ganey 2006 Health Care Satisfaction Report.* South Bend ID.

2. D. Maister, "The Psychology of Waiting Lines," *The Service Encounter,* J.A. Czepiel, M.R. Solomon and C. Suprenant, Lexington Books D.C. Heath and Company: Lexington, MA., 1985.

CHAPTER 8

The Patient Encounter

Key Chapter Lessons

➤ Realize the dangers of batching work – and how to avoid it

➤ Understand how a virtual patient can eliminate physician batching habits

➤ Learn the most effective steps to prepare for an encounter

➤ Recognize the value and components of pre-visit planning

➤ Understand the pitfalls of "service recovery" time

➤ Identify the characteristics of efficient physicians

➤ Facilitate your patients' interaction with your practice

➤ Enhance patient-physician communications

➤ Calculate the cost of physician and staff time per minute

➤ Recognize the importance of the tone set by the physician

➤ Identify new methods to assess patient satisfaction

The most important step

The previous chapter explained how to reduce the length of patients' wait time, or at least make their wait as pleasant as possible. The next step in patient flow – the actual encounter between the patient and the physician – is the most important step in the entire process. It is, in fact, what the customer – the patient – values most. According to lean thinking, the goal is to "pull" processes towards optimizing this interaction. Physicians need every tool possible to make this interaction of maximum value to the patient and to enable the physician to deliver the highest quality of care.

Make the most of the physician's time during the patient visit

Have you ever been focused on completing a complex task but then were forced to put everything aside to search for a tiny piece of important information you needed to finish? And did you also have 10 other tasks waiting at the same time? Now you know why physicians feel so frustrated when the patient flow process is inefficient and impedes their productivity. Sometimes, the interruption or logjam is missing information needed to refer a patient to the proper facility for a test, or a clinical assistant who can't be immediately located to complete an exam.

Add all those extra minutes that a physician spends each day tracking down paperwork before, during, or after a patient visit. Now, multiply those minutes by the cost of the physician's time per minute. Beginning to see why patient flow problems can cost big bucks to a medical practice?

Most importantly, these interruptions and logjams add no value to the patient's experience. Remember, our goal is to design the flow around the patient. Fortunately for us, accomplishing that can also help us reach our financial goals.

 THINGS TO CONSIDER

How much does your physician's time cost?

It's pretty easy to find out what it costs your practice per minute of physician's time. In order to demonstrate, let's assume the following:

Physician compensation per year: $200,000

Physician weeks worked per year: 46

Physician hours worked per week: 50

➤ 50 hours (physician hours a week) * 60 minutes = 3,000 minutes per week

➤ 3,000 minutes per week * 46 weeks (physician weeks a year) = 138,000 minutes per year

➤ $200,000 (annual physician compensation) ÷ 138,000 minutes = $1.45 per minute or $86.96 per hour

Now work through this formula using numbers from your own practice:

a = Annual physician compensation (_____)

b = Physician weeks worked per year (_____)

c = Physician hours worked per week (based on patient/physician interaction or communication; include operating room time for surgeons) (_____)

➤ Step 1: c * 60 minutes = d (minutes per week).

➤ Step 2: d * b = e (minutes per year).

➤ Step 3: a / e = cost per minute.

Stop all that batching

Although the physician's time is the most expensive factor, it's not a license to hire staff without considering functionality or teamwork. Indeed, making each function work well is the key to streamlining patient flow. Unfortunately, a critical ingredient to preventing streamlined patient flow is the habit of batching work – a behavior that is well entrenched at many practices.

Batching work – putting it off or organizing it to work on later – is sometimes appropriate but it has become an unhealthy addiction in some practices. It is much more efficient to process work on a real-time basis.

Take a hard look at how work gets done at your practice. Identify where work is batched and find a way to do it more quickly.

Set priorities. Some practices set specific hours for staff to work on certain tasks. For example, between 7:30 a.m. and 8:00 a.m., a clinical assistant reviews test results received via the Web portal from the prior evening. Abnormal results are flagged electronically or manually and can be presented to the physician. At 8:00 a.m., the clinical assistant is ready to assist the physician in the clinic. Then, from 1:00 p.m. to 1:30 p.m., while the physician is in with a patient for a procedure, the morning test results are reviewed. This strict time allocation may not be appropriate for your practice but some staff may need assistance in setting priorities – they may even have to be told when tasks are due for completion.

Review your systems and processes. Double-checking, highlighting, using intricate filing systems, and other organizational strategies can make sense, but the accumulated effect of adding too many steps to the workflow can be disastrous. Review which steps in your work process truly add value – and which ones just delay everyone from working on the task.

While super-organized processes boost efficiency, if taken too far, they can turn staff into full-time organizers who never get around to working. Take a step back and make sure the real work is getting done. Don't force staff to spend more time organizing work than they spend actually doing the work.

A virtual patient

Staff aren't the only batchers. Physicians who stay late every night to return phone calls, work down task queues, or complete documentation are probably batching too much of their work. Guide them into the habit of stopping after every third or fourth appointment to spend a few minutes with a "virtual" patient to complete the work that has built up.

It's quite tempting for physicians to batch their administrative work – reviewing tasks, filling out forms, signing documents, making calls, and dictating – until the end of the day. They want to focus entirely on seeing patients during office hours. You know who these physicians are in your practice because they are the ones who stay until 7:00 p.m. or later every night trying to dig out from the mountain of tasks.

High-performing physicians deal with this challenge by adding a virtual patient to their schedule each hour – or even between patients. The virtual patient has nothing to do with changing your scheduling template or adding another exam room to your office. It is a concept designed to help physicians develop better work habits.

After every third or fourth patient, an appointment with a virtual patient is designated just for the physician to deal with documentation, returning telephone calls, or handling other quick tasks. For optimal efficiency, a workstation for the physician should be positioned near the clinical space. The work to be handled during the virtual patient visit should be clearly delineated and prioritized (for a picture and description of a high-functioning workspace, see Chapter 1, "The Lean-Thinking Revolution") and staff must be trained on how to deliver the information.

The appointment with the virtual patient may actually be scheduled in the system, but more often, it is just integrated into the flow. This is not a scheduling strategy; rather, it's the way work is managed. An appointment with a virtual patient means stopping to handle the work that has just come in during the last 30 minutes to an hour.

Intuitively, it is difficult to believe that adding a virtual patient to handle administrative work won't harm clinical productivity. But the opposite is the case. Consider that batching work means that physicians must rely on staff to manage the batches. In addition to taking calls during the day and being unavailable to the physician, staff start every morning handling yesterday's batches. The virtual patient gets physicians and staff working in step.

Batching is destructive to efficient work and increases stress on physicians because it:

➤ Requires physicians to spend more time trying to "recall" the details of a patient visit while documenting their encounters;

➤ Leaves physicians with limited staff assistance during clinic because staff must spend time fielding calls from anxious patients and referring physicians. If physicians don't review and offer responses during the day, callers continue to call until they receive the information;

➤ Causes staff to spend more time organizing and managing out-of-office communication requests and callbacks; and

➤ Disrupts workflow by making staff begin each day dealing with the pile of work physicians left on their desks or electronic task queues from the previous night.

Physicians who use the virtual patient strategy find that they start and end each day on time. That is, physicians can actually start seeing patients at 8:00 a.m. as scheduled because their staff is ready to assist them, instead of trying to catch up with work left over from yesterday.

Notably, process delays can happen regardless of whether you have an EHR. Instead of piles of charts, there is an overflowing box of inbound e-mail alerts. It's not about the construct of the record; it's the flow of the work.

Silos

Sometimes we program our staff and physicians to batch work without knowing it. A significant factor leading to batching work in medical practices is how positions are allocated. Most practices, even small ones, tend to parcel out tasks to staff. They divide support staff by relatively narrow job functions, and each function becomes its own silo. Silos – the referral clerk, the document scanner, the triage nurse, the surgery scheduler, and so forth – promote batching.

Here's an example of how silos cause batching. A report on a patient is faxed from the catheterization laboratory (cath lab). The nurse puts the report at the physician's workstation, and the physician signs it after reading it. The nurse takes it along with dozens of other reports to the records room. Although the document scanner is free, the nurse places the report on top of the large pile of papers that awaits the designated document scanning staff. The report from the cath lab sits until the staff member assigned to scanning tasks is able to scan it. Meanwhile, the cardiologist needs the report because the patient is being seen today at the practice. No one can find the report, so the nurse calls the cath lab to fax another report so the cardiologist has it for the patient encounter. Eventually, the same report is reviewed and signed by the physician, and both reports are scanned and filed in the patient's EHR. Of course, this results in confusion – and wasted time — during the patient's subsequent visit as both reports have been filed.

Repeat this behavior with the dozens – or maybe hundreds – of tasks small and large throughout your practice and soon you'll see batching on a large scale. Work is either delayed or duplicated until the person assigned to handle the function gets time to take care of the task. Returning to our concept of lean thinking, the patient doesn't care if your practice has a designated scanner; the patient just wants the physician to have the correct record. Because the patient assumes record maintenance is a simple task that shouldn't and doesn't go wrong, the patient won't feel he or she is receiving any great value from your scanning process. What the patient values is the outcome, not your intricate process. If you are staffing strictly by function and it is promoting bad work habits, namely batching, then you are going to a lot of trouble to provide no perceived value to the customer. That begs the question of why you are maintaining those silos of responsibility.

Another benefit from avoiding batching caused by silo-structured staffing derives from the perspective of human resources. The generations in most staff positions (teenagers to mid-40s) don't value the distribution of jobs by function. In fact, both Generation X and the newer Millennial generation (sometimes called Generation Y) are most interested in a diversity of job responsibilities. Eliminating all of those separate, functional areas when it is appropriate to do so may make the best sense for your patients *and* your staff.

Cross-training

An alternative to staffing by silos is to cross train staff for more than one area of responsibility. Preparing an employee to handle multiple jobs might mean you need fewer employees overall. High-performing practices cross train to boost productivity as well as reduce downtime when some employees are out.

Cross-training promotes teamwork and performance improvement as employees learn from each other. As you employ more "Gen X" and "Generation Millennial" staff, you'll find that cross-training helps keep them engaged. Turn these two generations' characteristically shorter attention spans and needs for more variety and purpose into a positive through cross-training.

Try training medical assistants to answer the phones, nurses to schedule appointments, and receptionists to room patients. In addition to benefiting the practice, learning new skills is terrific for your employees and their careers. A bright, eager, and hardworking staff member will embrace cross-training as a path to enhancing his or her skill set – and resumé. Use your staff to support one another, and they can better support physicians in the office.

Cross-training is a good way to engage employees in their jobs, but there is a limit. Don't depend on it for every function every day. While it's wise to avoid allocating job functions too rigidly or narrowly – forming silos, that is – you do need some employees to develop special expertise in certain complicated or high risk assignments, or otherwise necessary as dictated by state or federal law.

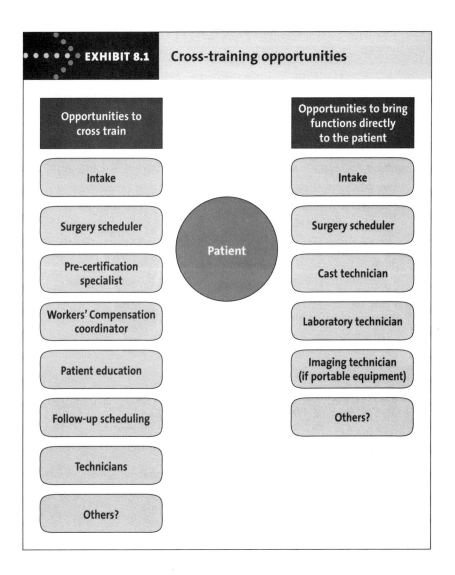

EXHIBIT 8.1 Cross-training opportunities

Opportunities to cross train

- Intake
- Surgery scheduler
- Pre-certification specialist
- Workers' Compensation coordinator
- Patient education
- Follow-up scheduling
- Technicians
- Others?

Patient

Opportunities to bring functions directly to the patient

- Intake
- Surgery scheduler
- Cast technician
- Laboratory technician
- Imaging technician (if portable equipment)
- Others?

Identify cross-training opportunities

Patients don't perceive value in the way we breakdown support functions. They expect the jobs to be performed correctly. As Exhibit 8.1 shows, there are two opportunities to pull value: (1) cross training staff to perform multiple duties and (2) bringing the functions to the patient instead of the patient to the functions. This latter opportunity is most appropriate when you must designate functions to certain individuals based on their specific job skills and/or based on state or federal requirements for the required level of training to perform or supervise the function.

BEST PRACTICES

Efficient clinic

High-performing practices use a three-prong approach to efficient patient flow during clinic:

1. Chart preview

2. Room stocking

3. Huddle

Adopt their workflow techniques to streamline your patient flow.

Pre-visit planning

Preparing for the visit is important to keep workflow on track. Without pre-visit planning, chaos reins – and staff try to control it by batching work – laying it aside to do later when there's more time. To avoid this non-value-added batching of work and foster real-time work processing, take the time to plan your day. You'll avoid chaos and reap the rewards of an efficient patient flow.

Pre-visit planning should start a day or two before the patient's scheduled appointment with these three steps.

Step One: Chart preview. A clinical assistant should check the patient's medical chart before the visit. Regardless of whether the chart is a paper folder or an EHR, it should be current with the patient's medications, test results, hospital records, operative reports, notes from consulting specialists, and so on. If the results or other missing information are not in the chart, get on the computer or phone and obtain them. Have them faxed or e-mailed, or find them online.

If the physician requested a test or other referral that has not been completed, ask a staff member to flag the chart to discuss with the physician a day or two before the appointment (but continue seeking that information through all other means). Evaluate whether the appointment should be rescheduled for a later date. If, for example, a patient was coming in to review the results of his or her liver biopsy but the biopsy hasn't been performed, then it's a waste of the physician's – and the patient's – time to keep the appointment.

Develop a protocol for missing information. Teach staff how to track down missing documents. If information remains unaccounted for when the final chart preview is done, make sure staff know to bring it to your attention. You'll want to know about it in enough time to possibly reschedule the visit if the missing information is especially critical to the visit. You're just setting yourself and your physicians up for an unhappy patient if you let staff wait until the patient is roomed to mention that the interpretation of her sinus CT is not available.

Also remember to electronically or manually flag important pre-visit reading materials, such as abnormal results that may have just been received and must be presented to the patient at the appointment.

Physicians who appear unaware of test results, consults, and other medical care of a patient will leave a negative impression with that patient. Even if a clinical assistant is called in to the exam room to retrieve the results and they are found during the encounter, the scene will inevitably leave the patient wondering just what other important information may be in limbo.

To make chart previewing easier, ask that the physicians state – or repeat a summary of – their orders at the end of their dictation. Make sure you are prepared for the patient's return visit by making a written summary of the physician's orders in a specific place in the record. Regardless of whether you use a paper or an electronic chart, this documentation can alert staff to check for results before the patient's next visit. That way, the clinical assistant can just look back to the last dictation to ensure that everything needed for the visit that is captured and previewed.

In addition to looking for records of past care, chart preview helps anticipate the physician's needs for the upcoming encounter. If the patient is making a follow-up visit, make sure the file folder (if you are using a paper record) contains all forms needed for that type of follow-up. This would include order forms for ancillaries, educational materials, pre-operative instructions, and so on. Do the same electronically if using an EHR. Go ahead and complete any appropriate standard information on the forms (patient's name, account number, date of service, etc.).

Although staff may complain that this preview process is unnecessary and takes too much time, the work is being done anyway. That is, they're finding the test results, hospital discharge summaries, forms, etc., but it's done in the middle of a busy clinic. More importantly, if staff waits until the physician discovers a missing result, it slows down the physician's productivity significantly. Without a preview process, the physician cannot be efficient and the value that the patient perceives is compromised.

Step Two: Room stocking. Pre-visit planning should also include stocking the exam room with all supplies that will be needed. Stock rooms at the start of each day and check them between patient visits. Exam rooms should be stocked for the types of patient visits that the physicians in your practice typically handle. Previewing charts daily can determine if special equipment or supplies are required.

Make sure that all of the equipment the physician needs is ready for the clinic. One way to prompt staff and hold them accountable for ensuring that equipment is in place is to hang hooks with labels for the equipment on the wall of the exam room. Or, try drawing the outline of the equipment in a drawer in each exam room. In addition to assuring the placement of equipment, assign a staff member to review the cleanliness of every exam room and start up every computer. Assign a clinical assistant to make a last-minute check of every exam room to make sure an adequate inventory of supplies is on hand before the clinic starts.

Often, the problems in inventory management are not running out of an item but finding it. Make sure items are available when and where the physician needs them. Use flags or pictures for a failsafe supply inventory system. It works like this: place a red flag or a picture of the supply (snap photos, use part of the packaging, or adopt an index card) on top of the final two or three units of the item. Write the exam room number on the back. When staff reach the flag or picture, they will put it in their pocket. At the end of the clinic, their pockets will contain the supplies needed per room to restock and/or order. This saves time and reduces uncertainty – no longer will you just have to hope that the staff responsible for restocking look in every drawer and cabinet. Although using flags or photos is an elementary approach, it's easy and very efficient. Try combining this daily management system with a more sophisticated software-based inventory management system.

The most efficient physicians never leave their exam rooms during the encounter. Why? Because they have the tools they need to get the job done!

Step Three: Huddle. Pre-clinic huddles that include the physician, nurse or clinical assistant, and appointment scheduler should be held before each morning and afternoon clinic. This three- to five-minute informal chat is a time to quickly review the upcoming appointment schedule. Use the appointment schedule as the "agenda." The purpose of the huddle is to give everyone a rundown of what's going to happen during that session or day, and review important issues that may have an impact on the day's patient flow. Staff should note if there is anything out of the ordinary or any issues that must be resolved immediately. For example, if three new patients were accidentally booked for the same slot, determine which patients can be rescheduled. It's also a good time to alert the physician to things that might throw off the whole day, such as the mother who typically schedules an appointment for one child yet brings in her other children, too. By getting ready for all of the family's children to visit, the physician and staff are better prepared. Finally, this is an opportune time for the physician to note which patients are likely to no-show (if, for example, they were admitted last night), and where patients with acute problems can be squeezed into the schedule, if necessary.

Make sure these briefings start on time, never run long, and are mandatory. Otherwise, it's just another meeting.

The pre-clinic huddle is like a football team getting ready for its next play. If every player is well-informed, the play will be executed effectively. Consider every clinic your "play"; if you're not coordinated, you'll never make a touchdown. Granted, even a huddle won't guarantee a touchdown (or an easy day), but you will be able to execute the play – instead of sitting back and waiting for the chaos to overwhelm you.

Previewing charts, stocking exam rooms, and huddling twice a day will help your practice function efficiently and your patients get the care they need at the time they want it. Let your patients pull value. Plan for the visit: control the day before it controls you.

STEPS TO GET YOU THERE

How to hold a pre-clinic huddle

Ask these questions during your brief huddles with staff before each clinic and you'll soon see results – smooth clinics, few mix ups and delays, and happy patients and staff:

Filling out the roster:

- ➤ Which staff are in today?

- ➤ Who's on call?

- ➤ Is there a clinical assistant assigned to the physician for the day?

- ➤ Who is responding to calls for the clinical team?

Planning the schedule:

- ➤ Do we anticipate problems?

- ➤ Do we anticipate any interruptions? Do any patients need to be rescheduled?

- ➤ Are there any likely no-shows on the schedule because of a hospital admission?

- ➤ Are there any patients with unusual needs?

- ➤ Do we need to ready the procedure room? Do we need any special supplies or equipment?

- ➤ Is information missing, such as test results?

- ➤ Are there any holes where patients calling in with acute problems could be fit in?

Avoiding fumbles:

- ➤ What went wrong yesterday?

- ➤ What's the solution to avoiding the same problem today?

WORDS OF WISDOM

What's the real reason you're here?

Finding out the real reason for the patient's visit can help the physician better prepare for the appointment. A handy way to do this is to have schedulers ask patients to describe their major symptoms when they call for appointments. The schedulers also can ask, "Since the doctor wants to make sure there is enough time to spend with you, can you tell us why you're coming in?"

Stagger lunch breaks so there is always a live operator to answer the telephone. The lunch hour may be the only time some patients can call. Some people do not have a private place to call from work and do not want to discuss medical problems in front of co-workers.

THINGS TO CONSIDER

Service recovery

Unconvinced about the need to reduce your waiting time to improve patient service? Consider the amount of visit time that is consumed when a physician walks into the exam room and must deal with a patient who is frustrated by an hour-long wait. One multispecialty practice measured its "service recovery" time at an average of three minutes per visit. With the high cost of physician's time, these precious minutes added up to significant muda (waste). Discuss this in your own practice; it may compel you to work on reducing waiting times.

When the physician waits

As we learned from Chapter 2, "The Physician's Time," the biggest hit on a medical practice's financial status comes from wasting the physician's time. Every additional minute that a physician spends trying to page a clinical assistant, locate a referral form, or find a chart is not just a minute wasted: it's money down the drain. More importantly, it's time away from what patients value most: a physician providing care to them.

Of course, no one wants to work in or be a patient of a medical practice where physicians step out of their exam rooms and scream for their clinical assistant to get there "on the double"! So, pressuring the physician to speed things up is not really the way to go either. Instead, look for ways that physicians and all of their support clinical and non-clinical staff can work smoothly without creating conflicts or wasting the physicians' time.

Flow sheets

One way to improve the flow process of the patient-physician encounter is to develop an electronic or paper "flow sheet." A flow sheet, a documentation of physician orders, can capture most of the verbal communication that physicians rely on and, often, must wait to receive.

Intended to capture communication regarding orders between the clinical team, the flow sheet should be designed to meet the needs of your practice. Consider the communications that take place in the hallway: "draw some blood on this patient," "let's send him down for a chest X-ray," "give him a sample of XYZ medication," "schedule his surgery," etc.

Put these communications in an electronic template or on a form that can stick to the record. If records are kept on paper, print the flow sheets in a bright color so they are easily distinguishable. I'm not advocating the elimination of all verbal communication, only to streamline flow.

Patient flow coordinator

The complex flow of staff, providers and patients is duplicated by other industries. Airports, for example, handle hundreds, if not thousands of planes, pilots, and customers every day, with efficiency and safety hinging on a well-designed flow process. Like a busy airport, some practices may benefit from an air traffic controller being in charge of patient flow. Hire a patient flow coordinator (PFC) to make sure rooms are turned over as soon as encounters have been completed, and to direct staff and providers to tasks. Frequently, there is no one person in the practice who has the global view of the day's events needed to identify and understand incoming work during a busy clinic. By filling that role, a PFC can help manage downtime by directing staff to perform duties that may otherwise not get completed in a timely manner.

Preference cards

Most people would readily cite the operating room as a shining example of efficiency in health care. Operating rooms run with little downtime, which is in the best interest of both the patient and the surgeon. Although several factors converge to create the efficiency of an operating room, one of the most important of these is a simple and easily replicable idea: preference cards. Surgeons are asked to reveal their "preferences" in terms of the set-up for the operating room. These preferences are translated into standing orders for how the room should be set. Equipment, materials, etc., are ready just as the physician ordered. When the surgeon enters the operating room, the surgery is ready to begin.

In the medical practice, the concept of preference cards can be replicated to garner the same value. See Exhibit 8.2 for a sample.

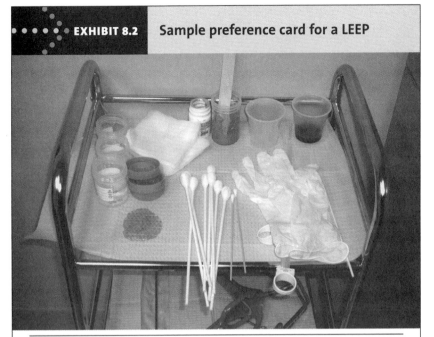

EXHIBIT 8.2   Sample preference card for a LEEP

ACTION: Offer 800mg Ibuprofen prior to procedure chart if given.

IN CHART	2ND SHELF OF STAND	SET UP ON STAND	COUNTER SET UP	ASSIST DOCTOR
➤ Leep procedure sheet ➤ Vitals stamp	➤ Blueteflon specula (1 sm, 1 lg)	➤ Blue Teflon forceps ➤ Small gloves (2) ➤ ECC (Kevorkian) ➤ KY squirt ➤ Biopsy jars, opened (3) ➤ Hurricane gel, opened ➤ Monsels solution, (opened and stirred) ➤ Acetic Acid in cup ➤ Lugols solution in cup ➤ Tongue depressor (1) ➤ Scoppettes (handful) ➤ Q-Tips (2) ➤ Pap brush (1) ➤ 4X4 gauze (1″ stack) ➤ Xylocaine with epi: 10cc control ➤ Syringe and spinal needle	➤ Zylocaine without Epi, 10cc control ➤ Biohazard can= out, left of stand ➤ Settings=65 cutting, 60 blend ➤ Machine= plugged in ➤ Grounding pad= plugged in ➤ LEEP pen= plugged in ➤ 5 LEEP electrodes (1 of each)	1. Turn on machine 2. Apply grounding pad to upper thigh 3. Adjust settings

As is provided in this example, the preference card should explicitly list the actions, documentation, forms, supplies, and assistance required for the procedure. Mistake proof the process by including a picture of the set-up.

Courtesy of Somer Shields, CMPE, Administrator, Portland, Oregon

The role of your clinical assistant

Clinical assistants – nurses and medical assistants – play critical roles in a practice's patient flow, yet very few practices dedicate sufficient training or orientation to this important responsibility.

An important role for clinical assistants is patient intake. Standard protocols for this critical function are often lacking as medical groups seem to depend on collective memory or unwritten rules to handle these important processes. The intake or rooming process initiates an efficient encounter that should not be left to chance.

In addition to escorting the patient and performing the steps listed above, rooming is the opportunity for the nurse or medical assistant to gather information about the patient to help the physician work more efficiently during the encounter. If the vital signs and history are recorded, for example, the time the physician needs to document the encounter can be reduced – and the physician can jump right into the assessment and plan. Without written protocols, training, and accountability for the process cannot be assured.

Think through the specifics of each step below to begin designing the rooming protocol that will best support the efficiency of your practice's providers – and add value to your patients:

Escorting the patient. When a clinical assistant is notified that a patient has arrived (see Chapter 6, "Reception Services," for tips on streamlining the arrival process), determine if there is an available exam room (or procedure room if a procedure is scheduled). If there is no available room, either communicate with the patient directly by walking up to the patient in the reception area or contact the front desk staff so they can inform the patient that there will be a delay.

If rooms and providers are available, then clinical assistants can room patients. They should walk to the waiting area and if they recognize the patient, walk up and say, "Good morning/afternoon, Ms. Jones."

If they do not recognize the patient, announce the patient's name in a voice loud enough to be heard by all persons in the waiting area but not sounding like they are shouting. Then, greet the patient, tell the patient their name and escort the patient to the exam or procedure room.

Rooming the patient. Assistants should be counseled to open doors for patients. It sounds like a natural form of courtesy but you should not leave even this small-but-meaningful behavior to chance. Assistants should inform anyone who arrived with a patient (e.g., family members) where to sit in the exam room and where to place their belongings. Tell patients the proceedings of the visit, including the assistant's role. Finally, patients should be asked if they have any questions about the visit.

Taking the chief complaint. Assistants should ask patients to confirm the reason for the visit and gather additional information about their chief complaint.

Reviewing medical history. It is important that patients are always asked about their medical histories. In many practices, patients will have already completed a medical history form electronically or manually which can be accessed or collected at this time. Make sure the assistant takes the time needed to review the history form with the patient and ensure it is complete. Patients should be told that the information on this form is important to the provider's management of care. Ideally, the medical history has already been captured electronically, thus allowing the clinical assistant to input any changes or additions.

Determining current medications. Unless instructed otherwise by the provider, the assistant should ask patients to state aloud their current medications. Reading from the history form or current medication list, and getting nods or shakes of the head is not good enough. (To improve this process, some practices ask patients to bring all of their medications with them, and the assistant reviews the bottles. This is a great idea for patients who take several medications and may not always remember names and dosages.) Patients should be told why this information is being gathered. Some patients won't understand why the physician needs this information. For example, they may not think an endocrinologist needs to know what their cardiologist has prescribed. Information about current medications should be documented or inputted into patients' records.

Assisting with other paperwork. There may be other paperwork that patients must review, complete and, perhaps, sign before the visit starts. Many of these forms may be required, such as an advance beneficiary notification (ABN). (See Chapter 6, "Reception Services" about finding a sample ABN and how to use it.)

Prepping the patient. Following the protocols outlined by the provider, the assistant should ready patients for the provider. These steps, which should be directed based on the chief complaint, may include:

➤ Asking patients to undress and put on a gown or drape a sheet over them. This may include instructing patients to remove only one article of clothing, such as shoes and socks, up to the removal of all clothing;

➤ Asking patients to provide a urine sample. Be sure to give specific instructions about the location of the restroom and the protocols for the urine sample, including how to mark the sample and where to place it;

➤ Asking patients to step on the scale to measure weight; and

➤ Placing the blood pressure cuff on patients and getting a blood pressure reading.

Other protocols may include a lab draw, an X-ray or other radiological image, blood sugar, pulse oximetry, and other measurements.

Reviewing. Using the chief complaint as a guide, the assistant should ensure that all the equipment, supplies, and forms that the provider will need for the encounter are present and placed on the provider's workspace in the exam room to be ready for use. Exceptions to this step would include placing equipment where patients – particularly a child – could be put in harm's way. Initiating form completion at this point can save precious time for the provider. For example, if patients need a Family Medical Leave Act (FMLA) form completed, the assistant should obtain the form and complete as many of the fields as possible. Then the physician only has to complete the sections that require a physician's expertise and signature.

After completing these protocols, the clinical assistant should ask patients to sit where the physician wants to "start." This will save the physician from having to wait for patients to scoot down from the exam table to the chair or vice versa.

Although this may seem like an overly detailed rendition of what should occur before each patient visit, the fact is that these steps may not be happening all of the time or in exactly the same way. A surprising number of practices have not carefully defined this process step by step nor drilled it repeatedly with their clinical assistants. These duties should not be left to chance; protocols establish the basis for promoting accountability and enabling the evaluation of performance.

The result of failing to set expectations for the rooming process? The patient waits – and waits. Efficient rooming is seeking out muda or waste – and eliminating it.

Room by complaint

You can't design a usable rooming process for every possible chief complaint but you can use your physicians' five or 10 most common diagnoses as a guide. To determine your physicians' most common diagnoses, pull a report from your practice management system with the top-10 diagnosis codes billed during the last year (based on volume). Gather the clinical team and discuss the preparations necessary for each diagnosis to streamline the clinical process. For example, body weight might not be gathered for all patients, but it must be measured for prenatal patients in an obstetrics practice. Decide what standing orders should be in place and how they'll be executed and documented.

Evaluation of rooming criteria

To make sure rooming criteria support the physician's efficiency while also giving maximum value to patients, revisit the process at least once a year. Even if your staff "knows" what to do, it doesn't hurt to discuss the process periodically. It will be an opportunity to accommodate different criteria for new services or physicians, as well as to reinforce to staff the importance of the process.

When evaluating your rooming process, make sure that you respect your patients' privacy. Don't, for example, have three scales lined up in a sub-waiting area for everyone to watch patients weigh-in. Although you may have to consider equipment costs or staff time, it's important to maintain your patients' privacy – and their dignity.

WORDS OF WISDOM

Assessing assistants

Members of the clinical team play a key role in improving the patient's experience. When assessing the performance of clinical assistants, don't stop at the physician's input. Ask also if clinical assistants:

> ➤ Present to the patient appropriately?

> ➤ Introduce themselves to the patient?

> ➤ Acknowledge spouses, partners, or other loved ones who are accompanying the patient?

➤ Discuss their role in the visit?

➤ Outline the 'agenda' for the encounter (e.g., who will come in next)?

➤ Ask patients if they have questions?

➤ Ask patients if there is anything that can be done to make them feel more comfortable?

➤ Thank patients for choosing the practice?

Follow these guidelines to establish expectations for the role of the clinical assistant.

Managing exam rooms

A key player in the efficient patient encounter is the exam room itself. The average physician uses three exam rooms; the average nonphysician provider uses two exam rooms. While this is interesting data, the key to knowing how many each physician *needs* (as opposed to wants) is to examine the workflow. Calculate the average time that it takes for a clinical assistant to room a patient, the time the physician spends to see each patient on average, and the time an assistant may need to spend on post-encounter education and instruction. Note that visit time is not necessarily the time slot set in your scheduling template, so you'll want to measure each function yourself.

If the clinical assistant takes three to five minutes to room a patient, the physician takes 12 to 15 minutes with each patient, and a clinical assistant returns to assist with post-encounter education and instructions, three exam rooms are plenty. Use Exhibit 8.3 to visualize room turns – using it should help you prove that three exam rooms are enough for a physician and clinical assistant who are working at the pace described above.

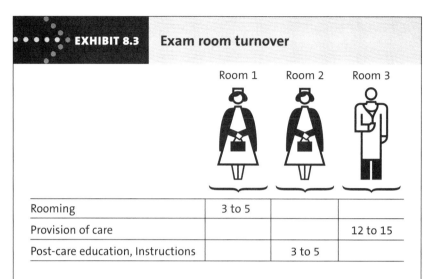

EXHIBIT 8.3   **Exam room turnover**

	Room 1	Room 2	Room 3
Rooming	3 to 5		
Provision of care			12 to 15
Post-care education, Instructions		3 to 5	

Measure the time that the physician and staff consume to perform their jobs. Then, make sure that you have enough rooms to turnover before the physician is ready for the next patient. In this example, the rooms are turned over every 18 to 25 minutes. In order to ensure there is always an available room for the physician, the range of three to five minutes must be maintained for each clinical support activity. This allows enough time for the physician, who spends 12 to 15 minutes per encounter, to move to the next room where a patient is ready.

Change the average time per patient, or the services you render to the patient (e.g., patient needs a cast removed and an X-ray) and you may need more or fewer exam rooms.

The efficient physician's primer

Staff and space are critical to an efficient patient encounter but they are not the only factors involved. Following are the steps that today's most efficient physicians complete each day so they can see more patients without staying later at work or taking administrative work home:

Review the next day's schedule by 3:30 p.m. each afternoon. Look for mistakes. Note any changes and give them to the front office by 4:00 p.m. so staff can immediately contact affected patients to reschedule. If the scheduling process works well (see Chapter 4, "Scheduling" for tips on enhancing your scheduling), these changes should be minimal.

Huddle with your core staff before each clinic session *everyday*. Never skip this meeting. Go over any changes or mistakes in the schedule, predictable no-shows on the schedule, patients who were admitted to the hospital, and messages that are expected and how they should be handled. Involve the scheduler in the huddle or give any changes to support staff immediately.

Stay on time. Empower support staff to help. Many physicians set their pager on vibrate-only mode and ask support staff to page them when they are with a patient for more than a specified period of time, such as 30 minutes. Or, staff are instructed to interrupt with the statement: "Dr. Jones is on the phone for you." The physician can ignore the signal that it's time to move on or use it as a polite excuse to wrap up.

Pull work into the day. Use the virtual patient, which was discussed previously in this chapter, to avoid work piling up.

Start on time. If you don't start the day on time, don't expect to run on time. Many physicians start late because of their scheduling systems. Perhaps, the appointment schedule is creating a problem. For example, if the first appointment is at 8:00 a.m., is there enough time for the patient to pass through the reception, registration, and rooming processes before being seen by the physician at 8:00 a.m.? Even in the most efficient practices, these pre-encounter steps take 15 or even 30 minutes. Set your schedule accordingly – if you want your physician to start at 8:00 a.m., have the first appointment scheduled at 7:30 or 7:45 a.m. Don't resort to telling patients to come 15 minutes early to 'fill in paperwork'. Decide whose time the appointment represents – yours or your patients' – and set your processes around your decision.

Position clocks. If you have wall clocks in your exam rooms, put them behind the patient. That way, the physician can face the patient and watch the time without having to look down at a watch. Moving the clock from the patient's line of sight also means they are less likely to stare at the clock while waiting for the physician.

Manage face-to-face encounters. Physicians who consistently score high on patient relations (bedside manner, that is) learn to greet patients with an appropriate touch, such as a handshake or a gentle touch to the shoulder, maintain eye contact, and lean towards patients while they talk. They also remember to acknowledge the partners, family members, or guests who come to the exam with the patient. When applicable, the physician should discuss their roles in the patient's care.

Set the agenda. Physicians can take the lead smoothly without appearing overbearing by quickly establishing the agenda of the exam at the beginning of the encounter. They can do this by simply paraphrasing the patient's description of the chief complaint and symptoms. For example, "Ms. Jones, we're going to address your stomach pain this morning. Is there anything else you want to discuss?" Get the patient's agreement on the agenda, and focus on it.

Offer patient education materials. The more you have to explain, the longer the visit will take. If patients present for a consult about an anterior cruciate injury, your staff can ask patients to review a brochure, video, or computer software on the topic when they are roomed. Educational materials cannot replace your clinical evaluation and decision-making but having them available before the visit may help you and the patient get down to the nuts and bolts issues faster.

Make exam rooms more efficient. Just about everything the physician needs should be within arm's reach. Set expectations with staff that rooms will always be stocked so the physician never has to leave to find the equipment, supplies, samples, forms, or educational materials needed. Moreover, with standard exam rooms, physicians can use any exam room in the practice, if necessary, without missing a step.

Review your practice's telephone medicine. Efficient physicians limit how much acute care management their staff provide over the telephone. Telephone medicine isn't always good medicine. Tell schedulers and telephone triage nurses that patients who call in with acute complaints should be scheduled for appointments. A quick office visit is often more time-efficient and medically effective than a lengthy telephone conversation. You'll also capture the revenue associated with serving patients' acute needs, instead of letting a nurse try to provide it over the telephone at no charge. (See Chapter 5, "Patient Access," for opportunities to improve appointment availability.)

Match young physicians with a mentor. Help new physicians adjust to your practice and understand what's expected of them. Residency and fellowship programs have not taught trainees the basics of efficiency. It's important to train physicians about efficiency before bad work habits set in. (See more about training new physicians in Chapter 5, "Patient Access.")

Keep the team on the same page. For example, maintain a written log of scheduled patients at the clinical station; as a patient is roomed, record the arrival of the patient in your EHR or mark the exam room number next to the patient's name, and electronically or manually check off the patient as the visit is completed. Take it up a notch by implementing an electronic tracking system to monitor patients as they move through various stages of the patient flow process (e.g., imaging, lab, cast room, etc.).

Stay focused. Limit interruptions during clinic, such as prolonged conversations with pharmaceutical sales representatives or telephone calls to your financial advisor. Schedule time for these activities before or after clinic. Physicians can make optimal use of transit time to and from activities by placing callbacks from their cellular phones.

Document during the visit. Consider documenting the encounter *during* the encounter with the patient (see below). Alternately, give physicians a way to dictate after each visit or, at minimum, record the encounter after every third visit if using the "virtual patient" concept. It's more efficient than batching dictation until the end of the day or the end of the week.

Teach physicians to become better closers. At the end of the visit, efficient physicians review the agenda that they and the patient agreed upon at the beginning of the visit. They review action items recommended. Another wise step is to write down the plan (or enter it into the EHR), or give the patient a copy of the documentation. This reinforces what is being explained about the next steps, such as a referral, a laboratory test, imaging, or patient education materials. They also use a team approach to close the visit by calling in a clinical assistant to complete the encounter. The clinical assistant explains the orders written during the exam and handles patient questions about directions to the testing facility, when to expect test results, and who will notify them so you can be on the way to the next patient in the next exam room.

Handling the "Oh, by the ways"

Your best efforts to improve your physicians' work styles can all be undone by four little words – "oh, by the way…" The patient may have just a minor question or comment but it's often a new, major issue that extends the visit.

Urologists, for example, find this to be commonplace. Male patients often leave questions about impotence until the end of the visit. They're embarrassed about it, but can't face their wives in the waiting room who will surely ask, "Did you talk to the doctor about *the* issue?" as soon as they see them.

The "oh, by the ways" can lead into an extended office visit that will put an already late physician further behind schedule. If you often hear the four little words, don't lose hope. There are strategies to help you:

Develop a better scheduling script. Instruct schedulers to get more information from patients when they set up appointments. For example, schedulers can say, "The doctor wants to have enough time to meet your health care needs; is there anything else that you want to discuss?" It won't work every time but setting expectations upfront adds value to the patient and the provider.

Postpone the concern. If the patient's last-minute concern is complex, but not acute, there is nothing wrong with asking the patient to schedule another appointment. For example, the physician can say, "Ms. Smith, the issue that you are raising is so important that I'd like to allow enough time to thoroughly discuss it with you. Since we made time today to address only your XYZ concern, I'd like to schedule another visit with you so we can have enough time to address this." Have patient education material ready for frequently asked questions so patients don't go home empty-handed.

Preempt. Set the agenda at the beginning of the exam. Ask the patient to confirm what you'll be addressing that day: "Ms. Jones, I'm going to summarize what you've told me, which is: . . . I'll be addressing those concerns today. Is there anything else you'd like to discuss with me today?" Anticipate frequently asked questions. For example, expect that a post-menopausal woman may have questions about hormone replacement therapy. Have written material on hand and direct the patient to credible Web sites. The physician can offer a brief summary of advice and ask a clinical assistant to discuss the issue further with the patient to see if another appointment is needed. Recognize communication differences between male and female patients. For example, male patients often leave the most important issues until the end. Draw the information out of them early with open-ended questions about sensitive issues relevant to the encounter.

Seize the opportunity. Sometimes, dealing with the "oh, by the way" comment today heads off more work tomorrow. For example, it may be possible to add a routine exam to an already scheduled follow up visit, which will open the physician's schedule to accommodate another patient. This strategy, commonly called "max packing," won't make sense if the extra work adds no additional reimbursement, creates inconvenience for the patient, or puts the physician hopelessly behind schedule.

Learn to code. Physicians who understand evaluation and management coding and the proper use of modifiers to indicate extra work can accommodate last-minute questions during patient encounters and get paid what they deserve. When counseling and/or coordination of care with the patient and/or the family member dominate the visit, physicians can bill by time.[1] You must record the time spent on this counseling. If you can't control the "oh, by the ways," at least get paid for them.

 THINGS TO CONSIDER

Combating the "doorknob syndrome"

Directly addressing the "Oh, by the way, doctor", three researchers published a sentinel article regarding preventing what they call the "doorknob syndrome." Noting that the syndrome occurs at the end of the visit, the authors write: "We believe that it has its origin at the beginning [of the visit], when agenda setting occurs. Although clinicians tend to blame the patient for this distressing syndrome, in fact it is frequently the result of defective interview technique: failure to elicit the patient's entire agenda early in the visit."

To prevent the doorknob syndrome, researchers suggest setting – and sticking to – an agenda for the patient encounter. Here are the topics and related questions they suggest asking:

What are the patient's main concerns for today?

[I need an MRI.] "So, we need to talk about your desire to have an MRI. What else?"

What are the clinician's concerns?

"I know I asked you back so I could recheck your blood pressure and listen to your lungs, and I heard you say that you were quite concerned about your sore foot. If it's OK with you, I think we can listen to your lungs again, discuss your blood pressure readings, and then take a look at your foot. Sound reasonable?"

What are the patient's most important tasks?

I see that you have several concerns today. Can you tell me what goes on the top of your list?

What must be attended to, and what can be postponed for future visits?

"I want to make sure I've heard all your concerns, and then we have to decide together what we can do today, which concerns to tackle, and perhaps which to save for another time."

What if further negotiation is necessary?

"I know you were concerned about your knees and the rash and the hoarseness, and I think I need to focus on the chest pain first. We may not be able to do justice to all these issues today, but I think that chest pain could be the most dangerous, so we should attend to it first. Does that sound OK?"

Source: L. Baker, D. O'Connell, and F. Platt. "What else? Setting the agenda for the clinical interview." *Annals of Internal Medicine*, Volume 143, (November 15, 2005), 10:766-770.

Dictating during the visit

Physicians can save time by dictating during the exam. That practice could eliminate the extra one to two minutes it normally takes per encounter to recall the details when dictating after the fact. For 30 patients, that recall time could be up to an hour – time the physician could use to see a few more patients and increase income, relax with family, or do personal errands.

Why to try it. Dictating in front of patients won't add time to the visit and requires no investment. Try for a week or two and then stop if it doesn't work for the physicians or their patients. True, some patients will interrupt frequently to ask questions or add comments. In those cases, note in their record: "no IRD (in-room dictation)" so everyone knows not to waste time dictating in front of them in the future.

It improves patient care. Many patients leave their physician's office with less-than-complete retention of the assessment and treatment plan, which is often delivered verbally and only once. Dictating in front of patients means they will hear the physician's advice more than once. Furthermore, it offers patients opportunities to clarify any points, which is particularly important if the misunderstanding would have led to an inappropriate treatment plan. If the documentation is complete in the exam room, a copy can be printed and given to patients as a visit summary.

It helps manage malpractice risk. Dictating in front of patients gives them more opportunities to clear up misunderstandings and contribute to making the record as accurate as possible. Recording the phrase "dictated in the presence of the patient" into the record provides an additional measure of risk reduction. This note in the record may make it harder for a plaintiff to successfully argue that the instructions and/or diagnosis were unclear. No longer will physicians have to admit during a deposition or in court that they had dictated the notes several hours after examining the plaintiff.

It's embraced by patients. Most patients want to participate in their health care. Exam-room dictation can lift some of the "mystery" of medicine for them. Physicians should first say, "I would like you to hear my assessment and treatment plan again as I record them for your medical chart. May I record them now? Please feel free to interrupt me if you feel there are any misunderstandings on my part." It will give patients a better sense of how much time and effort the physician is putting into their care. Infusing humor never hurts; your patients will surely get a chuckle if you start off by dictating the patient's name and date of birth, followed by "presented in the office today looking much younger than her stated age..."

Getting started. It doesn't matter if you have an EHR or still make notes on paper charts. You can use a small digital recorder, voice recognition software, or whatever other technology your practice transcription process requires. Put the recording devices in your exam rooms and start using them. If you still prefer to record patient encounter notes by typing or writing, then summarize aloud as you write or type the information into the record.

When you shouldn't dictate. If live dictation seems to intimidate a patient or perhaps raises some fears about being recorded, make the "no IRD" note in the record and go back to written notes. Other times to not dictate would include during procedures or when domestic violence, child abuse, or elder abuse is suspected. You might not want to announce opinions if the suspected abuser is present.

Physicians who adapt to dictating during the exam find that most patients love it. The additional benefit is no longer seeing that stack of charts waiting to be dictated at the end of the day.

Inefficiency: A vicious spiral

A little inefficiency can quickly lead to big problems. If you're struggling with inefficiency, see if this scenario sounds familiar:

Dr. Samantha Wilson struggles to keep up with her patient volume, and work begins to pile up. Messages come in, prescription renewals are requested, and forms stack up. In between rooming patients, her nurse, Judy, spends time organizing the growing stack into tasks that she sends to Dr. Wilson's queue in the EHR.

By 5:30 p.m., the clinic is winding down. Dr. Wilson tells Judy to head home; she already has worked a half hour of overtime. Judy mentions the 30 tasks that sit in her e-mail queue, and leaves.

Alone, Dr. Wilson starts returning calls to patients – even though the nurse could have returned the call earlier had Dr. Wilson instructed her to do so. She writes (or e-mails) instructions to Judy to handle the messages that can wait for morning, the prescription renewals, and forms. When Dr. Wilson finally leaves it is past 7:00 p.m.

Office hours start again at 8:00 a.m. and Judy makes it to the office five minutes early. She puts her personal items on her desktop and logs into the EHR. She enters her user name and password and sighs when she sees the 30 new e-mail tasks that sit in her queue.

*Here's where the inefficiency becomes a vicious spiral: Would any nurse in his or her right mind ignore the physician's assigned tasks and instead walk to the reception area to escort the first patient in to an exam room? Of course not. Faced with the tasks at hand, Judy will easily spend at least the first 20 to 30 minutes of her day prioritizing and handling a portion of them. In the meantime, today's messages, forms, renewals, and other work start to filter in. She is handling yesterday's **and** today's work. Her anxiety level increases and her morale decreases. It's not hard to conclude that Judy's productivity, in turn, declines.*

Thus, it's no surprise that the first patient isn't ready for Dr. Wilson until 8:45. The day is running late already.

You can see how a little inefficiency soon leads to a problem with staff productivity and turnover, and has a negative impact on patient satisfaction. It also means that physicians are rarely home for dinner with their families.

If your practice is in the vicious cycle of inefficiency, recognize that it won't get better until you take concrete steps to stop the cycle. Implement efficiency strategies before burn out becomes endemic to your practice.

Quality, not quantity is the key to a successful visit

I'm sure that there is at least one physician in your community with a terrific reputation among patients – yet that the same physician is rumored to see 40 or more patients a day and still finish on time. Held in high regard by their patients, these physicians have a special gift for getting the work done faster while making patients perceive that the visit was longer. That is, each patient leaves with the impression that the encounter lasted an hour when it was actually only six minutes. These special physicians may have personality traits that help them, but don't despair. There is much you can learn from these naturally efficient physicians – and adopt for yourself:

Make eye contact. Eye contact indicates interest and creates a connection between the physician and the patient.

Sit with the patient. Physicians who stand during a discussion with a patient may convey that they are in a hurry. Sitting down, leaning in, and crossing one's legs indicates an interest in what the patients have to say.

Reach out to the patient. It doesn't have to be a physical touch; even an introduction and a smile will work.

Make a little chitchat. A few friendly words regarding the patient's family or work gets the visit off to a friendly start and doesn't have to eat up precious time. Some physicians keep personal notes in the patient's record as a reminder.

Make sure the patient is comfortable. Patients who have been sitting in a chilly exam room for 30 minutes – naked, save a piece of paper wrapped around their hips – are not going to be in the best of moods when you enter. Make sure your patients are comfortable and you won't have to spend the first few minutes of the encounter "warming" patients up. Try upgrading to cloth gowns – and make them available in regular and extra-large sizes – to help you and your patients.

Listen first. Studies show that patients start off by discussing their least important complaints and build to the more intimate or distressing symptoms. Physicians who let the patient finish talking, while making notes or jotting down questions, get through interviews faster and make patients feel as if they were heard. Yet, research shows that physicians interrupt after only 16.5[2] to 18[3] seconds of listening. The bottom line: it's more efficient – and valuable to patients – to listen first.

Work in front of your patients. Start reviewing patients' charts at the nurses' station or in the hallway but consider completing the review of the chart and any test results in the exam room with them. It's a good opportunity to educate patients about what you're assessing, explain what the tests were for, and what the results mean. Often, patients don't see this extra time that you spend managing their care. Do it in front of them and they'll realize their time with you is really 15 minutes – not five.

Say "thank you." Patients will feel good when you express your appreciation because it acknowledges that you know they had a choice of physicians.

Be happy. If you're unhappy, everyone around you – including your patients – will feel the same. Happy physicians are not just more pleasant, they are more productive because their staff and patients respond to their optimism.

Some physicians are naturally gifted with good – and efficient – bedside manners, but with practice and the input of others, it is possible to learn these techniques.

STEPS TO GET YOU THERE

Popular, efficient physician Richard Honaker, MD offers his top-10 steps to optimize patient flow – and delight his patients

1. Communicate non-verbally with your support team when possible. Giving directions verbally might interrupt the nurse, are more easily forgotten, and worse, might not get documented. Written instructions translate into accountability. Plus, I usually don't have to spend extra time giving instructions when I walk between rooms. For example, I write: "Zocor® sample. NW." [Translation: Give the patient a sample of Zocor and send them on their way (i.e., "non-wait")].

2. Standardize exam rooms. Every room should be identical right down to the positioning of equipment and supplies. I also never leave a room idle if there's a patient ready for it. No physician should "own" an exam room.

3. Use written materials to educate patients – and to get you into the next exam room. If I diagnose patients with H-pylori and see their eyes are glazing over from information overload, I ask them to review some written material about H-pylori and the workup I'm recommending. While they are reading, I proceed to see a patient in another room. When I return, the patient with H-pylori is better informed. We can review our next steps faster and I have fit in another patient.

4. Be able to call the nurse without breaking eye contact with the patient. Each of our rooms has a nurse call light within my reach at the exam room desk. If I anticipate something is needed, such as an EKG, I press the button to call the nurse without losing eye contact and proceed to the patient's next symptom or complaint before the nurse arrives.

5. Make each patient feel like he or she is your sole focus. I introduce myself and immediately sit down. I cross my legs so I don't look like I'm ready to leave as soon as the patient stops talking. I lean slightly towards the patient and maintain eye contact. I touch the patient in an appropriate manner and time. Before I break eye contact to start writing, I always explain my action: "Ms. Jones, let me write this down."

6. Use patients' names over and over again during the encounter. This assures them that I haven't "checked out" and that I'm listening. If I sense that they don't think I'm listening, I say, "Ms. Jones, a minute ago, you mentioned...." It tells patients I am focused solely on them.

7. Apologize for being late. Even if I'm running on time, I start every encounter by saying, "I'm sorry that I kept you waiting." It demonstrates my respect for the patient's time.

8. Avoid open-ended questions. I never end an encounter by asking, "Is there anything else?" It invites a positive response. Instead, I ask, "Now, we have covered everything you wanted to discuss. Is that correct?"

9. Control the list. When patients have a written list, I ask to see it (or, if it's in their head, I ask them to take a minute to write it down). I ask patients to prioritize by circling the top-three things bothering them. We talk about every symptom of the top three. I find that just getting the whole list to me helps comfort patients because they know everything's "on the table." For the lower-ranked issues I might

say, "I want to gather my thoughts about your headaches and spend more time with you on that...." Then, I schedule another appointment.

10. Get to your next patient gracefully. If an encounter is running long but it's not an acute complaint, I will say, "I have a sick patient next door. I have to put a fire out there. I will be back in a few minutes. Is that okay?" Most patients take the cue that they are spending a lot of time but by asking permission to go, I am respecting their time. Most will take the hint to wrap up the visit.

Source: Richard A. Honaker, MD, Family Medicine Associates of Texas, Carrollton, www.texasmedicine.com. A full-time practicing physician and frequent speaker on efficiency, Dr. Honaker was named as a "Best Doctors in Dallas."

WORDS OF WISDOM

A personal touch

Patients are delighted when their physician remembers personal information about them. This personal touch not only represents great service – it can foster efficiency because patients feel a connection to their physician earlier in the encounter. That rapport delights patients. It also allows physicians to gather and discuss more information in a shorter period of time.

A little advance work by the staff can help bring busy physicians up-to-date on their patients and immediate families. Delineate a section in your patients' paper or electronic charts to note personal topics, like profession, spouse's name, and even hobbies. Or, record a line in the documentation of the encounter. So, if the patient brings you a small gift, like a book, you can express how much you have enjoyed the book when the patient returns for the next appointment.

Some practices in rural areas even have staff review the local newspaper on a daily basis, clip out any articles that mention or relate to their patients, and file or scan them into the appropriate patients' charts.

As with medical information, it's important to respect the patient's privacy, so keep all non-public information confidential.

• •

Reach out to patients now, not later

The telephone is a wonderful time-saver but it is not always the ideal way to communicate important information to patients. Instead of spending time trying to track down patients after their appointment by phone and risking the potential compromises in confidentiality that come with electronic communication, why not try to communicate as much information to patients during the visit? It's not only more valuable to patients; it saves you time in the long run.

Here is a checklist of information that every patient should be able to receive during a visit:

- ☐ When and how they will receive their test results?
- ☐ When and for what purpose is the next visit to be scheduled?
- ☐ What is the diagnosis (presented such that patients can understand)?
- ☐ What is the treatment plan?
- ☐ How and where can patients receive additional educational information related to the complaint/diagnosis?
- ☐ If applicable, written orders for employer (e.g., return to work), prescriptions, etc.

Follow through by allowing patients access to their personal health records, and offer other functionality through a Web portal.

Improve patients' retention of information

The average patient only retains part of the information that is communicated during the encounter. Although it may be routine for your practice, most patients are surprised to hear that a test, procedure, or surgery is in order. Shocked by the news, they often do not hear anything else you tell them.

When patients don't remember what the physician explained, they are more likely to call the practice when they return home. This, of course, requires that you dedicate staff time in answering these telephone calls. If you can communicate more effectively with patients during the face-to-face encounter, you can avoid some, if not all, of these calls.

Plus, with more insurance companies reimbursing physicians through pay-for-performance plans, it behooves your practice – financially – to improve patient compliance. Better communication pays off.

Print a copy of the encounter documentation from the patient's record, or provide the "discharge summary" your EHR creates from the findings, assessment, and plan you've documented. Provide patients with written material about their condition or procedure or write out the patient's treatment plan on paper or even on a flipchart. Direct them to specific Web sites for more information or support groups. Or, encourage access to a personal health record you make available through your Web portal.

When there is something more complicated at hand, say a surgery, some physicians provide educational videotapes or software about the surgery, as well as pre- and post-operative information for patients.

Others use simpler technology, including paper and pencil, which can work just as well. See Chapter 4, "Scheduling" for information on care notebooks.

If patients do not speak English, or if it is a second language for them, it is still the physician's duty to make sure patients understand what is said. Use of qualified interpreters or translated patient education materials may be necessary.

CASE STUDY

The flipchart tells the story

An oncologist in the Southeast uses a flipchart to outline the treatment plan for patients. When speaking to a patient, the oncologist uses a colored marker to draw a quick and simple timeline of the treatment process on a flipchart. What patients really seem to value is that they can take the oncologist's chart home with them to keep. Many refer to it often.

Patients who rely on visual learning are overlooked by office processes. If a flipchart doesn't float your boat, try hanging white boards on your walls or pre-print drawings of the body to write on.

Medical schools getting on the communications bandwagon ... finally

Training in patient-physician communication is also now objectively evaluated as a core competency in various accreditation settings, including the Comprehensive Osteopathic Medical Licensing Examination (USA) Performance Evaluation, the United States Medical Licensing Examination, and the American Board of Medical Specialties' certification.[4,5,6] As a volunteer for a medical school, I was assigned to role-play a patient who was receiving post-biopsy results that unfortunately determined a malignant carcinoma. In this exercise, the physician (played by a medical student taking the course) bravely told me just what the lab results stated: "malignant carcinoma of the spleen." Considering that more than half of the adult U.S. population reads at below the 8th grade level, many patients would have walked away with this dreadful news without really knowing how serious the problem was, other than it involved the spleen (whatever that was).

This type of miscommunication is even more serious due to the fact that many patients don't ask sufficient follow-up questions because they fear appearing ignorant. When answering questions, physicians should be coached to respond in the patients' non-technical language. Not only do miscommunications of this sort reduce the quality of care and seem to raise physicians' malpractice liability risks, they tend to increase the amount of work for the practice. Rest assured that when a patient doesn't understand what the physician said, it won't be long until the patient calls the office for better understanding of the situation.

As this chapter explains, the patient encounter is certainly the most important step in the patient flow process. It is at this point that the practice can fulfill the reason why the patient came to the practice in the first place – the value that the patient perceives – to receive quality care. While maintaining a focus on that value, efficiencies in this step can create a more valuable experience for the patient, the staff, and the physician.

The physician sets the tone

I was once pulled aside by a productive physician with more than 30 years of experience. He told me that he had *the* answer to physician efficiency.

"If I started complaining about appointments scheduled at 4:45 p.m., the employees would hear me. Even if I didn't ask for a different schedule, staff would stop filling the 4:45 p.m. slot. We'd all be home in time for dinner, but we'd lose money. Whether we acknowledge it or not, our staff is always listening," he said.

His lesson was simple, but incredibly powerful: the physician sets the tone for the practice.

It isn't just what you say at staff meetings, it's what physicians "say" to everyone in the office – staff, patients and other physicians – through their day-to-day actions. Whether or not the practice is physician-owned, the physician shapes the atmosphere and influences the long-term success of the practice.

Physicians who want to make their practices better places to work start with themselves.

Physicians put in long hours and work hard, and expect those around them to do the same. But if physicians come back from lunch an hour late every day leaving an office full of frustrated patients, it won't take long for staff to replicate the pattern.

Physicians set the tone; a hard worker will usually end up with hard workers around them.

Efficient physicians look for solutions, not scapegoats. Yes, declining reimbursement might be the fault of insurance companies, but short of single-handedly reforming the entire U.S. health care system or changing professions, we're stuck with them.

Efficient physicians seek out ways to improve performance. They focus on the big picture. They do whatever it takes to create a culture of problem solving. They refuse to engage in the behind-the-scenes gripe sessions and clique forming that are all-too-common in health care settings. When someone starts complaining about someone else, they simply change the topic. In time, that behavior earns the respect of peers and staff. Better yet, people spend more time thinking about patients and going home happy.

Although we often find excuses to blame the system (whatever the "system" is), there is no one stopping you from creating an efficient patient encounter in your practice. Embrace change and you will find your patients, staff, and even physicians more productive – and happier too!

The patient as "co-producer"

So far, we've focused on the physician as the main producer of revenue in the practice. Of course, that is true, but don't forget where that revenue really comes from: it comes from patients.

Many service industries realize that everything they do starts and stops with the customer. To gain maximum value from their interaction with their customer and give the customer a better experience; namely, more convenience at less cost, many service providers are integrating customers into their workforces. How? Consider these examples of how the customer becomes the provider:

➤ Automated teller machines (ATM);

➤ Online bill payment;

➤ Restaurant salad bars;

➤ Self-service cashiering at retail stores;

➤ Self-serve gasoline stations;

➤ Self-serve car washes;

➤ Self-serve parking lots; and

➤ Shopping on the Web.

True, the customer is doing more of the work in these examples. But the return (the value) for them is (ideally) faster service, more convenience, and lower cost. I am not suggesting that you insist that your patients self-diagnose, write their own prescriptions, or administer their own shots. But putting patients in charge where possible can save your organization time and money. Here are some ways that "co-production" can fit into your practice's operations, bring more value to patients, and reduce wasted time for you:

- ➤ Place pads of paper titled, "Issues I wish to discuss with the doctor today" in the reception area. This may help save time at the beginning of the visit when the patients recall all of their symptoms.

- ➤ Provide patient education materials or videos while waiting or after visits. These resources may answer many of the questions patients might have and allow better use of the time spent with the physician.

- ➤ Allow patients to complete and submit their registration paperwork via a secure Web site before the day of the visit.

- ➤ Give patients electronic access to medical history and intake questions to complete before the visit or while they are waiting.

- ➤ Offer online bill payment.

- ➤ Maintain treatment plans or logs online for patients to record test results and monitor their own care (with your guidance).

- ➤ Develop a Web portal for your practice, offering patients access to their personal health records, as well as a variety of other functions, such as online test results notification.

Consider your patients as co-producers and discover the new and innovate ways that *they* can help you.

Set priorities

Days are long in a medical practice and it's easy to get buried in the details. That's why some physicians carry a laminated picture of their family in a shirt pocket. Each time there is an extra chore, they can pull out the picture and ask: "Can I delegate this task to support staff so that I can continue with the day and get home sooner?"

Efficient physicians are centered people. They don't get trapped in their practices. They know that their patients may love them but studies show that many patients will switch to other physicians over as little as a $10 dispute. They know that caring for patients doesn't mean abandoning one's personal or family life. Most importantly, their motto is: Be good to yourself and you can be good to your patients.

References

1. Coding based on counseling and/or coordination of care with the patient and/or a family member is based on the coding rules at the publication of this book.

2. L Dyche, D Swiderski. The effect of physician solicitation approaches on ability to identify patient concerns. *J Gen Intern Med.* (2005); 20(3): 267–270.

3. HB Beckman, RM Frankel. The effect of physician behavior on the collection of data. *Ann Intern Med.* (1984);101:692–6.

4. FD Duffy, DH Gordon, G Whelan et al. Assessing competence in communication and interpersonal skills: The Kalamazoo II report. *Acad Med.* (2004); 79(6):495-507.

5. R Gimpel, DO Boulet, AM Errichetti. Evaluating the clinical skills of osteopathic medical students. *J Am Osteopath Assoc.* (2003);103(6):267-279.

6. G Makoul. Communication skills education in medical school and beyond. *JAMA* (2003);289(1):93.

CHAPTER 9

Prescriptions

Key Chapter Lessons

➤ Discover ways to reduce prescription-related paper, eliminate errors, and handle formularies more effectively for the patient's benefit.

➤ Learn to maximize the productivity of staff by reducing the time spent on prescription processes.

➤ Recognize the importance of protocols for telephone-based prescription management and for making refills and renewals.

➤ Understand safer ways to manage drug samples.

Managing prescriptions

Don't overlook how much time and money your practice spends – perhaps wastes – to manage prescriptions. Many practices dedicate staff exclusively to the management of the prescription process. From the medley of incoming telephone calls regarding prescriptions to the sample closet, prescription management is an important function in medical practice operations and offers opportunity for improvement.

Prescription management is a complex process, but one that is critical to the patient's experience – and care. Patients want fast access to their medications and they want the correct medications. Obtaining the right drug that works – and perhaps one that is affordable – is the primary value your patients can pull from your prescription process. With so much riding on this complex process, medical practices must be prepared to manage this flow of work well.

This chapter explores managing the workflow of various aspects of the prescription process to add value to your patients' experience.

Consider your protocols

Prescription writing is so commonplace in most medical practices that we tend to overlook its impact on practice operations. Carefully designed protocols prevent that quickly jotted-out script – done dozens of times each day – from adding up to significant costs, slowdowns and perhaps even putting the patient in harm's way.

A number of insurance companies have implemented requirements related to prescriptions, including pre-authorization requirements, formulary delineation, and monitoring, as well as limits on the time period. In the past, a physician might have given a patient a one-year supply of a medication. Now, that patient's insurer might approve medications for only three months at a time. This means that the patient will need to visit the pharmacy more frequently to obtain medications (and make copayments) and will need to obtain your approval for a renewal more often. This translates to more inbound telephone calls from patients unless you take other steps to manage the prescription process; namely, by defining the process and communicating with your patients.

Ideally, your protocol for the period of time for which you approve the medication is timed to the follow-up appointment. In the best situation, the patient comes in for an appointment and the prescription is renewed and/or alternative medications are prescribed during that encounter. If you've decided to try a new medication – or alter the dosage – at that visit, set a reminder for a member of your clinical team to call the patient to determine whether the medication should be extended and/or altered. The timing of the communication from your clinical team should be dictated by clinical protocols – it may be hours, days, or weeks after the patient has commenced the medication. By having your clinical team initiate the telephone call, your practice avoids the extra time and effort of handling an inbound call.

Evaluate the timing of the prescription renewal and the patient's appointment. If you provide a 30-day supply with two 30-day refills to a patient, but ask the patient to return in four months, you're guaranteed to get a telephone call from that patient in 90 days. If there is a clinical need to evaluate the medication in 90 days, then consider a 90-day return appointment. If there is no clinical need, and you're planning to automatically extend the renewal period for another 30 days until the patient comes in for the appointment, then three refills should have been written. If the formulary only allows a 90-day cycle, you may not be able to avoid doing a telephone renewal, but again, this can be conducted between you and the patient's pharmacy if it is medically appropriate to do so. Considering that nearly two-thirds of all appointments result in a prescription (71.3 percent of physician office visits include drugs that were provided or prescribed by the physician),[1] paying attention to timing the renewal cycle can help your practice avoid many unnecessary telephone calls.

Describe side effects

Patients often fail to read the side effects printed on the medication packaging. Be sure that the patient knows to call you if a side effect or something that feels like one should occur. Instead of waiting for those telephone calls from worried patients, review the most common side effects with them when you prescribe the medication. Many practices print off a list of common side effects in the exam room when prescribing a medication. An informed patient is less anxious, more compliant, and less apt to call you for advice.

THINGS TO CONSIDER

Charging for renewals

Some medical practices charge patients who renew prescriptions if they have been seen recently. This charge is levied to recoup some of the additional costs associated with renewing the pre-scription via telephone instead of during the patient visit. Consider enacting this charge only if you ask patients during office visits if they have renewals that need to be considered, have clearly spelled out the terms of your new policy in advance of the request, and ensure that you're not breaking the terms of any contracts you have with insurance companies.

Set telephone renewal protocols

Inevitably, some patients will run out of refills before their next appointment. They will call to request a renewal. Many practices, plagued by the overhead spent on nurses to process these requests, have established a policy to no longer provide renewals over the telephone and/or they limit them dramatically.

A number of different telephone renewal protocols have been imple-mented by medical practices to include:

→ Patients who have run out of pills are provided a small supply based upon their physician's direction and given an appointment to address the renewal;

→ Practices with patients on maintenance medications have developed written protocols about telephone renewals, with specific direction on a maximum time between face-to-face appointments depending on the patient's clinical issues (e.g., one year and what medications clinical assistants are authorized to renew without physician approval);

➤ Patients are asked to contact their pharmacies to request a written order identifying all details of the medication be sent to the physician who would be able to then approve or give an alternative direction;

➤ Patients are directed to the practice's Web portal to generate an electronic request; or

➤ Patients are asked to schedule appointments as soon as possible, during which the physician can discuss the renewal request face-to-face.

Regardless of the path you or your patient chooses, document all medication renewals. Recording your actions is important for patient care.

Out-of-office prescription management

Many medical practices try to get ahead of the volume of incoming prescription-related telephone calls by dedicating telephone lines to prescription renewals or integrating the process into their Web portal.

Over the telephone, the dedicated lines can have live operators responding, but many practices opt to feed these lines into voice-mail boxes. Unfortunately, by the end of the day, these mail boxes are brimming with messages such as: "Hi. This is Mary Smith. I need my little blue pills refilled." Thus begins another game of telephone tag as the nurse tries to figure out who Mary Smith is, how to contact her for more information, and what those "little blue pills" are.

A more efficient way to manage prescription requests is via a Web portal. Patients can be directed to the portal to generate an electronic request for a medical renewal. The request is legible and documented. Electronic receipt adds value to the practice because it can be managed much more easily than a telephone-based request.

Of course, the best route to manage out-of-the-office prescription requests is to avoid them altogether. What one question asked during a patient's office visit can help reduce your volume of out-of-office prescription requests? The question is, "Do you need any prescriptions renewed today?" Too many times, a request about a prescription comes from the patient who was in the office just the week before. Try printing paper tablets with the heading: "Medications I Need to Discuss with my Doctor Today." Leave the tablets and pencils around the reception area or in each exam room. Make the medication renewal question part of the rooming process.

Refill or renewal?

Another step you can take to reduce the volume of telephone calls, delays, confusion, and frustration surrounding prescriptions is to make clear to patients that there is a distinct difference between "refill" and "renewal." Most patients are oblivious to the difference. They just default to contacting the practice to obtain their pills whenever they run out because, after all, you are the place that originated the request. Make it clear to patients that unless there is a problem with the medication, they should never have to call your practice for a refill. Explain that a refill automatically means the next bottle of pills has already been approved and just needs to be filled by the pharmacist.

If a refill exists, ask your patients to call their pharmacies directly. If the prescription requires a renewal, consider the renewal options outlined in the section above.

Unless your practice refuses to renew medications over the phone or Web, some patients will still call about renewals, so train operators to take messages, create a voice-mail box in your telephone system with prompts for requests and questions or develop a secure, Web-based prescription request system.

Set up protocols about how your staff will handle those requests and questions.

Consider establishing specific times to take the messages and manage these out-of-office requests, for example, at 10:00 a.m., 12:00 noon, 2:00 p.m. and 4:00 p.m. Set the expectation that the requests will be managed within four hours of receipt. Alternatively, communicate to patients that prescription requests will be processed in 24 to 48 hours. This will require patients to anticipate their needs and it will ensure that the practice has sufficient time to effectively manage the process.

Make it a rule: prescriptions must either be renewed according to the expectations you established – or the patient must be advised why not as soon as possible. You don't want patients or pharmacists to feel like their requests are going into a black box never to be seen or heard from again.

Legibility

To avoid callbacks from pharmacies, scrutinize the legibility of all providers who write prescriptions. Often, illegible handwriting prompts a telephone call from the pharmacist to clarify the medication, dosage, or other instructions. If Dr. Scribble is out for the day, then that work will fall on the other physicians in the practice that day. Automated prescription software will eliminate these telephone calls, and perhaps an unfortunate compromise to your patient's safety, by printing prescriptions and/or transmitting them directly to the pharmacy.

E-prescribing

For more efficient prescribing, use an e-prescribing solution. Not only is it quick, but formularies, tracking of side effects, and interactions can be at your fingertips. The prescription request often can be routed directly to the pharmacy from your office. (Check state laws to make sure your state allows for electronic transmission of prescriptions.) If not, place a printer in each exam room to provide the prescription(s) script directly to patients. Don't load the printer tray with blank scripts but rather capture the form in an image file on your hard drive. That will avoid the problem of leaving blank scripts lying around unattended.

Although e-prescribing won't save the physician much time when first prescribing a medication to a patient, this method will streamline future prescriptions. You'll be able to automatically recall all of that patient's previous prescribing information. And most e-prescribing automatically allows you to check for drug interactions and formulary compliance. Many EHRs contain integrated e-prescribing solutions and several insurance companies are providing them at no cost to participating physicians.

Paperwork

Medication pre-authorization is an increasingly popular tool that insurance companies use to control rising pharmacy costs, especially for pricey name-brand medications. The insurance company requires physicians to record written certifications for each medication prescribed. The authorization process often requires documents exclusive to that insurer. Although some insurers take advantage of information technology, for many others, the process of completing those documents and gaining approval involves additional staff time to contact the payer by telephone or fax.

Pre-authorization itself shouldn't be so burdensome but many insurers make it so by requiring physician certification every 30 days. Unfortunately, directing the patient to handle this process at the pharmacy isn't adequate.

If patients choose health plans with a 30-day pre-authorization process for pharmaceuticals, then ask them to bring the insurance company's required paperwork. Because many patients don't know the details of their plan's prescription authorization process, or may just be forgetful, take the initiative by asking the provider representatives of the insurance companies with which you participate to give you the forms. Either way, file the documents so they are easy to retrieve and complete for the 30-day authorization.

Estimate the additional time prescription pre-authorization takes your staff to complete. Perhaps measure a few typical rounds of forms completion and faxing or calling. It may seem like just a few extra seconds but multiply that by all of the pre-authorizations that one insurance company might require over the course of a year. It will add up. Be sure to let the company's representatives know how much their pre-authorization processes are costing you. Use this fact to help negotiate for higher payments for evaluation and management codes, which are expressly meant to include medication management.

Many patients choose to order their medications via mail order. It is more convenient for the patient and less expensive for the insurance company and the patient. But mail order pharmacies will likely require paperwork to be completed. Encourage patients to bring this required information with them to routine appointments, or mail or fax it in. You cannot be expected to keep updated versions of all the forms you might need for the many insurance companies out there.

Regardless of what plan your patient is on, you can handle the prescription process much more efficiently if you can do the work while the patient is in the office instead of exchanging telephone calls and mailings.

Although it would be terrific for the bottom line to bring the patient back for an office visit just to complete that bothersome pre-authorization or mail order paperwork, it's not a visit for which you can expect to be reimbursed. Unless other medical issues are addressed in that visit the encounter wouldn't be considered medically necessary.

Prescription paperwork is inevitable and it is one area where you'll need to accept that there will be inbound telephone calls as you work with the patient to process the insurance company's paperwork.

Formularies

Don't forget to check whether the medication you're prescribing is on the formulary of the patient's insurance. A formulary is a list of medications by clinical indication from which you must choose if the insurance company is to cover the cost of the prescription. Often, these lists are tiered, with the insurance company charging the patient a nominal copayment for generics and higher copayments for the pricier, name-brand medications. Formularies tend to place the most expense and often newest drugs into higher copayment categories. Non-covered medications may come with significantly high copayments or offer no coverage at all, requiring the patient to bear the full cost. The intent, of course, is to encourage you to prescribe (or the patient to request) a cheaper alternative. Many formularies try to limit the number of refills, the maximum days supply purchased at any one time, and even the daily dosage in some cases. When a drug isn't covered at all but you feel it is justified, you may be able to request an exception. Expect to put up a fight. Most insurance companies have targeted prescription costs as a major area of cost savings.

Ideally, you should be able to integrate formularies for each insurer into your EHR or e-prescribing software. This information may be available from the insurance company electronically in a software format that's easy to load into your system. Otherwise, someone at your practice must type in each drug and its related information by hand, which could run to many pages and need to be constantly updated. If you aren't able to obtain information about formulary compliance automatically through an electronic system, maintain a master list of formularies sorted by insurance company for the medications you commonly prescribe. Check the list automatically or manually when you prescribe. It will save you and your patients a lot of time later on. And it will help reduce the confusion that often sparks multiple telephone calls between you, patients, and their pharmacies.

Prescription samples

Most pharmaceutical companies employ sales representatives who focus on a single medication or several that may complement one another. To avoid disruptions to patient flow, ask the representatives to schedule time with physicians rather than "popping in" and trying to catch them during a free moment.

The representatives – often called "drug reps" – provide samples for physicians to distribute to patients at no charge. Samples provide an easy means of trying medications to determine what works best for the patient's situation. Samples also can allow a busy patient to start immediately on a course of medication, giving the patient a day or two to get to the pharmacy to pick up the full supply. Finally, the samples can be a benefit to patients who need financial assistance for pharmaceuticals.

Most physicians dispense the free samples provided by pharmaceutical sales representatives to patients. Some practices allow the visiting pharmaceutical representatives to access the drug sample area and keep it stocked. Most practices, and all risk managers, recommend against letting outsiders have access to and control over any part of this vital area of your practice. Samples may be free but be assured there will be a price to pay if they are not handled correctly. Maintaining samples is a responsibility, not just a convenience for patients.

Due to the necessary complexity of handling samples safely and the business risks practices may incur related to sample offerings, some practices have either discontinued providing samples altogether, or have integrated sample dispensing with their in-house pharmacy.

Some practices find the sheer volume of samples difficult to monitor for expiration. Others find it burdensome to document all the samples' details (see Best Practices). Those details will be critical if there is ever a recall of a medication. Some practices are frustrated by the challenge of controlling access to samples, which is an essential step to preventing inappropriate use by their own staff. For some practices, the potential business risk associated with a drug sample closet is too great and they have discontinued distributing samples altogether. If samples are distributed by your practice, ask your malpractice carrier for its recommendations.

 BEST PRACTICES

Handling drug samples

Follow these guidelines to best manage prescription samples in your practice:

➤ Use a storage area that can be kept locked and is not subject to extreme temperatures. Develop an established protocol to verify temperature settings within the storage area;

➤ Follow a procedure to ensure that outdated and deteriorated samples are discarded. Be sure to do regular inspections and document doing so;

➤ Discard expired samples according to the recommendations outlined by your state Department of Environmental Services;

➤ Keep an up-to-date inventory log. Include lot numbers on the inventory in case a drug in your sample closet is recalled. (See Exhibit 9.1);

➤ Keep an up-to-date sign-out log, including patient name, date, provider, medication, quantity, and lot number with regular reconciliation between the inventory and sign-out logs;

➤ Recognize that only providers with prescription-writing authority may dispense samples. Require that all providers accessing the drug sample storage closet follow state and federal pharmacy regulations;

➤ Discuss and document potential allergies, administration, storage, and side effects of each medication with the patient when distributing a sample;

➤ Document in the patient's record the medication, date, dosage, frequency, route, form, lot number, and person responsible for dispensing the sample, as well as what instructions were provided and that potential allergies and adverse reactions were discussed;

➤ Don't allow staff to access samples or use them personally unless the staff member is a patient at the practice and follows the procedures as outlined for all patients. Incorporate these rules into your human resources policy;

➤ Have a written policy and procedure regarding how your practice handles samples. Take steps to ensure that your practice complies with your documented policy and procedure for sample handling – the business risk of mishandling drug samples is just too great to do otherwise; and

➤ Consult your malpractice carrier regarding its recommended protocols.

. . . .

Implementing just one of the processes described in this chapter – or hopefully most of them – will greatly lighten the burden on you and your staff so you can focus more on patient care.

References

1. Table 5. U.S. Department of Health and Human Services, Centers for Disease Control and Prevention, National Center for Health Statistics, National Ambulatory Medical Care Survey: 2005 (June 29, 2007) by E. Hing et al.

Inventory inspection log

Inventory log for pharmaceutical samples

Date of receipt	Medication	Lot No.	Quantity	Dose/ Concentration	Expiration Date	Staff initials	Date of Review

Use a manual or electronic inventory form to track your sample medications.

CHAPTER 10

Managing Test Results

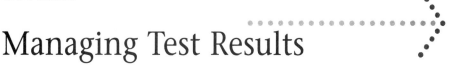

Key Chapter Lessons

➤ Evaluate your test results management process

➤ Analyze the test ordering process

➤ Evaluate the process of managing inbound results for physician review

➤ Identify methods to manage test results notification

➤ Integrate low-tech and high-tech solutions to improve test results management

Focus on patient's needs

Managing test ordering, reviewing, and results notification is a complex process for any medical practice. Whether you order one test a day or thousands, every one is important to a patient. Managing the testing process can be a chore but only if you let it. The solution? Let your patients pull the value from the efficient test result management system you create and maintain. The patients' stake in the process is threefold: they want the test ordered accurately, conducted accurately and timely, and they want to be notified of the results on a timely basis.

This chapter outlines the process of managing test results. There's no single way to manage results, but focusing on what the patient wants and needs – accuracy and timeliness – will allow your practice to create and sustain a system that works for your patients.

Whether you refer a patient to an external facility for a test or send the patient to your own ancillary service, you should have a mechanism in place to order, review, and report the results of each test ordered.

The ordering process

Traditionally, practices have relied on manual forms to order tests, and paper when the results are returned. Instead of letting the mounds of paper pile up, consider streamlining the order process.

Request direct schedule access to testing facilities, to include ordering laboratory tests and imaging studies. With electronic order entry the industry standard in hospitals today, electronic access for outpatient practices will be forthcoming. Schedule the patient at the point of care, ideally in the exam room, when the physician provides the orders. Because many tests require written orders, such as imaging, don't batch the work. Perform the ordering process during the encounter.

If you cannot schedule the patient at the point of care, discuss how orders can be received by the testing sites to which you refer. Instead of mailing or faxing an order, can the sites send you an electronic form to e-mail (securely, of course) or send to your fax server? Can the testing sites be integrated into your practice's Web portal? Develop similar paperless processes if you're referring patients to on-site testing.

Although this may seem like a "no-brainer," practices sometimes schedule tests but fail to document the order. Or, the physician verbally tells the clinical assistant or the patient to get the test but fails to document it in the patient's record. Be sure to record the order or use the test-order entry function in your EHR if you use one to document all tests ordered.

Ask providers to include information about each test ordered in their documentation of the encounter. This note in the record will serve as a "tickler" that staff will see when previewing charts before the patient's next appointment. Thus, they know to look for the results. It should be noted that if a patient never has a return appointment (and there is no other mechanism to track results), missing results may go undetected so don't rely on this method alone to be fail-safe.

WORDS OF WISDOM

Integrate advance beneficiary notifications (ABNs) with your test ordering process. Place the ABN on the backside of your test ordering form, if it's a paper form, or develop electronic flags for tests that are ordered that require an ABN. For a sample ABN, see Chapter 6, "Reception Services."

Receiving results

A paperless system is ideal to manage the mounds of paper sent to your practice by testing facilities. Unfortunately, you'll need to rely on the facilities to provide the method of receipt. Ideally, the results can be directly interfaced into your electronic health record or Web portal, creating a "tickler" for you to review. In addition to prompting your review, once you've signed off on them, the results are documented in the patient's record – with no paper involved.

If you can't interface with the testing facility, you'll need to review your alternatives. You can receive the results on paper, review them, report the results to the patient (see the next section for how to report results) and then file them.

If you have an EHR or a document scanning solution, scan faxes directly (i.e., no paper) into electronic form, tag them to be reviewed, and then file in the patient's record as a scanned document.

Patients with chronic illnesses may require constant testing. Diabetic patients, for example, test blood sugar levels several times daily. Decide on how you'll manage these results. It is ideal to accept results electronically from patients and maintain them in a personal health record that the patient can access through a Web portal and ideally, one that can be interfaced with your EHR. Alternatively, have patients print results on paper and bring it with them, and file or scan the documents into the patient's record.

WORDS OF WISDOM

Don't file test results until the physician has reviewed them. To ensure this process is followed, require a manual signature or electronic "sign-off" on all results. If you choose to vary from this protocol, discuss your process with your malpractice insurance carrier to ensure that your process meets its recommendations.

Reporting results to patients

There are many ways to monitor the test reporting process but it's important to choose one method and follow it religiously. Even one lost test result can have serious implications for your patients' safety.

Some popular monitoring methods – from low-tech to high-tech solutions are to:

Put charts in "timeout." If your practice maintains paper records, place charts waiting test results on a separate shelf or other specially designated area. File charts in date order using dividers to mark the day or week. Your staff can pull the charts off the shelf as test results come in and quickly spot any charts with outstanding results. Make sure to assign a staff member to review this shelf or rack weekly. If you don't like the idea of keeping some charts out of the central file, try putting a red jacket or similar identifier on charts awaiting test results. There's one critical drawback to filing those charts back with other records – it will be harder for staff to spot charts that are getting out of date. That's why it may be worth a little extra effort to keep a log, as the next tip explains.

Keep a log. Record test orders in a log. Also note the patient's name and a unique identifier, such as an account number. As results come in, highlight those entries with a color marker. Each week, scan the log for aging entries. Go another step by placing an asterisk or other identifier on entries after patients are contacted. A similar time-tested method is to use index cards or forms to record orders, and pull the cards or forms as results come in.

Use your PDA or desktop PC. This need not be a high-end program but merely a slightly higher tech version of the manual log. Record test orders and patients' names in a to-do list in a spreadsheet or word processing program. Mark patients' names off as results are received. Check daily for names that remain on the list after results were expected. A simple calendar program, an internal e-mail system, or your management system's scheduling module can serve the same purpose.

Keep a copy of each test order form in a date-ordered tickler file. Review this file daily to ensure that results are back when expected and that physicians are alerted.

Schedule a follow-up appointment. Make a follow-up appointment to review test results one to two weeks (or as clinically appropriate) after the patient's scheduled test. This is especially useful for biopsies, MRIs, CTs, and other major tests where results should be delivered in person, not by mail or over the telephone. Staff are "tickled" or reminded that test results have arrived or will soon arrive during the chart preview process before the upcoming appointment. If the patient doesn't show up for the follow-up appointment, you'll be able to see that the patient still needs to be notified of the test results.

Automate the system. There are numerous test results management systems to purchase. Some vendors specialize in telephone-based systems. Some vendors sell software that loads into your PC, while others use Web portals. You or your staff document verbally or in writing information about the patient's results, and ideally, provide some additional commentary. Patients are provided a unique identification number to punch or key into your telephone system or Web portal, where they can review their test results and your comments. Test results management via a Web portal allows longitudinal reporting of results, and most systems offer integration of test results with the patient's personal health record, which is a plus if your insurers have implemented pay-for-performance rewards. Whichever system you choose, make sure it allows you to monitor whether results are retrieved. Identifying which patients fail to pick up their results is important to know in order to proactively reach them.

Use recall. Many practice management systems feature an appointment recall function that identifies and sends reminders to patients recommended for future appointments. In addition to using the recall system for communicating health reminders to patients, use the function to recall yourself. Record the dates that test orders should be back based on protocols, such as one week for an MRI and so on. Then, direct all the appointment reminders to come back to your practice. The recall will identify the patient's name and the test you ordered. A staff member assigned to monitor the incoming reminders can check to see if results come in and if appropriate follow-up was made.

Embrace technology. Test results management should be a key component of any EHR. If you're shopping for an EHR, carefully evaluate this feature. It should be easy to use and incorporate all of the functionality of any manual system – recording orders and results, identifying outstanding results, and documenting, and possibly, handling patient notifications through an integrated Web portal. If an EHR is not on the horizon, consider building a simple-but-powerful database to perform the same functions. Call your local community college to inquire about an intern who could help build it. Unless the interface is built into your existing system, your staff still must enter the information about test orders. A simple database can easily identify outstanding orders. Plus, it can be programmed to "push" this information to you instead of you having to look for it. Alternatively, sign on with a vendor that offers connection to a customizable Web portal that can rapidly deliver a test results management solution to your practice.

Don't resort to telling the patient to "call back"

If you don't feel confident that your test tracking system works all the time, then you will be stuck telling your patients to call your practice if they haven't heard from you in a pre-determined time frame (e.g., two weeks). As mentioned in Chapter 3, "Telephones," this process will increase your volume of incoming calls. It also will increase the interruptions to your staff as they spend more time tracking down results that may have not yet arrived or been reviewed by a physician. Keep in mind also that the "call us back in two weeks" solution often leaves patients lacking in confidence about your operations, wondering whether your practice has the necessary systems to manage their care. Finally, you'll be hard-pressed to meet the quality standards being encouraged by pay-for-performance if you don't engage your patients in their test results. Don't rely on this so-called "solution" when there are so many new and affordable test results management systems that you can develop or buy.

No matter how you manage the process internally, awaiting test results can be a frightening experience for patients. To relieve their fears – and reduce the amount of unproductive communication that takes place before tests results are confirmed, give patients written materials about their tests. Make sure the materials describe – in simple terms – what the test is for, why it is important for the physician to have the test and when to expect test results.

Make sure that results are reviewed in a timely manner. Decide what your timeframe will be (24 hours for review and results notification, for example), and stick to it. Remember, every hour is precious to the patient. Always communicate abnormal results as per clinical norms would dictate. And make sure that your tracking system – whether electronic or handwritten – is kept secure and can be accessed only by those in your practice who need to know the information.

Regardless of how you monitor the results, it pays to be proactive. When the results come in and have been reviewed by the ordering (or designated) physician, place an outbound call, e-mail, or other pre-designated communication to the patient. Don't wait for them to contact you. If you've set expectations about the timing of your efforts and how you'll communicate, you'll avoid incoming phone calls (see why that's the best thing to do in Chapter 3, "Telephones") and you'll be sure to deliver great service.

No test results system is fail-safe. That's why it's important to hire employees who understand why medical tests are important. Staff who recognize the danger of letting test ordering, reviewing, or results – even one – fall through the cracks are the vital components to the success of any test results management system you deploy. Staff your practice with employees who truly care about patients and you will already be well on your way to efficiently managing the process your practice puts in place.

THINGS TO CONSIDER

Be flexible

A few patients may not want to go along with your preferred means of delivering test results. Anxiety about a test result can run high, even among the best-educated patient who is getting the most routine test. Seek to accommodate these worries by being flexible. If a patient doesn't want results delivered in your standard manner, offer alternative choices and have a means to manage the request if it is within reason.

BEST PRACTICES

Meet non-English speakers' needs

High-performing practices meet the needs of non-English speaking patients. If your patient population includes non-English speakers, develop your results notification verbiage in their language. In the case of an automated system, your vendor should be able to assist (be sure to check on this when you're evaluating systems), and manual forms can be translated by a professional interpreter, a patient volunteer, or perhaps a community resource. Not only do your efforts benefit your patients, but they also help the practice by reducing calls from confused patients.

CHAPTER 11

Practice Services

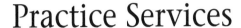

Key Chapter Lessons

➤ Evaluate your practice services process

➤ Identify the various components of practice services

➤ Learn charge entry methodologies

➤ Recognize the most efficient process for follow-up scheduling

➤ Identify the pros and cons of processing referrals and appointments for ancillary services and specialists

➤ Facilitate payment at practice services

➤ Learn to document more efficiently

➤ Identify the value of gleaning information from patients who have left your practice

Save time and money at the end of the patient flow process

Practice services is a much more accurate term to describe the many functions that occur at what has traditionally been called the "checkout" desk. Regardless of what you call it, this concluding step of the patient flow process should complete the patient encounter, not extend it. The interaction at practice services also is a time for staff to anticipate and meet the patient's needs for additional information. The tasks included in the practice services process vary from practice to practice, but I'll review those functions common to most medical practices.

GETTING STARTED

Practice services checklist

Use this checklist to find the gaps in your practice services process.

☐ Do practice services staff get the information they need about the patients' follow-up visits so they don't have to depend on patients to tell them when they are to return?

☐ Are patients told what ancillaries are required?

☐ Are patients told where to go for their appointment(s)?

☐ Are patients told how and when they will be contacted regarding test results?

☐ Do patients feel that all of their questions have been answered?

☐ Are patients given the opportunity to provide input regarding their encounter (e.g., a patient satisfaction survey)?

☐ Are fees collected in a courteous but firm manner?

☐ Can patients pay by cash, check, credit, or debit card?

☐ How quickly are charges entered into the system?

☐ What steps are taken to ensure that charges are accurate?

☐ Is there some meaningful communication at the patient's departure to conclude the visit?

☐ Do patients receive all of the educational materials that may be needed?

☐ Have patients had their prescription(s) renewed?

STAFF BENCHMARKS

Practice services

Practice operations task	Workload range
Check-out with follow-up scheduling, charge entry and cashiering	60-80 patients per day
Check-out with scheduling and charge entry	70-90 patients per day
Check-out with scheduling and cashiering	70-90 patients per day
Referral specialist (inbound or outbound referrals)	70-90 patients per day

Forget trying to staff practice services based on how many physicians they serve. The number you need depends on how many patients need to be assisted.

The workload range depends on what functions you assign to practice services staff, as well as patient population, information system, level of automation, and work processes utilized at the practice. The more information you gather and/or deliver during each patient served (thus, the higher the transaction time), the lower the productivity you should expect.

Given the multitude of variables, measure the time it takes your staff to handle each patient and apply that transaction time to reach your practice's ideal workload range.

Smooth practice services save time on the phone

Want to reduce the volume of unnecessary telephone calls to the practice and the time staff spends handling those calls? Then, make sure patients receive every piece of information they may need before they leave the practice after their visit is concluded. When a patient has to call back for more information after the visit, staff time is spent locating the information, researching the proper answer and, possibly, checking with a member of the clinical staff to make sure the right information is being provided. To reduce the volume of unnecessary callbacks, make sure that your practice services desk has completed the scheduling of appointments, tests, procedures, or surgeries – and collected payments and provided receipts – for each departing patient.

Make a list of the information you give out routinely to patients at the practice services desk. This list may include appointment reminders, prepping instructions for procedures, or directions to a lab or imaging facility. Next, take a look at the practice services area in your practice. Are there pre-printed materials (or materials that can be swiftly printed from your information systems) for staff to distribute? Do printed materials appear neat and legible? Are they located where practice services staff can easily find and reach them? Does the practice maintain a consistent and clear way (such as a paper or electronic check-off list) to instruct the practice services staff about what to schedule, how much to collect, which forms or other materials to hand out? It's easy to say you don't have time to sit down and think through and plan for each of these many tasks but consider that the alternative is to continue spending far more of your time repeatedly telling each staff member what to do for each patient. Like all of the other staff involved in patient flow tasks, practice services staff should be provided with the tools and resources they need to perform their responsibilities accurately and timely.

One of the most important processes to conclude the patient's visit is charge entry. This step enables the practice services staff to accurately collect payments. The process of entering charges can take many forms but the method of entry is either paper or electronic.

Electronic charge entry

Electronic charge entry, available through most EHR systems, offers the most streamlined process to enter charges. When physicians complete the documentation of the visit, they choose the procedure code(s) that best describes the services provided and documented. The selected codes then interface with the practice management system to become charges that will be billed to the patient and/or the patient's insurance company.

Paper charge entry

Manual charge entry features paper charge tickets (also known as encounter forms or superbills) on which a physician can record the services performed. The charge tickets should be concise, yet conducive to capturing all charges. The ticket should be designed to feature all of the physicians' commonly used procedure codes. The tickets may, for example, provide commonly used diagnoses codes on the back of the form and space to write out unusual services or procedures performed. It's important to update the charge ticket every year based on the annual updates by the American Medical Association to CPT codes used by physicians to code and bill. (An electronic system would accomplish this automatically.)

Ensure 100 percent charge capture

Regardless of how charges are entered, it's important to establish checks and balances to ensure no charges are missed. Most practice management systems and EHRs have "missing charge" reports that can make an electronic match between the appointment schedule and charges billed. Run these reports daily to identify charges that were accidentally overlooked, prevent filing incomplete claims with payers, or under-charging patients.

Of course, the appointment schedule-to-billed charges match is only an overview. Don't forget to also track down all charges as you check for missing charges. Sometimes, the type of visit can be clue. For example, although your management system tells you that an office visit for a routine preventive exam was billed for Mr. Jones, you also should ask: Was the EKG normally included for patients in this age group also included? If your system cannot automatically account for all services rendered, go back and audit the service logs against charges billed.

Avoid batching work

The mantra of "pulling work in" applies extremely well to charge entry. Whether it's done electronically or on paper, make sure that the charges are submitted by the time the patient leaves the office (versus the end of the day, or even worse, later that week). This step will facilitate the collection of the copayment, co-insurances, and the amount that is applied to the patient's deductible (the latter two of which are impossible for you to collect if you don't know what the charge is). Time-of-service collection is your opportunity to improve cash flow – and avoid spending precious practice resources on mailing patient statements.

 WORDS OF WISDOM

Accuracy or timeliness?

For charge capture, accuracy is paramount. If you have to choose between the accuracy and timeliness of charge entry, choose accuracy.

Charge edits

A real-time charge editing system that interfaces (or is integrated) with your practice management system or electronic claims clearinghouse will allow you to create a more accurate claim.

(Unfortunately, 100 percent accuracy cannot be guaranteed because the proprietary edits used by insurance companies are subject to change at any time.) An interfaced, or integrated, system can give you real-time feedback regarding charges that were posted inaccurately. Imbedded logic systems can be used to ensure the appropriate use of diagnostic and procedure codes and modifiers. More sophisticated systems, using medical necessity edits such as Medicare's National and Local Coverage Determinations, alert users to a diagnosis code(s) that won't be paid when billed with the procedure code. An electronic editing system allows the user to fix problems on a real-time basis. It will also alleviate the time-consuming rework that occurs in the business office (and often comes back to the physician days, weeks, or even months later to fix).

If automation is not an option for you due to the lack of products that work with your current practice management system or because of the expense, then create your own charge editing process. Train the practice services staff in coding. They don't have to know all 7,000-plus procedure codes, but they should be familiar with the top 50 or so that your practice's physicians always seem to use. Alternately, have a member of the business office who works insurance claims be assigned to review charges manually – the missed and incorrect charges that are caught will make it worth the effort.

Follow-up scheduling

The EHR, paper charge ticket, or a document designed exclusively for this follow-up scheduling, should include a place for the physician to indicate the time a patient may be asked to return for another visit, such as "two weeks" or "four months." The practice services staff can use this information to offer the patient date(s) and time(s) to return for the follow-up visit. Once the date and time are chosen, offer the patient written confirmation of the appointment. You can speed this process by printing a confirmation from the system, which will also create an electronic record showing that the patient was given the information, by whom, and when. Many practice services staff find it is convenient to continue writing appointment details on the traditional pre-printed appointment reminder cards. They might also offer to e-mail the information to the patient, but be sure to consider patient privacy and obtain written permission when transmitting information to them electronically.

BEST PRACTICES

Follow ups and medications

High-performing practices implement processes to compare the timing of follow-up appointments with any medications that were prescribed. If the patient is to be seen in three months, make sure that the patient's prescription and authorized refills extend for the same appointment unless there is a clinical reason not to do so. If the patient is trying a new medication, create an electronic or manual tickler to call the patient. It's always easier to place an outbound call versus waiting for the patient to call for advice. This "best practice" avoids the inevitable phone calls from patients who just need a few days worth of a renewal in order to get them through to the next appointment.

WORDS OF WISDOM

Scheduling follow-up appointments

Frustrated by the volume of patients that slams your practice each week? Your practice services staff can help. First, try to smooth out the peaks and valleys in patient demand for visits by scheduling all follow-up visits on Tuesdays through Fridays (unless the patient requests a Monday appointment). When a physician indicates a follow-up visit is to be scheduled in four weeks, ask your practice services clerk to look for an appointment slot that does not fall on a Monday. This policy will allow you to keep Mondays primarily available to acute visits, which should make your Mondays – everyone's nominee for the most hectic day of the week – much more manageable.

When scheduling patients for follow-up visits at the time of checkout, be sure to maintain scheduling templates three months out. If those templates just go 30 or 60 days out, your practice services staff will have to ask patients to "Just give us a call." By processing the work on a real-time basis, your practice can reduce the telephone demand.

Forcing practice services staff to say, "Just give us a call," not only delays the appointment scheduling process, it makes your staff spend more time to accommodate the patient. Why? Because the scheduler will have to ask the patient to repeat the physician's instructions for a follow-up visit, chief complaint, etc. Instead, pull in the work. The only word of caution is that scheduling too far out will create no-shows because many patients will forget about the appointment they scheduled six months ago. There's no hard and fast rule, but it's generally not a good idea to schedule more than three to six months out.

See Chapter 4, "Scheduling," for more tips about appointment scheduling.

Outbound referrals and ancillaries

At the end of the encounter, the physician may decide to refer the patient to a specialist(s) and/or for an ancillary service(s). Depending on the patient's insurance, a referral may also need to be processed. Processing referrals usually consists of obtaining an authorization from the patient's insurance company that a test, consult, or other service can be made. Ancillary services, such as physical therapy or MRI, almost always require a written request – often called an order – from the referring physician as well as an approval from the insurance company. Because outbound referrals are generally required for ancillary services, these processes are described together. These administrative processes may vary depending on your information systems, the systems used by the entities to which you are referring patients, and the systems offered by the insurance companies. Although your practice will need to account for these factors, you do have options as to when and where to perform the required functions.

Let's look at this process in terms of where it can take place:

At practice services: Patients who are to be referred to a specialist or to receive ancillary services are given the necessary paperwork in the exam room. Alternately, the instructions are noted on the patient's record (which is printed and given to the patient to keep), a charge ticket, or an internal routing form. The patient is directed to the practice services counter where a staff member (typically, a non-clinical administrative staffer) processes the paperwork and/or schedules the appointment(s). Some of these functions can be set aside or batched later in the interest of the patient's time. However, if there is time, it is best for staff to call or electronically query the physician, ancillary facility, or other provider to whom the patient is being referred and make the necessary appointments for the patients. For a courtesy referral (e.g., an OB/GYN suggests a dermatologist to a patient who complains about postpartum hair loss), the patient may be requested to schedule the appointment.

Pros: The practice services function is completed in a single process. The patient is moved away from the clinical area without any further distraction to the physician.

Cons: The physician originating the request may have to provide additional information before the appointment can be made. If so, the practice services staff will have to leave the workstation and find the physician to get the necessary clarification.

It is generally not cost effective to employ staff with clinical training at a practice services desk. However, handling these requests does require some proficiency in clinical terminology to make sure the proper appointments are made with the appropriate providers. That may require staff members who have no clinical training to ask many questions of other staff and slow down the process in order to complete this step accurately and efficiently. One way around this is to hire a medical assistant or nursing assistant for the position.

Another disadvantage of handling referrals and appointments at the practice services counter is that these workstations are typically located where the patient's and staff member's conversations can be overheard by others, especially if there is a line of patients waiting to check out. Few medical practices can afford to have several semi-private counters as many hospital emergency departments do for admissions.

An additional disadvantage of handling referrals at this counter is that patients typically want to leave as quickly as possible after they complete their visit. The referral task is just one more thing that can lead to considerable queues, particularly if there is only one staff member to handle the checkout duties at the practice services counter. So, how else can you handle these post-visit processes?

 KEY CONCEPTS

Key referral concepts

The details of the referral process, to include the existence of, type of, process, etc., are established by insurance companies. Fortunately, many insurance companies have automated the referral process, thus easing the administrative burden on practices submitting and/or receiving them. Depending

on the patient's insurance coverage, they may or may not
be required.

Outbound referrals: The practice refers the patient out of the
practice to a specialty physician (e.g., orthopedic surgeon)
or other services provided outside the practice (e.g., physical therapy). Outbound referrals are generally made by primary care physicians but many specialists refer out for
ancillary services and/or for consults with other specialists.
Outbound referrals are processed at the end of the visit.
They can be done in more than one way (see "Outbound
referrals and ancillaries" earlier in this chapter). This
allows the patient to promptly receive information regarding the referral to another provider or facility.

Inbound referrals: The practice accepts the outbound referral
(as just described) from another practice. Inbound referrals
are generally received by specialty physicians, and should
be processed during check-in or preferably on a pre-visit
basis; that is, the referring physician or patient should
communicate the inbound referral prior to or at the time
of the patient's visit. The referral is necessary for the specialty provider to receive appropriate payment.

To summarize: Outbound referrals are processed at the end of
the visit or at checkout; inbound referrals are processed at
check-in or preferably on a pre-visit basis. Outbound referrals
are made to specialists or ancillary providers, and become
inbound referrals for those same providers.

• •

In the exam room: Conduct the referral and scheduling process in
the exam room. It is certainly private, but a telephone or computer
connection must be available for the staff member to use in securing
the referral and/or making an appointment.

Pros: Work is processed on a real-time basis. A clinical assistant can begin the process immediately after the visit is concluded or, possibly, before the physician has left the exam room. There will be fewer mistakes, such as ordering the wrong test or failing to recognize a timing issue (e.g., a lab test that must occur two weeks before the specialist's consult). Patients won't have to repeat information to more than one staff member, and they will be able to immediately pose any questions to the physician. This method also allows for maximum privacy and confidentiality.

Cons: Exam room referrals tie up exam rooms. Think twice about using this process if space is at a premium in your practice. This method could cause your physician to be idle while waiting for an available exam room – remember: a physician's time is the most expensive thing to waste in your practice.

At the nurses' station: Have a clinical assistant conduct the referral and/or scheduling process at the nurses' station. A suitable telephone or computer connection must be available.

Pros: The clinical expertise of the clinical assistant will be helpful to ensure an efficient referral or appointment scheduling process. From the nurses' station, a nurse or the physician can usually be located quickly if there are questions.

Cons: Nurses' stations are not the places to create lines of patients waiting to be served. You do not want patients hanging out in the clinical area because this will create a distraction for the physicians and other patients. It increases the opportunities for a patient to waylay a physician to ask more questions and, potentially, have an impact on the physician's productivity. Ideally, all of the patient's questions should have been answered during the clinical encounter.

THINGS TO CONSIDER

Preparing the patient for the test

Some hospitals and testing facilities give practices the necessary items to prepare patients for their tests when they occur on the same day as the referral. With the preparatory materials on hand, the practice can then send patients directly to the testing facility. For example, the practice will have on hand the oral contrast necessary for certain CT scans. Patients are given instructions to drink the contrast and then are directed to the testing facility. By the time patients reach the facility, they are ready for the test.

In an electronic system: Technology may allow your practice to process most – if not all – referrals and authorizations automatically. Many insurance companies offer a portal through which to request and monitor referrals. There also are vendors who contract with insurance companies and practices to manage the same process for a fee. If you have an EHR and/or Web portal, you could even automate the request process directly from the physician's orders.

Technology may also allow your practice to automate the scheduling of ancillary services and appointments with specialists. Many integrated health systems give access to their member practices to schedule appointments online or accept requests electronically at the offices of their ancillary facilities and specialists.

Or, you can program your own EHR and/or Web portal to automate the paperwork for you and even send an electronic request automatically when the physician chooses to refer a patient for a test or to a specialist.

Pros: Automating the referral and scheduling process can reduce the time spent performing the transaction(s), thus reducing patients' wait time and improving their satisfaction. The process will also improve workflow and eliminate staff time.

Cons: The technology to process the referrals and schedule the appointments may not be cost-effective or even possible at your practice. Your practice is at the mercy of the insurance companies, hospitals, laboratories, imaging facilities, and specialists' offices – until they can accept and process the request automatically, you may be tied to the fax or the phone.

In a hybrid system: The best approach for handling referrals and appointments may be a hybrid model in which follow-up appointments and referrals are processed at checkout while all ancillaries and specialists' appointments are scheduled in the clinical area, either at the nurses' station or in an exam room, depending on the space and technology available. By using the time the patient is dressing after the exam, you can reduce the lines that are created by patients waiting and serve your patients promptly.

No matter how it happens, processing referrals and appointments can be an operational headache; so why not deploy automation and technology in every way possible to streamline this process.

 THINGS TO CONSIDER

Scheduling referrals and risk management

If you have concerns about whether you are required to schedule the appointment(s) with facilities and specialists to whom you have referred your patients – or whether you have to make sure that patients actually keep their appointments – check with your malpractice carrier. Some practices have stopped scheduling appointments with testing facilities and specialists and just give instructions to patients to make their own appointments, but there may be risk management issues for you to consider depending on the situation.

THINGS TO CONSIDER

Help your patients

If you are referring the patient for a test that requires preparation, be sure to give the patient instructions about preparing for the test. Give the patient a map to the facility if it's not at your practice's offices.

Collecting payments

The practice services desk – checkout, that is – is the appropriate time to collect any monies owed to the practice that you did not collect before the time of service (at the front office). Be sure to request and collect these copayments in addition to any co-insurance.

Make sure you've previewed the patient's account at least a day before the appointment. This will allow your practice services staff to know what portion of the patient's deductible has been used to date and what portion of the allowable charge can be collected on the date of service. More patients are paying higher deductibles these days and a small-but-increasing number are paying medical expenses via health savings accounts (HSAs) that might not have any copayments.

This is also a good time to ask for payment (in full or partial) on any outstanding account balances the patient may have from previous visits. Don't just ask for past-due balances; collect on new accounts. It will save your practice from sending out statements, and avoid the possibility of never collecting the funds. Of course, this must be done in a polite, but appropriate manner. Staff may need a little training to hit the right balance of firmness and courtesy.

In addition to patient balances, consider setting up payment plans at checkout for patients scheduled for procedures, tests, or surgeries your physicians are scheduled to provide.

Don't wait until the patient gets to the practice services desk to ask for payment. Asking for copayments or payment for scheduled procedures can certainly be done at check-in. High-performing practices are starting to collect a deposit at reception services from certain patients. These patients may be self-insured, subscribers of high-deductible plans, have histories of late payments or nonpayment, or they may be about to receive non-covered or cosmetic services. If so, then at the practice services counter, the patient would be asked for the remainder of the payment or immediately credited if the charge turns out to be less than what was collected upfront.

Make sure your practice has the ability to accept credit cards, debit cards, and personal checks, in addition to cash. Yes, credit card companies do collect a fee, but it will still be less money than you'll lose in billing costs if you have to pursue that payment after the patient leaves the office. If there are extenuating circumstances, such as patients who routinely write bad checks, then limit your options accordingly or take measures to prevent problems.

Don't rely on posted signs that say you "expect payment." Instead, instruct your staff to ask for payment politely but firmly, such as: "Ms. Smith, how would you like to take care of your charges with us today?" Instruct your practice services staff to start writing out the receipt as they ask the question to demonstrate that payment is expected – now. Make sure that your practice's policy to collect charges at the time of service also is mentioned prominently in all new patient registration materials, on your practice's Web site or portal, on billing statements, and wherever else is appropriate.

Although the emergence of more high-deductible health plans is causing more practices to collect monies owed to the practice for the services rendered, be aware that some payers require participating providers to wait until the claim has adjudicated, and they have instructed their covered patients to wait until insurance pays.

BEST PRACTICES

How to ask for money

High performing practices script time-of-service collection requests for staff to use. Try these to start.

> ➤ "Ms. Jones, will it be cash, check, or credit card?"

> ➤ "Ms. Jones, how would you like to take care of your balance?"

> ➤ "Ms. Jones, your insurance company requires us to collect your copayment. How would you like to take care of that today?"

Remind your staff to stop talking, and start listening once they ask the question. It's all too often that we talk ourselves out of collecting.

Document encounters in real time

The documentation of the patient encounter – described in detail in Chapter 8 – doesn't occur at the practice services station – but several critical steps must occur just after the encounter is completed. While the patient is being checked out, the physician is often in the back of the office documenting the encounter with the patient. If this isn't occurring – or you're looking for ways for the process to be more efficient, there's help for you.

Most practices have at least one physician in the practice who finds the schedule so overwhelming that the only time available to dictate notes is late at night or on a day off. But delaying dictation raises the likelihood that the physician might forget to document a provided service or procedure or note an important clinical question. The consequences can include increased chances of inaccurate coding and improper reimbursement, particularly if the charges were submitted without documentation. And, the more serious consequences of failing to document an important finding or aspect of the treatment include compromising the future care of the patient and, potentially, a malpractice complaint. If you can find ways for the overwhelmed physician to document more efficiently, you'll help your practice to improve cash flow and lower the chances of physician burnout, in addition to reducing risk and improving patient care.

Try these tips to help physicians who can't find time to document daily:

Develop documentation time savers. Ask physicians to write down the typical questions asked of patients suffering from the five most common complaints treated at the practice. Create a checklist of those questions with room for notes below each question. Based on the patient's chief complaint, put the appropriate template into the patient's chart when it's pulled for the next day's appointment. The checked-off items and notes on the template will help physicians save time later when dictating. EHRs can automate this process – and make it more efficient – by electronically pulling templates and checklists based on the patient's risk factors and complaints.

Ask physicians to dictate notes more often. An efficient time to dictate a note is after each patient or after every two or three patient visits at a maximum. Using this "virtual patient" (described more in

Chapter 8, "The Patient Encounter") the information remains fresh in mind and the physician spends much less time trying to remember or look up details about the patient's visit. Physicians who delay dictation until the evening or weekend will spend about 60 seconds per patient to recall the relevant details and assemble the notes of each patient. For a daily workload of 25 to 30 patients, that can add 30 minutes to each day's dictation duties.

Dictate during the encounter. It is possible for physicians to document encounters in real time and do so in a patient-friendly way. Physicians can explain that they are documenting the visit and would like the patient to hear what will be put into the record. Physicians must not turn their back to patients or mumble into the recorder. Few patients understand all of the medical terminology, but most will appreciate hearing the details of their visit and the plans for treatment. Dictating in front of patients further reinforces the physician's assessment and plan, which can improve patient education and compliance. See Chapter 8, "The Patient Encounter" for more details, including the pros and cons, of dictating during the encounter.

Physicians who dictate in real time or after each patient visit are ready to focus on the next patient or task. And they have one less reason to feel overworked by long evening or weekend hours.

Following up on records transfers improves service, boosts retention

Are your physicians or staff doing something that drives away patients? And if you are, how would you ever know?

Most practices survey the satisfaction of current patients, but I rarely see anyone survey the patients who could provide the most valuable feedback of all: the patients who leave for another practice in the same community.

Surveys indicate that fewer than one in 10 dissatisfied customers ever tell the merchant, company, or service provider why they are taking their business elsewhere. While many types of businesses don't have the ability to track down the customers they lose, we do. That's because in health care, most patients ask their former medical provider to transfer records to their new one. Instead of looking upon a transfer request as another time-wasting, money-losing cleri-cal task, consider it a potential gold mine of unvarnished commen-tary that can lead to improving the satisfaction of current and future patients.

Doing the survey

One of the hardest tasks in preparing a survey is finding a suitable survey population. That's no problem here. Your staff already gath-ers and files each written request to transfer a patient's medical record. Instead of dumping the fulfilled request forms into a file drawer in the records room, take the following steps:

Sort requests. Don't call patients who ask for records to be sent to practices outside your community; do call those going to providers within your community.

Recruit an interviewer. Ask an experienced staff member, preferably at the management level, to call any transferring patients who do not leave the community. Pick someone who has an excellent phone manner. This is not a job for the newly hired receptionist.

Write a script. For example, start by saying, "Our practice is working to make improvements for our patients. We are contacting you because you transferred your records to another practice, and we hope that you might be able to provide us some feedback regarding that decision."

Seek information. Keep the conversation short and focused on gathering basic information and commentary about why the patient left.

Create a check-off form to categorize patients' comments. Most patient complaints fall into two categories: those within the practice's control and those that are not. In the former category are patients' complaints about access (e.g., appointment availability), facility, staff, physicians, telephone service, and general operations. Other complaints such as a change in the patient's insurance or relocation, are outside of your control. Placing patients' reasons into standardized categories will allow you to compare trends over time and pinpoint opportunities for improvement.

Don't get defensive. Don't get flustered if the patient's complaint is based on an unreasonable expectation or is about something that you know wasn't a problem. Just listen. Although you may not agree with the basis of the decision, the fact is that you didn't meet that patient's expectations.

Compile and review results. Track transferring patient interview results by date and, possibly, other demographics. You may find that patients of certain demographics, such as age, sex, or race, are more likely to transfer. You might find one provider or one location has more problems retaining patients. Review results at least quarterly.

Act on the information. If you're losing dozens of patients because your practice dropped a payer, take another look at that decision. If location is always mentioned, then you should cultivate new patients in the nearby community or consider relocating, too. If patients complain about an operational process, analyze that process for performance improvement. The same goes for complaints about staff, your facility, and so on.

Following through on this information not only will improve your knowledge base regarding patient satisfaction, it will send a clear signal to current and former patients that you are on the pathway to improvement.

A smooth and efficient practice services function allows your practice to complete the patient encounter on a positive note. Use this opportunity to leave an indelible and positive impression of your practice on every patient.

CHAPTER 12

Technology

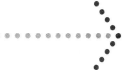

Key Chapter Lessons

➤ Evaluate your practice management system

➤ Harness the Internet to help patient flow

➤ Develop a Web portal to improve practice operations and patient education

➤ Determine the advantages of document management

➤ Utilize personal digital assistants (PDAs)

➤ Deploy e-prescribing

➤ Implement electronic health records (EHRs) to benefit workflow

➤ Learn to be a wise purchaser of technology

➤ Assess vendors

Technology offers bold innovation, but be careful to avoid obstacles

Buying the right information technology and using it correctly will make medical practice operations more efficient. Technology, however, cannot be a replacement for effective work processes. Layering automation on top of inefficient processes will only create more inefficiency. Get the core processes right – and then use technology to increase value to the patient. Don't automate for the sake of automating.

This chapter presents an overview of many technologies that can be used in medical practice operations, how to choose these technologies wisely, and how to implement them successfully. This is not a primer on the hardware and software required to make your practice function; instead, this chapter serves to supplement your current knowledge and highlight the technology applications that can positively affect your operations.

The practice management system

Although there are still a few practices out there holding on for dear life to their pegboards and appointment books, most now have practice management systems that offer automated solutions for billing and accounts receivable, scheduling, and registration. "Practice management system" is a catch-all term. There are hundreds of practice management system vendors and many nuances to these systems. At the very least, make sure that your practice management system – or the next one you buy – can:

➤ Manage all of your billing and accounts receivable, scheduling, and registration functions;

➤ Share a master patient registration database;

➤ Transmit insurance claims and produce billing statements;

➤ Produce robust management reports;

➤ Allow upgrades to improve functionality and meet new regulatory and payer requirements; and

➤ Integrate with other software products and services – including those produced by other manufacturers.

Speaking of vendors, the company that sells you your new practice management system should be capable of providing more than a good product that works well for the moment. Since so much of your day-to-day operations will depend on the practice management system, it is wise to seek out a vendor that:

➤ Offers timely, accurate, accessible, and cost-effective customer service;

➤ Supplies updates or technical improvements necessary to fix system shortcomings or glitches at no cost;

➤ Produces upgrades that are reasonably priced and provide improved functionality;

➤ Offers you ways to contact and share experiences with other users through users' conferences, networking groups, and online forums; and

➤ Responds appropriately and promptly to assure that the product – and the functions you perform with it – comply with regulatory requirements, such as HIPAA.

Think of your technology vendors as important stakeholders in your practice's success.

Once you have chosen your core practice management system, your vendor can help you define your hardware needs. Be sure to revisit this topic annually to make sure that your hardware keeps up with the demands of your software.

The majority of practice management systems now in use are based on client-server technology. That is, you buy the system in a "box" and the software that makes it run resides in your practice. A growing number of medical practices are opting for systems that are Web-based or are provided by an application service provider (ASP) that is accessed via the Internet. There are many advantages to this model. The vendor tends to the software and you need not be concerned about disasters destroying your data. But if you do opt for a Web-based or ASP model, make sure your vendor complies with HIPAA regulations and offers state-of-the-art security. Using ASP technology is acceptable under HIPAA. However, reasonable safeguards must be in place to ensure that your patients' information, the network connections between your practice and the ASP or Web-based service, and your practice management system itself are secure.

WORDS OF WISDOM

Portability and password safety

As computer storage devices become more portable – a single thumb drive can contains thousands of patient records – it's more important today than ever to ensure that your systems are secure. Make it a policy that laptops, CDs, thumb drives, and any other portable device containing confidential information cannot be removed from the office. If storage on such a device is necessary, use devices that can be protected with passwords. It's just too easy for these portable devices to be taken in the midst of a vandalism or theft. And, don't forget to create and enforce a sensible password policy, such as not posting vital passwords on sticky notes on computer monitors, and changing important passwords periodically.

The Web

New research indicates that the majority of patients access the Web for information about health. This trend relates to the concept of value discussed throughout this book – patients perceive value in finding information on the Internet because it is ample, free, and easy to access. Unfortunately, while there is ample information on the World Wide Web, there also are no restrictions and little guidance to help patients differentiate between the many Web sites that provide accurate health information and the many more that do not. You can't hold your patients by the hand as they browse the Internet, but there are ways you can guide them to the more reliable information. A Web site is a must-have for your practice to educate your existing patients and market your practice to new ones.

At minimum, use your Web site to offer potential and existing customers information about your practice. Treat your Web site like an online telephone directory advertisement. Include your practice's name, providers' names and backgrounds, practice location(s), driving directions, nearby public transportation, if it is available in your community, and how to contact your practice for more information. Consider also putting your practice's policies for financial obligations, prescription renewals, telephone calls, and appointment scheduling on your Web site.

Designing for the Web

Remember that your Web site doesn't exist in a vacuum. Patients will view it alongside of other sites that may have invested more money into their design than your practice produces in several months. Therefore, be sure that your practice's Web site is graphically appealing when it first loads onto the user's computer screen. There are many templates now available that can help assure that your site has a professional look.

Because visitors may not see the entire first page, depending on how their monitors are set up, Web designers recommend testing a newly designed page from several different computers. Another tip is to avoid overloading your Web site with photos, animations, sounds, and graphics – they will make your site load onto a visitor's computer much slower. Make sure the template you use, or the designer you hire, places the navigation bar (which viewers use to find other parts on the site) on the left or top side of the page – never at the bottom. You'll lose many customers right off the bat by getting these basics wrong. In addition to essential information, such as how to contact your practice and a description of the providers, your Web site can engage current patients. Create a frequently-asked questions section and post material about your providers' services. Often, text from existing printed brochures can be modified to use on the screen but remember to keep sentences and paragraphs short – onscreen reading becomes a chore when documents are very long. While it may be helpful to give viewers a link to a major reputable Web site (such as the Centers for Disease Control, National Library of Medicine, etc.), avoid posting too many links to other Web sites – you'll just be sending patients away from your Web site. Links to other Web sites also become a maintenance issue because you will have to frequently update those links when the target sites change (which they frequently do). New and current patients also will find it helpful to see a list of the insurance companies with which your practice participates.

Developing a Web portal for improved efficiency

Take advantage of the Web's potential to help reduce practice costs and increase operating efficiency. To do so, it's time to transition your Web site to a Web portal. Although you can use your existing Web site as a platform, a portal creates a single, customizable point of access to applications and information. To start, consider what types of incoming telephone calls could be better handled via the Web. Test results, prescription renewals, and statement inquiries are just a few. Try to shift some of the many customer questions that historically come in via the telephone – and often during peak clinic times of 9:00 a.m. to 11:00 a.m. and 1:00 p.m. to 3:00 p.m. – to arrive via your Web portal. Unless the inquiry is about an urgent medical matter, many patients will appreciate getting the information they want via your practice's Web portal.

Regardless of the functionality, patients perceive a Web portal as a value because they feel like they are participating in the process and have been given a greater choice. A Web portal can also streamline access to your practice through offering patients the ability to self serve to:

> ➤ Practice information. Although your Web site delivers basic information about your practice, use a portal to take it up a notch. Deliver information about new services (e.g., your practice now offers bone densitometry) or changes in service (closed for inclement weather). Consider posting virtual tours

(via a downloadable video stream) so that patients can get a bird's-eye view of your practice.

➤ Appointment requests. Patients can schedule appointments directly, or make a request whereby you assign a staff member to contact those patients to set a specific date and time. In addition to handling appointment requests, a portal can manage reminders, cancellations, and recalls.

➤ Online registration and medical history. Using a Web portal to take care of the registration process and gather a patient history can streamline the administrative check-in process, and save precious minutes when patients actually show up.

➤ Online bill payment. This easy and cost-effective feature can offer immediate cost savings, improve your cash flow, and provide convenience to patients.

➤ Test results. Delivering routine laboratory or other test results via secure Web access can dramatically reduce the staff time needed to manage inbound phone calls.

➤ Prescription management. Requests for renewals of maintenance medications can be made via the Web portal, and your practice can target which patients to alert when there is a drug recall. A portal can streamline the prescription process for you and your patients.

➤ Referral management. Request and receive information from consulting specialists, which can cut the time and costs that a paper-based referral system requires.

For practices that serve as a medical home for patients (see Chapter 5, "Patient Access" for more information), a Web portal can streamline the coordination of the patient's care.

If you extend any or all of this functionality to your patients, be sure to maintain the staff and resources you need to manage it on a timely and accurate basis. If you fail, patients won't return.

Finding revenue on the Web

Your Web portal can lead the way to future practice revenue through online patient care and improving patient compliance.

After a procedure code for "online consults" was introduced by the American Medical Association in 2004, some payers jumped on board to reimburse these online consultations. Discuss coverage with your payers, but don't get discouraged if coverage for online consults has not been extended to beneficiaries. As more patients rely on the Web for medical information, their willingness to pay for personalized care is rapidly increasing. You'll know if you can indeed collect from patients directly to reviewing the definitions of "covered services" in payer contracts. The goal should be to make sure that any charges for answering patients' questions online falls under the payer's definition of a "non-covered service."

Offer secure messaging with patients or online consultations for an additional charge. Many patients will see this as a valuable option that is worth the cost. Implement a per-use charge or establish a fee to cover unlimited messages with your practice's physicians. Several vendors offer assistance with – or complete management of – online care management. (For more information on online consults, see Chapter 4, "Scheduling".)

Your practice might not immediately gain a great deal of revenue from online messaging and consults, but you may discover that your practice becomes better equipped to attract more self-referred patients who will improve the practice's overall payer mix.

The advent of pay-for-performance (P4P) means that patient education and compliance, in essence, becomes an avenue for financial gain. Use your Web portal to offer patients access and ability to manage their personal health record. Maintaining personal medical information puts patients in charge of their health. Deliver materials to educate patients on your portal. In addition to directing patients to your portal to save practice costs, your practice can control the content to ensure your patients are getting sound information.

As payers develop reimbursement mechanisms via performance standards (i.e., P4P plans), improving patient education and compliance will not only benefit your patients' care, but your practice's bottom line.

THINGS TO CONSIDER

Technology helps meet P4P demands

Many insurance companies have established designated quality measures for physicians to report on for their beneficiaries. Additional reimbursement is earmarked for practices that achieve and report the quality measures, which have been formulated to provide evidence of physicians' clinical outcomes. Thus, the term, "pay-for-performance" is associated with these reimbursement methodologies. Identifying the quality measures put forth by the insurance companies with which you participate will be your first step, followed closely by determining what measures relate to the care you deliver. Internal discussions must be held about how to achieve the measures, to include alerting staff and physicians to patients who meet the criteria for the measurement and the expectations set forth by the insurance company regarding quality management. Of course, it is everyone's hope that the measurements will be consistent among insurance companies and a true reflection of quality care. Under these circumstances, practices can establish clinical protocols for all patients.

For many practices, the most challenging aspect of P4P is tracking and reporting the quality measures. For practices on paper, you'll need to develop a paper-based system to identify encounters that need to be tracked, and a monitoring system to track

outcomes related to your care. An EHR enables a practice to integrate the quality measures automatically. The practice can collect, track, and deliver reports on each measure and for the
applicable payer. Regardless of the tools you have to monitor
your performance, don't wait until the end of the reporting
period. Develop a methodology to provide feedback to your
physicians and staff on a consistent basis.

Patients will be an important facet to P4P. Many quality measures require positive self-care. Enhance techniques to exact better compliance, to include face-to-face and post-care patient
education and personal health records.

A sample of the quality measures chosen by CMS for Medicare
beneficiaries are as follows:

> Hemoglobin A1c Poor Control in Type 1 or 2 Diabetes Mellitus
> Description: Percentage of patients aged 18-75 years with
> diabetes (type 1 or type 2) who had most recent hemoglobin
> A1c greater than 9.0%.

> Beta-blocker Therapy for Coronary Artery Disease Patients
> with Prior Myocardial Infarction (MI)
> Description: Percentage of patients aged 18 years and older
> with a diagnosis of coronary artery disease and prior myocar-
> dial infarction (MI) who were prescribed beta-blocker therapy.

> Cataracts: Assessment of Visual Functional Status
> Description: Percentage of patients aged 18 years and older
> with a diagnosis of cataracts who were assessed for visual
> functional status during one or more office visits within 12
> months.

> Screening or Therapy for Osteoporosis for Women Aged
> 65 Years and Older
> Description: Percentage of female patients aged 65 years and
> older who have a central dual-energy X-ray absorptiometry

(DXA) measurement ordered or performed at least once since age 60 or pharmacologic therapy prescribed within 12 months.

Source: Centers for Medicare and Medicaid Services, 2007 Physician Quality Reporting Initiative (PQRI) Physician Quality Measures

Imagine the time your staff might spend trying to track this important information by hand with a paper record. Now consider the assistance that technology, especially an EHR, can provide with this effort. Develop the infrastructure to support these initiatives in order to position your practice for pay-for-performance.

BEST PRACTICES

Web portals

High-performing practices use a Web portal to improve their ability to allow patients to pull value from the practice by offering:

➤ Comprehensive information about physicians, hours of operations, policies, etc.;

➤ Information about new or changing services;

➤ Appointment requests, reminders, cancellations and recalls;

➤ Pre-registration;

➤ Medical history;

➤ Prescription renewals;

➤ Drug recalls;

➤ Test results management;

➤ Personal health record;

➤ Patient education;

➤ Secure messaging;

➤ Online consults;

➤ Online bill payment; and

➤ Referral management.

High-performing practices make the Web work for them – and their patients.

. . . .

Benefit from a portal

Go beyond having a static Web site. Design a practice portal to encourage interaction with patients, enhance your practice operations and improve patient care. Ultimately, physicians must stop viewing patients who go online to obtain information about their medical conditions as bothersome. If patients can be directed to accurate information, then that knowledge can help them become more likely to comply with physician-recommended treatments. Better compliance can help speed recovery and reduce the volume of clinical questions that often come in by telephone. As this self-knowledge promotes more responsibility, patients will rely less on what, at times, seems like trying to maintain constant communication with your practice.

Electronic mail

Here are some ground rules to follow if you use e-mail or the Web to communicate private information to patients:

➤ Implement encryption strategies in compliance with HIPAA and current industry standards;

→ Develop clear parameters about what – and what not – to e-mail;

→ Set expectations about your response time;

→ Discuss whether and how you'll handle e-mail 'volleys'; and

→ Establish processes to manage e-mails, to include recording both the e-mail and your response.

Because of the several risk management issues involved in e-mailing patients about their health, think through the entire process before opening the door to e-mail.

WORDS OF WISDOM

Guide your employees' Internet use

Concerned about giving your staff Internet access? Many practices worry about staff spending too much time surfing or shopping online. Yes, abusing Web access privileges is possible, but the demands of most staff jobs are so significant that most people can find few spare moments for online foolishness. If you think that e-mail or Internet access will help patients or will help the office improve its productivity, then don't let fears of Web abuse stand in the way. That said, establish a clear policy for personal use of the Internet while at work.

Sample Internet use policy:
Because of the business implications and potential for misunderstandings as to employee conduct, no employee may use the practice's computers for their personal use unless the employee's supervisor grants approval. This includes accessing the Internet, playing computer games, or using e-mail. The policy is in force at all times: before work, during work hours, after work, or during lunch or breaks. Even if approved by your supervisor, personal use of the Internet should be

infrequent, of short duration, and may not interfere with work duties. The practice may monitor, measure, and track the use and performance of its systems for technical or other reasons at any time, and may access any information contained in its systems.

If you wish to prevent employees from making any personal use of the Web site through your practice's connection, use readily available software that locks users into only the Web sites you designate.

Document management

Document management systems offer a wide variety of automation options for medical practice operations. Use these systems to store and retrieve information from documents electronically. Electronic storage and retrieval of documents also can create a "quasi" EHR.

Here are some ways that your practice can use document management:

Re-organize. Take your transcribed office notes – if you receive them in an electronic format such as a Word document – and organize them by patient identifiers. Using a database program, you can put the notes on a local area network (LAN). Each note will be accessible to the physicians who have passwords to your internal network. This is a great solution for physicians who are on call and wish to review notes of a patient's recent office visits. On a day-to-day basis, you can provide clinical staff with passwords and they may be able to answer triage calls without a costly chart pull. By writing a policy describing who has access and the process for maintaining logins and passwords, you can make this database system HIPAA-compliant.

Scan everything. Scan every piece of paper that comes into your office, from lab results to operative notes. Add the scanned images to the document management database (described above). Scanning patients' insurance cards and explanation of benefits (EOBs) will help improve efficiency in the business office (staff will no longer have to search for EOBs to submit claims for secondary insurances).

Convert faxes. Use an electronic tool to translate all incoming faxes directly into electronic files for easy filing. Use patient identifiers to index and upload faxed lab results, radiology reports, nursing home patient status updates, and more to the correct patients' files. Be sure to think through your indexing system before you start scanning. You don't want it to become too complex, but you also don't want to be forced to scan through hundreds of pages to find what you need.

Use databases. Use business card scanning software to scan vendor and other business contact information into an electronic database that all staff can access whenever they need to call for supplies, repairs, or services.

Scan and scan again. Scan patients' insurance cards and driver's licenses at registration. Use your current information systems to facilitate this process or build an interface with an automated system to transfer the image to an electronic file that can be imported and attached to patients' accounts.

Document Image Management Systems (DIMS) are bundled software and hardware solutions that index scanned patient charts and associated documents. These applications often include message routing (for phone message handling) and e-prescribing functionality or an alliance to an e-prescribing solution. DIMS are a less costly entry point on the road to the EHR and can typically be integrated into a future EHR.

Picture archiving and communication systems (PACS) are more sophisticated – and more expensive – types of document management systems. Most practices that rely heavily on images, such as radiology and orthopedic surgery, use PACS because the radiological images that they must store and retrieve contain a massive amount of digital information – far more than a mere word processing document system could hold. As the cost of PACS decreases, expect more practices – maybe yours – to take advantage of these powerful storage systems.

WORDS OF WISDOM

Document management saves money

Have you looked at the cost of storing the hundreds – maybe even thousands – of old records that you must maintain to comply with record retention laws? Some medical practices are beating the high cost of document storage by using CDs or thumb drives to hold thousands of scanned document images. You'll need a high-speed scanner and some staff time, but the reduction in storage fees often pays for the scanner within the first 12 months. Instead of stressing out your existing staff, save money by hiring high school and college students to do the scanning after hours or in a back room. (Be careful about who you hire and enforce the same level of confidentiality that you require from your staff.)

If you do scan old records, check your state records retention laws for how long you need to keep records and make several copies of each CD or drive. Better, yet, upload the files to a reputable document management firm that provides Internet access, or store the duplicate copies in different locations – at least one of which should be off-site – in case of an emergency.

Personal digital assistants

Personal digital assistants (PDAs) became popular in the 1990s, and can now be found in the pockets of many physicians. Although some are just for personal use, PDAs can offer a host of opportunities to automate certain functions to improve efficiency:

Charge capture. Encourage physicians to use their PDAs to capture charges, particularly in the hospital, nursing home, and other non-office locations. If you don't capture all those charges, it means you don't get paid for them. Place PDA docking stations where physicians can quickly download the charge information when they return to the office from surgery or after hospital rounds. Most charge capture software now interfaces with the practice management system through a wireless connection, thus allowing you to ditch the docking station. Remember, however, that someone must key the charges into the PDA in the first place. If you have a physician who never remembers to record charges on old-fashioned index cards, then don't expect the PDA to magically solve this forgetfulness. (This is a good example of getting the core work processes right before you automate; embracing technology just to automate, without improving the process that's being automated, won't offer a positive return on investment.)

Address book. Use as an address book for referral sources. Send them office notes, hospital discharge summaries or operative reports by routing the documents through an online connection in your PDA directly to their fax numbers or e-mail accounts. Only route documents if the communication is secure.

Calendars. Keep everything from the physician's operating room schedule to medical staff meetings on the PDA. Physicians can keep their personal schedules on the same PDA, too. (See Chapter 2, "The Physician's Time" for time management tips.)

Prescriptions. PDAs can help the prescription process in several ways. A PDA-based prescription system can help physicians keep track of which drugs are on which formulary and reduce the number of calls from pharmacists suggesting substitutions. It also provides appropriate dosing and contraindications. Best of all, these systems allow physicians to send electronic prescriptions directly to the pharmacy – no more calls from patients who lost their paper scrip or pharmacists who can't interpret the physicians' handwriting. (Note that your practice will need to check on your state law regarding e-prescribing. Some states still require manual signatures for all or certain categories of medications, such as narcotics.)

Coding and documentation. Accurate coding and documentation are critical to getting paid appropriately. PDA-based coding software offers coding edits and guidance, note templates and more.

Reference. Reference materials, such as Harrison's Textbook of Medicine and Physician's Desk Reference, are only two of the many useful resources available for use with some PDAs. Even better, these texts can be queried through key word searches to help you find what you need more efficiently.

Knowledge. Database tools can help when the physician is on call in the middle of the night and can't access professional assistance from colleagues. These tools, many of which are free or available at a low cost, support clinical decision-making and can access a host of resources. Those who use PDAs with Internet connections can find services that regularly abstract pertinent medical literature.

Point of care. Choose from dozens of point-of-care medical calculators, algorithms, and checkers designed for PDA users.

Call schedules. Keep call schedules on everyone's PDA so you can eliminate the ubiquitous "master calendar" that physicians and clinical staff have to stop by the office to look at, or call an already busy staff member to check. Add information about hospital rounds, and notes about patients in-house to help the physician to whom you're signing off.

Today's PDAs can combine telephone, messaging, e-mail, video images, Internet connections and other functions in one device.

Before you trade in your pager, phone, e-mail account, fax, voice mail and even your computer for a single, all-purpose hand-held PDA, evaluate the functionality of the device carefully – and how it integrates into your other technology-based solutions.

EHRs

EHR is a term that means taking everything that is contained on paper in a patient's medical record and automating it. But it's more than just getting rid of the paper and automating the information. Practices that have found the most success with EHRs are those that use their systems to get information to the users faster and with less hassle.

THINGS TO CONSIDER

EHR vs. EMR

The terms EHR and electronic medical record (EMR) are often used interchangeably; however, the term "EHR" includes health information for a patient across multiple provider organizations whereas an "EMR" is that patient's information within one provider entity.

YOU KNOW...

you need an EHR when...

➤ Your practice's multiple sites are close enough in proximity that patients go to either facility and your staff must spend hours each day pulling patient charts and faxing them between sites;

➤ You pack up a rolling suitcase with patient charts each morning for a staff member to drive to a satellite clinic for that day's appointments. When an additional patient walks in, staff at your central facility must break from other duties to find and fax the walk-in patient's charts to the satellite;

➤ Your practice does not respond to its large volume of triage calls for hours because the messages are recorded and callbacks must wait until the patients' charts are found. Many hours of staff time are wasted taking and routing messages, as well as pulling and filing charts needed for them;

➤ Charts that your physicians need for prescription renewals or to answer triage questions are often found at the bottom of a stack on the desk of the physician who is notoriously behind on dictation;

➤ The business office's appeal of an insurer's claims denial is delayed several days until, finally, the patient's chart is located on someone's desk. In it is the documentation that can support the appeal for payment;

➤ The administrator has to go to the office on Saturday afternoon to let in the physician who is on weekend call so he or she can find the chart of a patient who is being admitted to the hospital;

➤ A physician must be paged at home because the colleague covering that day cannot read the illegible handwritten note of the patient's last office visit – or the treating physician just makes a guess;

➤ Despite your best efforts, many of the hundreds of patient telephone calls your practice's triage nurses and staff receive each day are never charted;

➤ A physician receives a call from an out-of-state hospital emergency department where one of the patients was injured while on vacation and the physician needs the patient's records quickly;

➤ A physician realizes months later that the results of a patient's biopsy was never received; or

➤ Drug recalls require countless hours of staff time pouring over paper records to determine which patients should be contacted regarding their medication.

An EHR can resolve all of these problems — and more!

● ●

Although it's not an all-inclusive list, here are the benefits of an EHR for your practice:

➤ Integrates national standards of care and payer-based P4P criteria;

➤ Puts updated, complete, and legible information about the patient in the physician's hands at the point of care;

➤ Enables real-time access from off-site computers;

➤ Delivers and monitors health maintenance initiatives;

➤ Stamps the signatures of users, as well as times and dates, electronically;

➤ Facilitates correspondence with referring physicians, hospitals, nursing homes, and other providers;

➤ Assists the practice in managing office workflow by monitoring patients from registration to the conclusion of the encounter;

➤ Decreases space, staffing, and supply costs related to medical records;

➤ Potentially reduces or eliminates transcription costs;

➤ Improves physician's ability to manage care while on call because information is accessible;

➤ Identifies candidates for treatment based on new clinical guidelines;

➤ Facilitates drug recalls;

➤ Enhances compliance with privacy regulations by restricting access to designated users only;

➤ Identifies and reviews candidates for clinical trials, as well as monitoring trial participants;

➤ Allows multiple users to access records simultaneously from separate locations;

➤ Records phone, e-mail, and other non-face-to-face communication seamlessly, allowing the user to identify the nature of the issue, the action to be taken, who is responsible for it, and documents the communication;

➤ Identifies and monitors coding patterns;

➤ Facilitates the coding and capture of charges;

➤ Improves ability to document all services, capture charges to represent them, and code appropriately for them;

➤ Documents and queries orders, medications, allergies, etc., with ease;

➤ Transmits patient records to remote providers in an emergency;

➤ Monitors tests ordered and prompts for missing results;

➤ Facilitates reporting of quality measures recommended or required by insurance payers with which the practice participates; and

➤ Permits data mining to identify classes of patients for preventive health reminders, seasonal services (e.g. flu shots), potential candidates for new services, etc.

An EHR can streamline your practice into a more efficient office. However, it's not enough to have an EHR – you need to make it work for you. If your practice still takes phone messages on pieces of paper, which then float around the office and get lost or if you still print patient records from your EHR and drag them in a suitcase to the satellite clinic, then your EHR isn't doing you any good. To be successful, an EHR should eliminate duplication and streamline workflow.

Before you sign a contract, consider these tips about your purchase:

➤ Get the scoop on the company's financial position by asking the company for its financial statements, a history of the product line, and list of its other EHR users that are similar to your practice in size and type. Be extra diligent by also getting a full business profile that lists the company's key contacts, employee count, officers, competitors, and key fiscal numbers.

➤ Get the vendor's commitment to provide several days of staff training, as well as to train a staff member or physician to monitor and fix routine issues, and to follow up six months post-live implementation to assess the adoption and use on a day-to-day basis.

➤ Make sure the vendor updates the system's medication, clinical content, and coding-related information at least quarterly.

➤ Carefully review all aspects of the generic templates and those that are specific to your specialty, and determine whether you'll need to allocate resources to refine or develop templates that meet your needs.

➤ Be careful about buying an EHR that has no track record of smoothly interfacing with your practice management software; alternately, the EHR that you're considering may come packaged with a practice management system that could replace your current system. If you replace your practice management system as a result of an EHR purchase, be sure to evaluate the functions of that software from start to finish, and how you'll transition your system into a new one. It won't do much good to improve the medical documentation portions of your workflow if you have to make big sacrifices in automating billing and collecting for your services.

➤ Make sure you know about every new hardware, software, upgrade, and interface that you must purchase to make the EHR work.

➤ Negotiate the terms of training, customer support, upgrades, and service before purchase.

➤ Estimate the drop in productivity, and if necessary, the financial impact of it.

➤ Plan for the system to go down – and ask how the vendor handles disaster recovery – in detail.

➤ Make sure that your practice has clear ownership of all of its practice and patient data that are stored on the servers, backup tapes, etc., of vendor or other business partners.

➤ Negotiate what will happen if the relationship ends, to include if the vendor goes out of business or fails to perform, what notice of termination is required, how and when the data will be transferred, as well as liquidated damages for non-performance.

EHR costs vary tremendously; prices are dropping, and system capabilities are expanding. It's time for your practice to discover the future – now.

 GETTING STARTED

Look for certified EHRs

In 2006, the Certification Commission for Healthcare Information Technology (CCHIT) started issuing certifications for EHR systems using more than 300 criteria that focus on the products' security, interoperability, and functionality.

CCHIT's certifications are drawing attention because this non-profit organization was formed by three leading health care information technology (HIT) associations – the American Health Information Management Association, the Healthcare Information and Management Systems Society, and The National Alliance for Health Information Technology. Although there have been many national rankings and awards for EHRs, CCHIT is unique in that it was awarded a three-year contract by the U.S. Department of Health and Human Services (HHS) in

2005 to develop and evaluate certification criteria, and to create an inspection process for HIT in three areas. These areas include:

1. Ambulatory EHRs for the office-based physician or provider;

2. Inpatient EHRs for hospitals and health systems; and

3. The network components through which EHRs interoperate and share information.

The CCHIT certification process is a response to the HHS goal of improving health care through information technology called for by President Bush in his 2004 State of the Union address in which he announced the goal of providing the majority of Americans with an EHR by the year 2014.

In the event of a disaster

The upside to paper is that it was relatively hard to destroy unless there was flood or fire, of course. Consider that with an electronic system, your entire patient database – and all important clinical records – can be wiped away in seconds with a computer virus, power surge, or major hard disk failure. Although your practice may not be in any immediate threat of a natural disaster, it pays to be alert to natural, man-made and computer-caused disasters.

To ensure your practice is disaster-ready, follow these tips:

➤ Store important documents – or images of them – electronically, and maintain originals of important documents in a fire- and water-proof safe off the ground;

➤ Dump storing backups on tapes or other storage modalities, and use a secure online backup system;

➤ Buy insurance, namely, business interruption and recovery insurance, sufficient enough to cover your costs and keep you in operation during the recovery period after the disaster;

➤ Keep contact information for all of your business partners and staff handy in a central database;

➤ Prepare checklists of actions and persons responsible for preparing the practice for a disaster (in the event that you receive an alert), and post-disaster recovery of operations;

➤ Establish protocols for handling patient care and staff notification during a disaster, as well as post-disaster communication;

➤ Stage a drill if a natural disaster is a real possibility; and

➤ Engage federal, state, and local resources to educate your practice about the consequences of natural disasters – and where you can seek help.

Remember that even if your practice is not in an area susceptible to earthquakes, hurricanes, floods, tornados, or other known natural events, your data and electronic systems are not immune from localized events, such as building fires, broken pipes, damaging electrical surges and so on – they can occur anywhere at anytime.

Preparing your practice for new technology

Use careful judgment when it comes to adopting any technology, whether it's for patients, physicians, or staff. Practices often read about a new piece of technology and introduce it without considering the effect on workflow or somehow expect it to magically create efficiency. Let your patients pull the value to them rather than you pushing it on them. Always ask, what value will this technology bring to my patients? Technology can significantly change processes and not always for the better; if you're not prepared for change or haven't thought it through, disaster can result.

When you consider a piece of technology, planning is in order. Even if the technology looks great and adds value to your patients' experience, consider how it will work on a day-to-day basis in your practice. Gather a workgroup of everyone, or at least representatives from several departments, who will be affected by the technology. Then, create two flow charts: one showing the workflow as it exists today and another one showing how it will change with the new technology. Remember, don't apply technology without reconsidering the process itself. Don't just replicate the process as you managed it with paper. Develop the flow chart based on the new process driven by the new technology. What are the implications for your physicians, your staff, your facility, and your patients?

Don't overlook even the smallest item: Physicians who never learned to type will have trouble keeping up with their patient load if they must suddenly switch to an EHR that requires the use of a keyboard. Will you give typing lessons? How long will it take them to peck at the keyboard? Will you hire a scribe? Will you allow these physicians to continue to dictate? Is there an affordable electronic tablet system that will recognize handwriting? What will accommodating these needs cost the practice?

Physician productivity could decline over the short-term while a new EHR system is implemented. To minimize that impact, develop templates, pull-down menus, and other features that will mesh your physician's work style with the system's requirements. Most of all, dedicate individual training for physicians using their paper-based notes as a starting base. Contract for on-site support to fix glitches or respond to users about problems immediately. A day of on-site support won't do; contract for several weeks. The cost and quality of this support will also be a point on which to evaluate potential vendors.

Conduct a financial proforma. It doesn't need to be anything fancy, but make sure that you measure what the technology costs (including service) and what you will gain. The benefits may include increasing revenue, reducing costs, or simply giving better customer service. The point is to know exactly what you're getting into so there won't be any surprises.

Deciding on a vendor is difficult. Since every practice is different, you can only rely on yourself. That is, just because a vendor's product works for the practice next door doesn't mean it will work for you. Do your own homework. In addition to interviewing vendor-provided references, find at least two practices using the system that are not on the vendor's reference list. Queries to online discussion forums hosted by national, state, or local practice managers' or physicians' organizations may help you locate users whose views haven't been screened by the vendor. Talk to those practices, and if possible, visit them. Your extra efforts will pay off in getting the real story behind the product and its maker.

After you've decided on the technology and the vendor, train, train, and re-train. Don't assume anything. People are often embarrassed to admit that they're technologically challenged, so start the instruction process at a basic level. As you hire more staff and physicians who have grown up with the information superhighway, the basic training won't be a necessity. Until then, make sure you allow everyone to start at a basic level.

Easy ways to avoid a bad technology purchase

Don't fall in love with the new technology's bells and whistles. Do this and you could end up with a system that does a great job of solving problems you never had while creating many new ones. Instead, buy technology that will improve your margins and expand your capacity. Buy technology that will help you manage your operations more efficiently and effectively. Buy technology that will get the job done.

Don't forget about your people and processes. Practices that make this error are the ones that buy systems that require a busy physician to hunt through multiple screens for patient information during the visit. Instead, keep in mind that the software you buy will affect the way your practice works and even the way your physicians practice. Understand your patient flow processes inside and out before making a purchase. Know before you buy if your physicians can be trained and accept typing, pointing and clicking, or using a voice-automated program.

Don't give everyone in the practice – or your vendor – equal ownership of the project. Expecting that your vendor will handle every implementation concern or that problems can somehow resolve themselves is asking for trouble. Make sure that one member of your staff takes leadership on the project and can make the day-to-day decisions about the issues that will inevitably come up. Rely on this person for troubleshooting and advice for related software purchases.

Don't ignore your current technological infrastructure. Ignore these details before buying and you may end up with downtime that is detrimental to your practice and your patients. Of course, your operating system is critical, but don't forget to also assess your current system's processors, memory, and disk space. Read the software vendors' "minimum technical requirements" to find out if your computers, servers, network, and other software programs are compatible with and capable of handling the new technology. Explore what "minimum" means to determine if it's going to mean that your practice can operate at optimal speed.

Don't give the vendor control over your buying process. If you don't define what you want out of the new system, then the vendor will. Instead, figure out what you are trying to accomplish by buying the new system. List the capabilities you expect from the system before interviewing vendors.

Don't evaluate vendors only on technical capabilities. Instead, ask vendors if they provide customer support during your working hours. Ask them if ongoing training is available. Have they dealt with physician practices or your specialty before? Is their software installation and customer service handled by their staff or by contractors? How long will it really take to get the system working? Is there an extra charge for support, training, and implementation? What happens when the system goes down?

Don't forget to ask for references. Software is a complex purchase. Buying software like an EHR is the beginning of a partnership with another business. It's a partnership that your practice will have to rely on to deliver quality patient care. It's in your best interests to ask technology vendors to give you the names of several references. Be sure to ask for references that are medical practices of similar size and the same specialty or specialty mix as yours. Supplement the vendor's list by calling around to colleagues at other practices, and hop on a practice managers' e-mail forum to ask for feedback about the system.

WORDS OF WISDOM

Use the student connection

If you are interested in integrating technology into your practice but don't think you can afford it and can't do it yourself, consider calling the information systems department of your local community college or university. Speak with a professor about sponsoring a team project or intern, or post a listing for a part-time position to assist you or even do some custom programming for you. Give them your ideas, and see what they can do. It's a cost-effective way to get the job done.

Use technology to get results

If you just want to integrate new information technologies in a limited fashion in your practice, or supplement your high-tech office with additional automation, try some of these ideas.

➤ Offer in-office kiosks at which patients register and make payments as they arrive at your office. In addition to offering patients more convenience, these kiosks can save significant time for receptionists, and perhaps allow them to shift to other check-in duties.

➤ Use e-mail to reduce telephone traffic. Set up e-mail accounts with names like triagenurse@yourpractice.com or billing@yourpractice.com to help users direct their messages. Not only will redirecting inquires to flow through these e-mail boxes reduce telephone demands, it also can help you track where these messages go, who responds to them, and what people are asking about.

➤ Sign all of your staff and physicians onto instant messaging (IM) through an online service. Instant messaging works well for everything from reminders about staff meetings to announcing the arrival of patients for their appointments. Notably, many IM programs are not secure. Before your staff starts using a program downloaded from the Internet or your Internet Service Provider, do some homework to make sure your IM system is secure enough to handle patient arrivals and intra-office communication.

➤ Use online calendars and reminders (e.g., Microsoft® Outlook calendar) to manage appointment waiting lists, tickler files for everything from insurance appeals to lab results, staff events, and other tasks.

➤ Offer online bill payment. Send patients a link to your secure online bill payment system. On the form listing your practice's privacy policy, include a check off box next to e-mail address so they can give you permission to send notifications of their balances via e-mail. Link them to your secure Web site, and allow them to pay their bills online.

➤ Use electronic, biometric time clocks that allow staff to clock in and out at their workstations each day with a simple brush of the thumb (using a thumbprint to identify the employee). These systems are more affordable than ever and can monitor arrival and departure times and download that information directly to your payroll system.

➤ Network with other practices through chat rooms or e-mail forums offered by your professional association, specialty society, and state or local medical societies.

➤ Sign up for a coding advice service so that you can e-mail tough coding questions to a coding expert – and get accurate answers fast.

➤ Access the online products, services, and practice management information of professional organizations like MGMA.

➤ Look for the current clinical findings and management research through Internet search engines, such as www.google.com or www.pubmed.gov.

➤ Buy medical and office supplies, equipment, furniture, and other office necessities through online group purchasers or Internet-based discount retailers.

➤ Save time and money on continuing medical education (CME) by taking classes or finding CME-accredited articles online instead of always attending on-site conferences.

➤ Participate in webcasts for CME, management, and staff training.

➤ Take advantage of online insurance coverage and benefits eligibility verification, as well as claims status inquiry services that many insurance companies offer online through direct access or Internet portals.

➤ Deploy a telephony-based predictive dialer to help manage patient collections. Use the predictive dialer for patient responsibility balances, pre-registration, referrals and pre-authorizations, bad-address clarification, and communicating with patients when their insurance company rejects a claim and you need more information to re-file it.

➤ Use direct claims submission whenever insurance companies offer it. Post charges and – voila – transmit them directly to the insurance company via the Web for faster payment.

➤ Use electronic payment posting and funds transfer to eliminate manual posting staff and get money in the door faster.

➤ Use human resources-related Web sites like www.epraise.com and www.hrtools.com to help manage employees and to boost morale.

➤ Buy gift certificates for employee rewards from thousands of online retail establishments.

➤ Manage documents better through services like www.efax.com, which transforms incoming faxes into e-mail messages. Test results and other reports can be easier to store and locate when they are in a digital format.

➤ Get free reminder e-mails about important dates, like employees' birthdays and employment anniversaries using Web sites like www.hallmarkreminder.com or www.birthdayalarm.com.

➤ Post your employee schedule, policy manual, managed-care manual, call schedule, hospital rounds list, and other pertinent information on a secure Web site so you or your staff can access it quickly.

➤ Manage credentialing tasks online.

➤ Utilize an online bill payment service offered by your bank to save on postage and increase the efficiency of your accounts payable process.

➤ Access online interpretation services if a non-English speaking patient presents to the office without an interpreter.

➤ Throw away the little dictation tapes and use digital transcription. Use secure Web sites to transmit transcription files online to vendors who can turn around your dictation faster and cheaper.

➤ Try the latest generation of voice-recognition systems for dictation.

➤ Establish online connections to your practice management system and EHR for employees whose duties are conducive to working at home or off-site.

➤ Use a digital camera to take pictures of patients or their physical conditions. Use photos to identify patients by sight instead of just name, store pre- and post-procedure photographs, or paste photographic images in correspondence to referring physicians.

➤ Use a tablet PC to deliver patient education in the exam room or take hand-written chart notes electronically that can be integrated into your practice's records system.

➤ Develop a Web portal for your practice to deliver value to your patients (for more information, see information on Web portals).

Technology continues to offer vast rewards for practices willing to redefine their own processes and deliver better outcomes in practice operations.

As new, technology-dependent physicians and employees enter the workforce, and patients demand more automation to enhance access and convenience, integrating technology into your practice won't just be fun and games – it will be essential. There are so many ways to integrate automation into your practice; it only takes a creative mind, and some careful planning to harness technology to work for you.

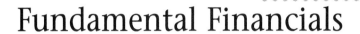

CHAPTER 13

Fundamental Financials

Key Chapter Lessons

➤ Identify key financial concepts

➤ Learn about fixed and variable costs

➤ Calculate your overhead rate

➤ Analyze your break-even point

➤ Understand how expense reduction can backfire

➤ Discover effective strategies to cut costs

The fundamental financials

When patient flow runs smoothly, a practice's revenue and physician productivity improve. So, now that we have presented the details of patient flow, let's look at what can happen – financially – when you improve it.

When you subtract the practice's operating costs from the total revenue collected by the practice, the result is net operating income. Practices owned by physicians call this net operating income: physician income, or physician compensation. A practice that has other types of owners, such as a hospital or a physician management company, might just call this net operating income: income.

No matter what the ownership structure is, achieving a positive net operating income is critical to sustained financial performance. By increasing your revenue and/or reducing your expenses, your practice can increase operating income. This chapter focuses on understanding the impact of patient flow on your bottom line.

Controlling cost is at the heart of running operations more smoothly and profitably in any type of business. Costs (called expenses when costs are incurred to generate revenues) measure the use of the resources, or assets, that the practice uses to produce revenue. Resources that your practice uses everyday to bring in revenue will likely include clinical and non-clinical staff, equipment, supplies, and the facility.

An often-quoted statistic is the overhead rate, which is a measure of your practice's ability to use non-revenue-producing (operating) expenses to leverage your assets (physicians and nonphysician providers). The overhead rate is determined by dividing your operating expenses by your net revenue (collections).

In this chapter, we will examine how the operating and staff resources of the practice are used to leverage physicians' (or any billable providers') time to produce revenue.

 KEY CONCEPTS

Key financial concepts

Contribution margin: The revenue generated by an additional volume of services minus the variable costs to produce the volume equals the "contribution margin." For example, an in-house lab generates $20,000 in revenue and incurs $5,000 in variable expenses to perform an additional number of tests. Thus, the lab has produced a contribution margin of $15,000 to help cover fixed expenses. In general, when the contribution margin is positive, performing additional services is a good financial decision.

Fixed cost: An expense that remains the same without regard to change in volume.

Leverage: The ability to use a resource to increase the value of an asset. For example, leveraging a physician's time by having a nurse return a portion of the calls allows the physician to spend more time with that day's patients. While the nurse answers the telephone calls, the physician can generate more revenue by seeing the next patient. (This definition simplifies the twin issues of operating and financial leverage. Operating leverage refers to the extent a business commits itself to higher levels of fixed costs. Financial leverage refers to the extent to which a business gets its cash resources from debt as opposed to equity.)

Overhead rate: Operating expenses divided by net revenue (collections). A measure of a practice's ability to use non-revenue-producing (operating) expenses to leverage its assets (physicians and nonphysician providers).

Provider: Anyone who can bill third-party payers for services (generally, physicians and nonphysician providers, such as physician assistants and nurse practitioners). Third-party payers maintain different rules governing the billing of services provided by nonphysician providers, which often depend on the type of provider.

Variable cost: An expense that fluctuates in direct relationship to a change in an activity associated with the generation of revenue. For instance, each time a physician sees a patient, a quantity of medical supplies is used. Thus, medical supply costs vary directly (up or down) with the number of patients seen.

Volume: The number of patients the practice's providers handle.

WORDS OF WISDOM

"We pay attention to our costs, but we put our energy and our passion into growing our revenue."

– Administrator of a profitable pediatric practice,
southeastern United States

Fixed cost: Get to know it and how to measure it

There are two broad categories of costs: fixed and variable. Let's first focus on fixed costs – expenses that remain stable regardless of volume.

Fixed costs can include:

> ➤ Support staff, wages, and benefits;
> ➤ Information services (computer and telecommunications);
> ➤ Furniture and equipment;
> ➤ Building and occupancy (utilities, housekeeping, grounds, etc.);
> ➤ Professional liability and other insurance premiums;
> ➤ Promotion and marketing; and
> ➤ Miscellaneous operating costs (e.g., administrative services) that do not depend on patient volume.

These fixed costs do not vary with the volume of patients. That is, if the volume of patients at your practice is 20 patients on Monday and 19 on Tuesday, your practice doesn't pay 1/20th less on Tuesday for its rent, telephones, support staff, liability insurance, and so on.

A subdivision of fixed costs is a step-fixed cost. This represents the costs that remain fixed until the volume of whatever activity they are supporting increases or decreases significantly; then the cost of that activity – the resources it uses – adjusts up or down accordingly. An example of a step-fixed cost would be the cost of hiring an additional clinical assistant to help a physician handle higher volume when the schedule of patients changes from 15 to 30 patients a day.

Here are two important things to remember about fixed and step-fixed costs:

> ➤ Fixed and step-fixed costs do not change because of minor fluctuations in the volume of services provided or in the number of patients seen. That is, if your patient volume increases from an average of 18 per day to 19 per day, you won't run out to hire another clinical assistant.

> ➤ Fixed and step-fixed costs together account for more than 85 percent of the total operating cost structure in most medical practices. (We'll look at the other 15 percent – variable costs – in the next section of this chapter.)

GETTING STARTED

Fixed and step-fixed costs to track

➤ Support staff wages and benefits

➤ Information services (computer and telecommunications)

➤ Furniture and equipment

➤ Building and occupancy

➤ Professional liability and other insurance premiums

➤ Promotion and marketing

➤ Miscellaneous operating costs that do not depend on patient volume

WORDS OF WISDOM

Specialties with high variable costs

Some medical practices have higher variable costs than others. In an oncology practice, chemotherapy drugs alone can represent a significant portion of the practice's total operating cost. Because chemotherapy is used on a per patient basis, it is a variable cost.

Variable costs

Although the majority of your expenses are fixed, or stable, without regard to volume, you will have certain other expenses that occur only when your practice provides a service. These are the variable costs.

A variable cost is an expense that goes up and down in relation to fluctuations in the activity that caused the cost to occur in the first place. The activity, or resource consumption, that causes the majority of the variable costs that occur in most medical practices is physicians seeing patients. That is, if a physician did not see a patient, these costs would not occur.

To demonstrate what generally makes up a variable cost, let's assume the service is a patient visit. When a patient walks in your door, your practice generates a form(s) for the patient to sign. The patient is given a gown to dress for the visit. Certain medical supplies may be used during the visit. After the patient leaves, a claim is generated, followed by one or more patient statements. All of these items – form, gown, medical supplies, claims, and billing statements – are expenses that occurred solely because of that patient's visit. These are variable costs.

Unlike fixed costs (rent, computer system, clinical assistant, etc.), if the patient cancels the visit, you do not incur the cost of consuming the resources included in the variable cost category.

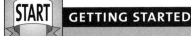

GETTING STARTED

Variable costs to track

➤ Administrative supplies and services

➤ Medical supplies and drugs

➤ Laundry and linen

➤ Miscellaneous operating costs (lab supplies, laundry and linen, etc.) that depend on patient volume)

Using total practice cost

Your overhead rate describes the resources you must use to generate revenue. The higher the rate, the less there is to contribute to physician income. Your overhead rate will largely depend on your specialty. In surgical specialties it may be as low as 30 percent, while in primary care, overhead can be as high as 65 percent.

Surgical specialties have the benefit of using the hospital's resources (operating room nurses, hospital floor, and unit nurses) with relatively small office staff while primary care groups bear all of the costs of an office, typically seeing patients five days per week. Although surgical specialties still have receptionists, billers, telephone operators, etc., they have proportionately lower costs than their office-based colleagues.

However, the percent of total costs for any practitioner, regardless of specialty, is typically 50 percent personnel expenses and 50 percent operating expenses. That is, out of $100,000 in total practice costs

STAFF BENCHMARKS

Medical practice overhead by specialty

Specialty	Overhead rate
Pediatrics	61.42%
Obstetrics/Gynecology	52.87%
Internal Medicine	55.32%
Family Practice	57.90%
General Surgery	43.44%
Cardiovascular/Thoracic Surgery	34.51%

Source: *MGMA Cost Survey for Single-Specialty Practices: 2006 Report Based on 2005 Data*, median data reported.

Overhead varies greatly from specialty-to-specialty, so it's important to benchmark against your own specialty.

(exclusive of the provider's compensation), $50,000 is spent on personnel and $50,000 on operating expenses.

Revenue also impacts the overhead rate. Since the overhead rate is a ratio of costs to revenue, if revenue (the denominator) is higher, than the rate falls. Therefore, because surgical specialties have higher revenue than other physicians, their overhead rates are lower.

KEY CONCEPTS

Overhead rate

The overhead rate equals all the costs that are used to support the providers in a practice to generate revenue. These expenses do not include the physician's income or benefits or nonphysician providers' income and benefits. The rate captures the practice's ability to turn operating costs (the numerator) into revenue (the denominator).

• •

STEPS TO GET YOU THERE

What's your "Total Practice Cost"?

List your practice's costs on an annual basis.

Your annual fixed costs

$_____ Support staff wages and benefits (medical, vacation, sick leave, retirement contribution, employer's FICA contribution, etc.)

$_____ Information services (computer and telecommunications)

$_____ Furniture and equipment

$_____ Building and occupancy (utilities, housekeeping, grounds, etc.)

$_____ Professional liability and other insurance premiums

$_____ Promotion and marketing

$_____ Other miscellaneous operating costs that do not depend on patient volume

= $_____ Total fixed costs

Your annual variable costs

$_____ Administrative supplies and services

$_____ Medical supplies and drugs

$_____ Laundry and linen

$_____ Other miscellaneous operating costs that depend on patient volume

= $_____ Total variable costs

Total fixed costs + total variable costs = total practice costs

Once you've completed the "What's your total practice cost?" work-sheet, it is a simple step to determine your overhead rate. To com-pute your overhead rate, you will also need to know your practice's total annual practice revenue (unless you choose to calculate this on a quarterly basis, in which case you would divide quarterly operat-ing cost by quarterly revenue). Divide total annual practice costs by the total annual practice revenue from the worksheet (include both fixed and variable costs) and the result is the overhead rate, which is expressed as a percentage.

[total practice costs (fixed + variable) ÷ total practice revenue] * 100
= overhead rate (%)

Since the majority of a practice's costs are fixed, or stable, almost regardless of volume, it is critical to determine the level of volume your practice must handle to cover its fixed costs (see Exhibit 13.2). The revenue brought in from any volume achieved after this break-even point (and after variable costs are subtracted) is profit. Profit adds to the net operating income that is critical to the practice's financial success.

Once you calculate your overhead rate, you will know how many dollars are being expended on operating costs per dollar earned. For example, Rheumatology Associates calculated its operating costs at $456,955 and its revenue at $985,001. Using the formula, the over-head rate is 46.39 percent. For every dollar earned or collected by the practice, $0.46 is spent on overhead costs.

We would presume that the majority (if not all) of the remainder ($0.54) is consumed by the physician(s) as income. The goal is to have as low an overhead rate as possible (that is, you would rather spend $0.40 on operating costs for each dollar collected than $0.50, as that would leave more money to distribute as income).

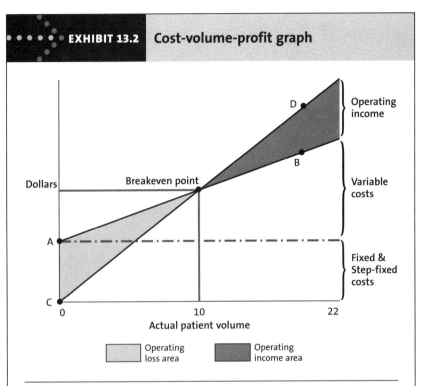

EXHIBIT 13.2 Cost-volume-profit graph

A = Fixed costs + step-fixed costs
  Fixed costs and step-fixed costs include rent, staff, utilities, malpractice insurance, information systems, furniture/equipment.
B = Total costs (variable + fixed) at 20 patients per day
  Variable costs include administrative supplies, medical supplies, drugs.
C = Revenue at 0 patients seen
D = Revenue at 20 patients per day

Assumes that the step fixed costs are "fixed" for this level of patient volume. For example, the nursing and administrative staff remains constant for 25 patients per day; if the level of volume rose to 50 patients per day, the fixed costs would rise.

^Note that this model does not account for capitation; in order to account for it, point C would need to be moved up the x axis.

The Cost-Volume-Profit graph describes the relationship between cost, volume, and profitability in a medical practice.

But don't forget that overhead is a ratio of costs to revenue. Don't just focus on cost-cutting opportunities when trying to reduce your overhead rate. Increased revenue also affects the overhead rate. If you narrow your focus to cost reduction without understanding the impact on revenue from your efforts, you may leave the overhead rate unchanged, or worse, even higher.

CASE STUDY

Decreasing overhead the wrong way

Rheumatology Associates (RA) was disappointed at its overhead rate of 46.39 percent, based on annual operating costs of $456,955 and annual revenue of $985,001. They decided to take action by leasing out one of its exam rooms at the prevailing market rate to an urologist in the suite next door who needed extra space. RA reduced its lease expense by $4,900 per year, which dropped its operating expenses to $452,055. However, the loss of the exam room also reduced the volume of patients that RA was able to see. Because the physicians had one less exam room from which to work, RA's revenue declined by 2 percent ($19,700) to $965,301.

Recalculating its overhead rate, RA divided its new expenses of $452,055 by its new revenue of $965,301. With this cost-cutting method, its new overhead rate actually increased to 46.83 percent. RA failed to recognize that its overhead rate consists of costs and revenue. Simply reducing its costs was not the answer to reducing its overhead rate, particularly because it actually decreased its revenue, thus increasing its overhead rate.

What's your volume/cost break-even point?

At some point during the average month, your practice will handle enough volume to break-even. But when? A practice needs to know whether this break-even point will occur earlier or later in the month, or if it will occur at all. The following exercise demonstrates how to determine the number of patient visits needed to break-even in a typical month.

Let's assume the practice had one physician. Let's also assume that each visit the physician provided produced an average of $100 in revenue. Based on a review of a few previous months' invoices and other records, the variable cost (linen, administrative supplies, and medical supplies used per visit) was calculated at $5 per visit. The $5 per visit is based on the total variable costs incurred during the months in review divided by the number of visits during that month. A quick glance at the practice's readily available records (office rent, insurance premiums, administrative staff salaries, equipment leases, etc.) showed that its total fixed cost was $20,000 a month. The physician sees approximately 400 patients per month, and wants to know if this is adequate to break-even.

Revenue per visit:	$100
Total visits per month:	400
Total revenue per month:	$40,000 ($100 * 400)
Desired physician income per month:	$15,000 (or $180,000 per year)
Fixed cost per month:	$20,000
Variable cost per month:	$2,000 ($5 per visit * 400 visits)

To determine the volume of patients needed to break-even, we must observe the total costs that the physician would like to cover, which is the fixed cost plus the desired physician income, which together equal $35,000. Because some of the revenue per visit, which totals $100, must be used for variable expenses, which are $5 per visit, we know that we can use $95 per visit to allocate toward the fixed costs and desired income. $95 is the contribution margin expressed on a unit of service basis. Therefore, we can divide the sum of the fixed cost plus the desired income per month ($35,000) by the unit contribution margin per visit ($95), which equals 368 patient visits per month – the break-even volume.

We can see that 368 patient visits per month allow this physician to break-even; that is, cover the operating costs incurred and receive the desired income. With 368 – or the 400 reported – patient visits per month, in sum, the physician covers current costs and receives $180,000 in annual income.

How many patients needed to support physician income?

Now, let's approach the break-even question from a different angle. Suppose you start out knowing that each of your physicians wants to earn $240,000 per year, and you know what it costs to run the practice. Your question is: how many patients do each of the practice's physicians need to see to achieve their desired $240,000 in annual income ($20,000 per month) per physician?

ANALYSIS

WORKSHEET
Visits needed to support income goal

What is the number of patient visits that your physicians need to meet their income goals?

Patient visits: ?
Fixed expenses: $20,000 per month
Variable expenses: $5 per visit

Assuming the physician wants to receive $240,000 in annual income, we know that we need to average $20,000 a month in physician income. We also know that the fixed expenses are $20,000 per month for a total of $240,000 per year. We also know that we are receiving $100 per visit, but we have to use $5 of that to pay for our variable expenses. Therefore, we have $95 left over for fixed expenses and physician income.

How many visits do we need per month? Divide the $40,000 in fixed costs and physician income by $95 and you arrive at 421 visits per month.

Fixed cost ($20,000/month) + physician income ($20,000/month) = total fixed cost

Revenue per visit ($100) – variable expense per visit ($5) = unit contribution margin per visit ($95)

Fixed cost + desired income ($40,000/month) / unit contribution margin per visit ($95) = visits needed per month (421)

The Answer: If your physician wants an income of $240,000 per year, he/she needs to see at least 421 visits per month.

Of course, this calculation also raises the issues of altering the other variables, such as fixed cost, variable cost, or revenue per visit.

Although many physicians focus solely on cost reduction to improve income, don't forget that you can alter your revenue per visit by changing your payer mix or range of services to a more favorable reimbursement, in addition to capturing all billable services and coding them correctly in order to collect all that you deserve.

ANALYSIS

WORKSHEET
What's your break-even point?

Use this worksheet to determine the number of patient visits your group needs to meet its physician income goals. To figure the break-even point for your own group, use the data you gathered in the "What's your total practice cost" worksheet. To complete this worksheet, you'll also need to know the level of income or physician compensation your physicians or practice owner(s) want to achieve. In the typical physician-owned medical practice, this income amount is called, "physician compensation." If you want to invest some of the revenues in the practice, such as for a new computer system, or a facility expansion, then determine the amount of investment to make.

Input your data (write in your practice's amounts in the spaces provided and then transfer the amounts to the blanks according to the letter per category). For this analysis, use annual data for each category.

(a) Desired physician income: _____

(b) Fixed cost: _____

(c) Investment: _____

(d) Variable cost per visit: _____

(e) Average revenue per visit: _____

Fixed cost + investment + income = total fixed cost

(b)_____ + (c)_____ + (a)_____ = (g)_____

Average revenue per visit – variable cost per visit = unit contribution margin per visit

(e)_____ – (d)_____ = (h)_____

Fixed cost / unit contribution margin per visit = visits needed per year

(g)_____ /(h)_____ = _____

Expenses: The bottom line

Intuitively, we know that the more patients a physician sees, the greater the revenue for the practice. We also know that per-visit revenue can vary and that variable costs and step-fixed costs also increase as volume increases. But what if your physicians already work long hours and see as many patients as they feel they can handle? What if their revenue enhancement options are somewhat limited? What if they also want to maintain or, possibly, raise their income goals? Since most physicians – like most people – want to control how many hours they work and meet their income goals, reducing fixed costs can be a good route to increasing income or, at least, maintaining it when reimbursement rates are static or declining. Attacking fixed costs can be an especially advantageous strategy if your physicians are experiencing declining reimbursements or increased competition for patients and cannot easily capture a more favorable payer mix or expand into more profitable service lines.

If you can reduce your fixed-cost base, you can reduce the number of visits your practice needs to break-even and achieve the physician's desired income.

STEPS TO GET YOU THERE

25 ways to cut costs

Evaluate these 25 proven methods to cut costs in your practice:

1. Reduce lease or rent payments by moving, reducing workspace, and/or renegotiating your current lease(s). If you leased your office space when the real estate market of office space was booming, you may be able to get a much better deal now. Or, you might consider subleasing the space you don't need.

2. Reduce support staff expenses by re-evaluating staff positions and duties. Maybe improved processes and

automation mean that some staff positions can be combined or eliminated without any loss in overall productivity? Could an employee with lower skills (and a lower wage) be able to handle certain functions?

3. Evaluate your vendor contracts annually, including those for business insurance, professional services, medical and office supplies, and equipment. Check competitors' prices and consider switching vendors. Don't forget about the smaller contracts, like those with your collection agency or electronic claims transmission carrier. Review service contracts every year to make sure that you're not paying for services that you don't need – or if you're paying high hourly rates when you could have a cheaper capitated service plan.

4. Watch out for vendors that are increasing prices due to regulatory compliance (e.g., transcription services that hiked their rates because of HIPAA). Shop around for better pricing before you agree to pay their increased rates.

5. Evaluate vendor value. Don't just price shop – make sure that you are getting what you pay for. Did a vendor "adjust" a fee or add a service charge without telling you? Has the quality or timeliness of their service dropped?

6. Review telecommunications costs, including local, long distance, and wireless telephone carriers. Carefully review bills to make sure you're not paying for services (like extra telephone lines or services) that you didn't ask for. Do the physicians need the cellular telephone plans' 1,000 "free" minutes-a-month or is there a plan that costs less? Are you paying more than seven cents a minute for long distance when you could pay less? Is there a vendor who will bundle your Internet connection, long distance, cellular telephone services, or other services for a reduced fee? Do you have the best available rate for cell phones and pagers? Do you still need a pager?

7. Reduce the expenses allocated to your information system – or at least free up money to be used for other technology improvements – by moving to an application service provider model for registration, scheduling, and billing.

8. Scrutinize your employee benefits structure as well as the service of the benefits agent with whom you work. Can you pass along health care insurance cost increases to employees? Survey employees to see what benefits they value the most. If personnel management is draining your practice, evaluate the option of a professional employer organization (PEO) to outsource all aspects of employee management, to include benefits.

9. Consider different options to reduce the impact of malpractice liability insurance premium hikes. Can you change deductibles? Ask your malpractice insurance carrier if it offers a discount if physicians take risk management courses. How about if you use an EHR or computerize prescriptions? Is your practice large enough to self-insure?

10. Look for free continuing medical education (CME) on the Internet or in journals. Consider low-cost, no travel options like webcasts and audio conferences if travel expenses are eating away at your CME budget.

11. Think about outsourcing billing, transcription, and even some front desk operations. Every few years, reassess whether handling these processes in-house or outsourcing them is cheaper. Research a vendor's performance carefully before making an outsourcing decision.

12. Utilize scanning and digital imaging to capture and store documents from patients' pictures to insurance cards. Reduce storage costs, paper supplies, copier equipment, and service costs.

13. Keep up with technology trends. Would an automated reminder system save staff costs? What about automated

referral processing? Automated charge entry? Automated lab results system?

14. Evaluate your overtime costs monthly. If you often pay for overtime, you may need to hire or reorganize. If you often pay billers overtime at the end of each month to catch up on claims filings, stop batching those claims and ask providers to submit charges by the end of every day. It will improve cash flow and eliminate overtime.

15. Do a better job of retaining staff. The expenses of hiring, training, and lost productivity make replacing an employee cost you three to six months of that employee's salary. High turnover costs money. Make sure your orientation and training processes, workload, and office culture help keep employees around, not drive them off.

16. Decrease statement mailings. More practices mail no more than three patient statements – instead of six or eight – before taking other action. Cutting mailings in half saves more than $1.50 per patient – it will make a big difference over time. Do a better job of collecting payments at the time of service and you can eliminate most statement mailings. Eliminate statements altogether by offering online bill payment.

17. Cut out the middleman. For example, submit claims directly to insurance carriers – or their Internet portals – at no cost instead of sending everything through a clearinghouse. Even though a clearinghouse may charge only a few pennies per claim, those pennies quickly become big bucks in today's busy practices.

18. Dig for bargains. Need medical or office equipment for your practice? Try shopping at Internet-based retailers or used equipment stores. Keep on the alert for a local business that is closing its doors and selling its furniture and equipment. Maybe another practice in your community is shutting its

doors or consolidating. "Retro" is all the rage in interior design, and a quick paint job on old furniture and equipment will bring accolades from patients. Buying used can save you thousands.

19. Track expenses. Introduce an inventory system to track all expenses, even "little" things like toilet paper. Keep tabs on volume and price of what you use so you can comparison shop. You may discover, for example, that it's well worth it to join a membership discount club, and stock up on printer paper and paper towels four times a year, instead of paying top dollar for these items through your current supplier who delivers these items to your door.

20. Give employees rewards that come from the heart, not just the checkbook. Instead of a nominal annual cash bonus, consider giving time off with pay as an alternative reward. It costs you nothing as long as you don't have to bring in a replacement. In these time-starved days, employees may actually prefer a little free time to a small cash reward.

21. Assess your professional advisers. Are you paying a retainer to anyone whose service you do not use or rarely use? What about bringing back in-house certain outsourced duties, such as bookkeeping? Is there a bright and eager person on staff who would happily take over bookkeeping duties in exchange for a small promotion?

22. Explore exemptions. If the expense of a managed-care or referral clerk is bogging you down, ask your payer for an exemption. Many payers have dropped some or all of their referral processes. The payers are realizing that the vast majority of referral requests are never denied, and this process costs them staff time, too.

23. Go electronic. Electronic claims submissions means better use of staff and faster cash flow. Electronic payment remittance means less staff time spent on payment posting,

more staff time spent on other duties, such as insurance follow up, and faster cash flow.

24. Save on transcription. Balance the costs, savings, and hassles of in-house versus outsourced transcription. Newer versions of voice-recognition software actually work for most people, and the start-up costs are well within the realm of most smaller practices now. If you are still using cassette tapes, shop around for digital solutions that allow physicians to dictate via telephone. For physicians who enter their own notes, create macros — single keystrokes that replace several tasks normally done with a mouse — in a word-processing program or EHR. And, of course, consider transcription savings when you are calculating the return on investment for that future EHR purchase.

25. Reduce your storage costs. Scan all of the old records that you have to keep, and pay to store, such as medical records, explanation of benefits, charge tickets, sign-in lists, telephone messages, etc. The storage cost of several dozen CDs or thumb drives are exponentially cheaper than a storage facility for thousands of records.

With creativity and determination, you can find ways to cut costs in your practice.

• •

Lowering fixed costs to break-even at lower volume

Here's one way to project the effect of a fixed cost reduction. The physician in this practice wanted to have a few more hours off each month for activities that did not bring in income, such as volunteering at a free clinic, attending CME classes or attending a child's school activities once in a while. How could this physician still achieve an income goal of $240,000 annually ($20,000 per month) and continue to break-even in the practice?

To reduce fixed costs, this physician plans to move from a facility that costs $4,000 a month in rent to one in the same neighborhood that costs $2,000 per month (50 percent reduction in occupancy expenses). This move would reduce the practice's fixed cost from $20,000 to $18,000 per month. However, before signing the lease on the new facility, the administrator wants to determine the effect the fixed cost reduction would have on the number of patients the physician has to see each month to meet expected income goals. The practice currently receives an average of $100 per visit, which is not expected to change if the practice decides to move.

Pre-move
Fixed cost: $20,000 per month
Physician income: $20,000 per month
Variable cost: $5 per visit
Patient visits: 425 per month

Post-move
Fixed cost: $18,000 per month
Desired physician income: $20,000 per month
Variable cost: $5 per visit
Patient visits: _____ per month?

With the reduced rental expense, the practice must bear $18,000 per month in fixed cost plus the $20,000 the physician wants to earn, for a total of $38,000. We know that the practice receives $100 per visit, but has to use $5 to pay the variable cost for each visit. That leaves the practice with $95 (unit contribution margin) to pay its fixed cost per visit, plus what the physician wants to receive in income. So, how many fewer patient visits can the physician see per month to continue achieving those goals at the lower rent?

We can determine the number of patient visits needed per month by dividing fixed cost plus desired physician income per month ($38,000) by unit contribution margin per visit ($95) to get 400 patient visits per month.

$$[\text{Fixed cost per month (\$18,000)} + \text{physician income (\$20,000)}]$$
$$\div \text{unit contribution margin per visit (\$95)}$$
$$= 400 \text{ patient visits per month.}$$

By reducing the fixed costs by $2,000, the physician could see 400 instead of 421 patients per month (21 fewer patients per month), and still achieve the desired annual income of $240,000. The exact number of hours freed up would depend on the time per visit.

Increasing income without cutting costs

During a discussion with a very profitable medical practice, I was struck by the comment of the manager: "We keep our eye on expenses, but we put our energy and passion into increasing our revenue."

While cost reduction is important, improving the revenue stream offers equal, if not more opportunity, to boost income. Of course, most physicians cringe when they hear of this focus, thinking of it only to stand for seeing more patients. Hopefully, you've learned some ways to improve workflow in this book, but there are more options to enhance revenue. Revenue improvement, however, can be a function of other variables under your control:

Coding. The coding system for physician services is complex and well-scrutinized by regulators. It is no wonder that several studies of physicians' coding patterns reveal under-coding. It's time to right-code. Current studies have focused on coding based on documentation; there's undoubtedly even more opportunity if physicians learned to document comprehensively to support the level of codes they use. The difference between levels of evaluation and management codes (such as 99212 and 99213) offers a significant differential in reimbursement – up to 25 percent. Learn to code, and you'll be rewarded with the payment you deserve.

Payer mix. As discussed in Chapter 5, "Patient Access," it's time to discern where the balance of provider supply and patient demand is in your practice. If your practice has more demand than you can accommodate, rebalance the equation by dropping participation with one or more insurance companies. You can positively influence your payer mix, thus improving your per-unit reimbursement, and you can gain operations benefits (by reducing the patient communications you have to handle out-of-office).

Contracting. Whether you're on the fence about dropping participation with a contract or not, evaluating your contract terms can benefit your revenue stream. Negotiate higher per-unit reimbursement. If this proves unsuccessful, focus your efforts only on a few heavily-used codes, or getting reimbursed for the codes that the company flat out denies (e.g., surgical assists, modifiers, unlisted codes, and bundled services). Or, negotiate with them to shorten the credentialing process, extend your appeal timeframe, develop procedures to avoid timely filing denials, and eliminate being forced to refund old credit balances, among others. Remember, it's your choice to participate with an insurance company. You've signed the contract. You're part of the relationship; take a stand. They can always say no – or yes!

Billing and collections. Establish processes to ensure capture of 100 percent of all charges, and make sure that clean charges are submitted to avoid back-end rework. Lean thinking even applies to billing: do it right the first time, and you'll avoid the rework. Then, evaluate your business office to ensure that collections are optimized, and write-offs minimized. Don't leave money on the table: it just means that you have to work harder.

An understanding of the fundamental financials, combined with a solid comprehension of patient flow opportunities, will allow you to implement operations changes in a cost-effective manner.

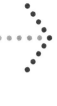

CHAPTER 14

The Patient-Centered
Practice of the Future™

Key Chapter Lessons

> ➤ Develop an understanding of the need to innovate

> ➤ Learn to change your patient flow to be patient-centered

> ➤ Discover the patient-centered practice of the future

> ➤ Identify case studies of innovative practices

> ➤ Recognize the benefits of a micropractice

> ➤ Understand what a "green" practice is – and why it's good
> for the environment

Rethinking the model

This book has provided a comprehensive look at practice operations from every significant aspect of patient flow. Although every process has been outlined and lean thinking has been emphasized to improve patient flow, we have yet to journey toward true innovation. Ask any patient about the value of a medical practice and they'd remark about the physicians. Yes, we understand that the provider's time is our most valuable asset, but have we built our practices around just that – the relationship between the patient and the provider? Have we used technology to replicate our paper processes or are we truly integrating automation to improve the patient's experience? Have we accounted for the shift in the generations at work? Are the solutions we currently apply merely perpetuating a model that doesn't work anymore for anyone? Isn't it time for us to rethink the entire model of how we practice?

Let's take a journey of opportunity and change the way we work. Allow me to present the patient-centered practice of the future.

The patient-centered practice of the future

The new model is formulated around the *patient*. Because of the variety of needs created by each specialty, the tactical plan may differ from practice to practice. However, the following themes and opportunities of the patient-centered practice are consistent regardless of the physician practice's specialty, locale, or business structure:

Front desk problems. Here is a key opportunity for redesign. Practice customers – patients and referring physicians – derive no value from the front desk; rather, they consider it a barrier to reaching the clinical team. A large portion of the practice's revenue cycle hinges on accurate information gathered here, yet front desk staff are usually the least compensated, most poorly trained, and most highly pressured to be fast and accurate while multitasking. All things considered, it's a disaster waiting to happen.

The tasks conducted at the front desk often require close coordination with other practice functions; but other practice staff frequently find the requests the front office staff make on them to be burdensome. These feelings are exacerbated by heavy workloads and a general lack of understanding about the entire practice operations process. It's not unusual for tension to be present between the "front" and the "back" office; in fact, it's unusual to see a practice where this tension is absent. Practice managers report that they feel consumed and distracted by the responsibility of managing the front desk, including its interactions with other functions. Managers are pressured by the turnover that seems to plague the front desk, and often devote so much time to front desk-related issues that they take their eye off of other critical responsibilities, including managing patient flow – and cash flow.

Silo-driven behaviors. For a variety of reasons, medical practices employ staff to perform functionally-based job duties. Employees are divided into silos – narrowly defined job roles. Referral clerks just process referrals; surgery schedulers just schedule surgeries; etc. In large part, it is the complexity of the external environment characterized by the array of regulations and rules imposed by insurance companies that causes managers to structure jobs so narrowly.

The challenges of this model are two-fold: (1) the functions rarely match the value that patients want from a practice (patients value the product – their appointment – but not the scheduler, the scheduling template, nor the many other behind-the-scenes efforts that make appointments possible), and (2) the approach is meeting resistance and resulting in employee turnover. The newest generations at work – Generation Xers and Millenials – are branded by some as lazy but in truth they crave diversity and meaning in work. They find little stimulation in narrowly defined, repetitive, non-creative jobs and know that in this vibrant economy, they can go elsewhere to find those qualities in a job.

This same sense of restlessness, search for stimulating work, and confidence in testing the job market elsewhere also extends to physicians. They, too, are Generation Xers and Millenials. Reflecting the characteristics of their generations, physicians leaving large practices to start micropractices is a growing trend. Tired of trying to provide comprehensive care to patients in an environment of narrowly assigned responsibilities and rigid walls between occupations, these physicians yearn to be back in control. At first glance, this quest to find more control at work may seem at odds with the desire of many younger physicians to achieve a better balance between the spheres of home and work. Having professional control offers these physicians better management of their personal lives – perceived or realistic. If your practice is seen as a player in the conflict by preventing physicians from feeling in control of their professional and personal lives, then those physicians will move on.

Seek solutions to meet the changing needs of your staff and physician workforce and your practice can become a desired place to work.

Space. Although we all recognize the value of the physician/patient encounter, the space in our facilities dedicated to it represents a minority of what we have invested into our practices. Need evidence? Consider that in many medical practices, more square footage is dedicated to patient *waiting* than to patient *encounters*.

The new model

To implement the patient-centered practice of the future, embrace the following principles:

➤ Promote cross-training of job functions;

➤ Institute technology to facilitate administrative processes;

➤ Extend technology to the patient to improve education and compliance, as well as patient flow;

➤ Bring resources and tasks— to the patient;

➤ Increase space dedicated to the patient/physician encounter;

➤ Enhance efficiency by doing today's work today; and

➤ Deliver timely access to patient care.

The model may take different forms based on your specialty, but the example presented in Exhibit 14.1 shows what can happen. Renowned medical architect Richard Haines, AIA, founder of Medical Design International (MDI), formulated a facility space plan based on the pillars of the patient-centered practice of the future.

Applying the principles of the patient-centered practice of the future and using MDI's space plan for a three-physician practice that we will call Medical Practice Associates, see how the staffing structures shown in Exhibit 14.2 change as the dimensions about the staff change. And, thus, a traditional practice transforms itself into the new model of a patient-centered practice of the future.

Medical Practice Associates wants to make the transition to the patient-centered practice of the future Currently, the three-physician practice has a maximum capacity of 18 patients per hour, based on its three physicians each seeing an average of six patients per hour. Let's review the changes they made to operations and staff and what transpires.

Front desk changes

Before their appointments, patients are encouraged to pre-register through the practice's Web portal or through a practice-initiated telephone-based pre-registration process with a business office staff member.

Upon arriving to the practice's facility, patients are received by a greeter who is positioned behind a small desk. The greeter electronically notifies the patient's care team of the patient's arrival. A report has already been generated by the business office regarding the patients whose insurance cannot be verified. These patients are greeted but politely asked to proceed to a nearby kiosk to complete their check in and obtain necessary insurance information online from their insurance company. If patients prefer to be assisted in person or if time doesn't permit, patients are advised that the registration process will be handled upon entering the exam room, whereby it will be completed by the associate assisting them. (Note that patients who need additional assistance for registration, i.e., their insurance could not be verified, will be visited in the reception area or exam room by a business office staff member.)

As a result of the deployment of a greeter, a kiosk for patient self-service as needed, and the new practice of completing registration functions in the exam room, the traditional check-in area now requires one staff workstation (for the greeter) instead of two.

EXHIBIT 14.1   Facility space plan

The following space program is a room by room listing of the space required to fulfill the goals and objectives for the facility as determined by Medical Design International. In developing the spaces, areas shown are considered to be from centerline of wall. Walls are 6" thick.

A room listed as 144 square feet might be 12'-0" by 12'-0" from centerline of wall to centerline of wall. After subtracting the thickness of the walls we would have a clear inside dimension of 11'-6" x 11'-6".

Clinical areas

Description	Traditional Practice				Patient-Centered Practice of the Future			
	Square feet	Qty	Area	Total	Square feet	Qty	Area	Total
Reception								
Patient/Family loads								
3 physicians x 6 patients/hour = 18 patients/hour								
18 patients/hour + 27 family (1.5 family/patient) = 45 people/hour								
Traditional waiting								
45 patients/hour – 9 exams = 36 seats	20	36	720					
Waiting-room-less waiting								
45 people/hour – 30 patients/ family in exams = 15 seats					20	15	300	150
Patient toilet	55	1	55		55	1	55	
Subtotal				775				355

EXHIBIT 14.1
(continued)

Facility space plan

Description	Traditional Practice				Patient-Centered Practice of the Future™			
	Square feet	Qty	Area	Total	Square feet	Qty	Area	Total
Business Office								
Greeter/Check-in	64	2	128		48	1	48	
Real-time check-in	48	1	48		48	0	0	
Checkout area	64	2	128		64	1	64	
Sub-waiting area	20	0	0		20	3	60	
Scanner area	24	1	24		24	1	24	
Phones	48	1	48		0	0	0	
Office manager	80	1	80		80	1	80	
Locking cabinet	12	1	12		12	1	12	
Business office staff	48	3	144		48	3	144	
Mail/Work/Copy	24	1	24		24	1	24	
Computer server	24	1	24		24	1	24	
Subtotal				**660**				**480**
Lab/Nurses' station								
Lab/Nurse station								
w/ U/C refrigerator	80	1	80		80	0	0	
w/ blood pressure	12	1	12		12	0	0	
Patient toilet w/ pass thru	55	1	55		55	0	0	
Scales alcove	12	1	12		12	0	0	
Subtotal				**159**				**0**

EXHIBIT 14.1
(continued)   Facility space plan

Description	Traditional Practice				Patient-Centered Practice of the Future™			
	Square feet	Qty	Area	Total	Square feet	Qty	Area	Total
Clinical area								
Exam rooms	108	3	324					
Medical assistant (MA) station	48	1	48					
Physician's workstation	36	1	36					
Subtotal	*408*			*408*				
Physician exam modules		3	1,224	**1,224**				
Care team practice space								
Patient-Centered Exam Rooms™					135	4	540	
Care team station, 2.33 Associates, U/C refrigerator					96	1	96	
Physician's workstation					36	1	36	
Subtotal				0	*672*		*672*	
Care team practice suites					672	3	2,016	
Patient toilet					55	1	55	
Subtotal								**2,071**

EXHIBIT 14.1 (continued) Facility space plan

Description	Traditional Practice				Patient-Centered Practice of the Future™			
	Square feet	Qty	Area	Total	Square feet	Qty	Area	Total
Procedure suite								
Procedure room	192	1	192		192	1	192	
Storage	48	1	48		48	1	48	
Subtotal				240				240
Physician area								
Physician consultation/office	120	3	360					
Physician office					80	3	240	
Physician toilet	55	1	55		55	1	55	
Subtotal				655				295
Staff and miscellaneous areas								
Staff lounge	144	1	144		144	1	144	
Staff toilets	55	1	55		55	1	55	
Bio-hazard storage	24	1	24		24	1	24	
Storage	144	1	144		144	1	144	
Subtotal				367				367
Subtotal				3,841				3,808
Hallway circulation 25%				960				952
Total gross area				4,801				4,762

		Highlights of the Patient-Centered Practice of the Future
•••••• EXHIBIT 14.2		

	Traditional practice	Patient-Centered Practice of the Future
Personnel		
Physicians	3	3
Care team staff (formerly, MAs)	3	7
Front office staff	3	1
Practice services staff	2	1
Practice manager	1	1
Operator/Records	1	0
Business office	3	3
	16	16
Space		
Exam rooms	9	12
Lab/Nurses' station	Yes	No
Team workstation	Yes; small	Yes; large
Physician office	Yes; rooms to fit consultation	Yes; small offices
Other		
Patients per hour	18	18
Patients/visitors in waiting area	36	15

Exam room adapts

The following activities which were traditionally performed at the front desk and after the patient exited are now all performed in the exam room:

> ➤ Completion of registration;

> ➤ Height and weight, as well as vital signs;

> ➤ Patient and family waiting;

➤ Language interpretation (if necessary);

➤ Blood draws and injections;

➤ Post-encounter patient education; and

➤ Post-encounter test and surgery scheduling.

Of course, the exam room needs to change to accommodate the additional work processes being centered there.

The new patient-centered exam room (PCER) (see Exhibit 14.3) features a moveable screen that is paneled with wood or another visually tasteful material, and which can easily slide between the two sections of the new multipurpose patient-centered exam room. The front section of the exam room has different flooring (carpeting, for

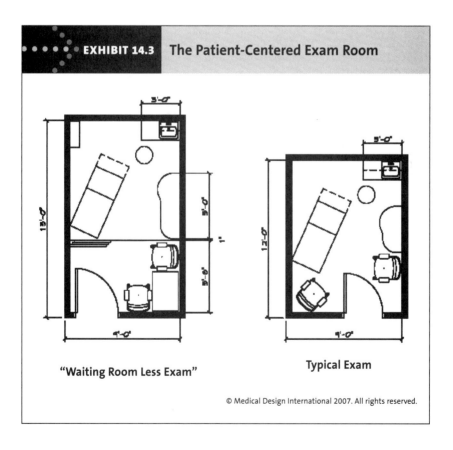

EXHIBIT 14.3 **The Patient-Centered Exam Room**

"Waiting Room Less Exam"

Typical Exam

example) with a comfortable chair for the patient. The room divider performs the following:

> Merges the comfort of a consult room with the necessity of an exam room;

> Allows the patient to dress in privacy and permits additional functions serving the patient to be performed during the encounter (workstations on either side of the divider); and

> Accommodates family members or friends accompanying the patient so they have adequate room, but the physical exam can be performed out-of-sight.

In the PCER, the physician sits at a workstation and can pivot easily from the consult "area" to the examination "area" of that room. The workstation features a desk that can accommodate an EHR.

To share images, graphs, and other information with patients, the EHR's display can be flipped onto the screen on the wall when desired so patients and visitors can see what the physician is explaining. A flat-screen monitor accommodates viewing patient records during the encounter so that physicians can show test results, images, etc. Technology not only serves a multi-functional purpose but facilitates the EHR as a two-dimensional tool to assist physicians and patients. The monitor can also be used for patients to access the practice's Web portal, to provide patient education, or to offer a selection of television channels while patients wait for the care team to arrive.

The exam room includes a small wall unit in which patients can store their clothes during exams. The storage unit and the furniture are placed so that immediately after undressing, patients can step directly up to the exam table where physicians can perform the examination.

While the productivity of the practice is assumed to be stable, having three extra exam rooms, and larger rooms overall, allows the practice to accommodate more patients within the practice. The exam rooms were increased from three to four per physician, for a total of 12. This increase in exam rooms allows for a 30-minute-per room-turnover, as demonstrated in Exhibit 14.4. Adding an additional exam room per physician gives the practice more flexibility to see additional patient volume.

Even though the number of exam rooms has increased, Medical Practice Associates still needs a reception area. The practice currently has nine exam rooms; thus, nine patients can be accommodated in the exam rooms while remaining patients must be given sufficient space in a waiting room area. Because the patient-centered practice of the futureoffers more exam rooms, which are slightly larger and offer sitting space within them, the reception area needed for Medical Practice Associates is reduced from accommodating 36 patients and visitors to just 15 patients and visitors. (The practice follows the national average for its specialty, which indicates that each patient is accompanied by 1.5 visitors, on average; thus, every patient appointment equates to 2.5 people needing accommodation.)

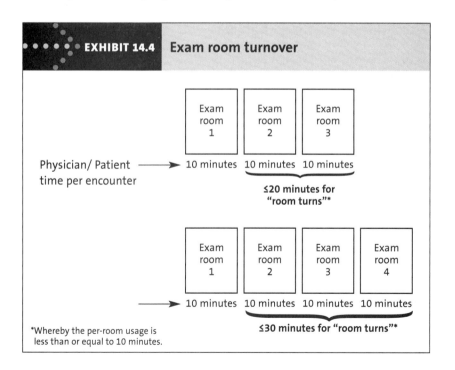

EXHIBIT 14.4   Exam room turnover

Care team associates

The exam room also facilitates the new role of a care team associate. Associates – medical assistants, nursing assistants, licensed practical nurses, registered nurses, and depending on the tasks required by the specialty, administrative staff trained in basic intake processes – now serve as a team instead of a particular role. In the patient-centered practice of the future, the care team associate is cross-trained to perform all aspects of the patient's clinical care. This cross functionality includes providing education, arranging for tests, and scheduling procedures and surgeries.

With a place at the workstation in the exam room, a care team associate can access the EHR and Web portal, serve as a scribe for the physician, provide interpretation, and if applicable, facilitate actions as instructed by the provider, such as ready equipment, pull educational materials, or retrieve items outside of the PCER.

Work hours, staffing changes

Another important change at Medical Practice Associates was to schedule care team members, including the newly designated care team associates, to work four nine-hour days and to work a half-day when patients are not seen. The work week remains at 40 hours, but flexibility improves morale and offers more flexibility in terms of staffing. One associate, for example, starts early and the other stays late.

The new "nurses station" (now called a care team work station) accommodates two associate team members per physician plus a shared associate. Formerly, Medical Practice Associates physicians had only one team member in the clinical area. A care team associate escorts the patient to the exam room, completes the registration process (if needed), performs rooming duties, draws blood, administers medications, and schedules follow-up appointments and tests as needed. (Notably, some duties may be limited according to scope of practice or state law.) All of these functions can be performed in the newly configured PCER. With more exam rooms, patient flow can only be positively impacted. The new configuration permits the work to be conducted efficiently in one exam room by one associate, minimizing process hand-offs and rework.

Each team member, on average, takes care of 24 patients each day (12 in the morning, and 12 in the afternoon, which is half of the 48 patients seen by that provider that day). In a 9-hour work day, that equates to 23 minutes per patient. Notably, some of those visits are performed exclusively by the nurse, and some, such as phone- or Web portal-based advice, can be more easily transitioned into reimbursable, face-to-face-based advice because the practice now has the capacity to handle more same-day appointments.

Impact on telephones

An additional associate, who formerly worked in a medical records/telephone reception role, now serves all of the teams. Scheduling is handled at each team's workstation. Every effort is made to keep the duration of calls to a minimum. Patients who call are almost immediately asked, "Ms. Smith, do you want to be seen?" and given appointment times. As a result, much less time spent on the telephone discussing symptoms, chief complaints, and so forth, and no permission is required for associates to schedule appointments. In fact, patients are trusted partners in the practice, and encouraged to make their own appointments through online scheduling access via the practice's Web portal.

Because follow-up appointments are made while patients are physically in the practice (in the PCER), the number of phone-based requests from patients is further reduced. Team members encourage patients to access and use the practice's Web portal to make their appointments directly. Online consultations are offered (as a non-covered service) to patients for whom face-to-face appointments are inconvenient or unnecessary. In the event that a care team associate speaks with a patient over the telephone and recommends that the patient be seen, the associate schedules the appointment. Call transfers are minimal.

Telephones are handled by each team, but most calls come directly to the additional associate who serves all of the teams. Care team associates also have their own direct telephone numbers, which they respond to between rooming patients.

The volume and duration of incoming phone calls at Medical Practice Associates is now much lower than at a traditional practice because patients can reach the same person who is taking care of them.

By making it easier to get appointments, patients feel they have better access to the practice and its services. Medications are renewed at appointments, test results are provided via the practice's secure Web portal, and return appointments are made for positive test results. Patients are provided a personal health record to improve access to information, enhance compliance, and encourage the patient to "self-serve." Nurse advice is performed at the practice (with oversight by the provider, and included in the six per hour cited for this practice), not over the phone.

Because the team cannot always answer the telephone, the incoming calls roll over to a practice services (checkout) staff member. A personal communication system alerts the associate to a telephone call, and/or a new message is taken in the EHR and added to the team's task queue. Tasks are reviewed and responded to between patients.

Because time-of-service collections remain important, both the kiosk and a practice services (checkout) workstation are able to accommodate this function. The practice services area includes a small reception area to accommodate post-encounter overflow. For example, when encounters run long and exam rooms are needed, care team associates can direct patients to this small reception area adjacent to the practice services workstation instead of completing post-encounter tasks (e.g., scheduling a complex imaging study) in the exam room.

These steps have reduced reception and practice services positions from five to two. The practice's head count was not reduced because those positions are now focused on greeting, helping answer the practice's two main phone lines and backing-up certain complex post-encounter tasks. Although the teams are cross trained to the fullest extent reasonable, all care team associates practice within their particular scope of practice.

Other space and staffing considerations

Because each PCER functions as a consultation room in the new facility design, the size of the physicians' private offices was reduced from 120 to 80 square feet. These offices no longer have to double as the physician's personal space and a consultation room. To enhance collegiality, the new down-sized offices were placed in a large work area divided by partitions.

A major value in the new design is the flexibility to meet staffing needs. This flexibility is especially valued because depending on the volume of patients, the scope of practice of the various staff, and the patients' needs, each team can have a licensed nurse, or may share one with another clinical team. The practice also has the flexibility to assign other ancillary positions, such as phlebotomists, ophthalmic technicians, registered dieticians, psychologists, and others, to support the teams.

The time is now

The description of this medical practice is very different from the traditional medical practice. It is patient-centered. It is innovative. And it makes effective use of three important practice resources to deliver value to the patient: the provider's time, support staff, and space.

The time is now for patients to pull value from us. Whether following the lead of Medical Practice Associates, the three case studies presented in this chapter, or forging your own direction, let's resolve to make the patient-centered practice of the future the practice of today.

THINGS TO CONSIDER

When being a little green is a good thing

The patient-centered practice can also be an environmentally friendly one. Informed design practices can make a difference in lessening the environmental impact of the facility. Sustainable building practices consider five fundamental design and construction practices that contribute to the impact buildings have on the environment.

1. **Sustainable site planning and development.** Reducing the project's impact on the natural environment through site selection and planning. Strategies include decreasing the building footprint, minimizing land disturbance, reducing storm water runoff and contamination, and minimizing the amount of heat the project emits (the "heat island" effect) into the nearby environment.

2. **Safeguarding water and water efficiency.** Minimizing water use by utilizing low-flow fixtures, harvesting rain water, using low-water use plants, and safely recycling grey water.

3. **Energy efficiency and renewable energy.** Reducing the ground level ozone, smog, and contributions to global warming by making improvements in the building envelope, incorporating highly efficient mechanical equipment, and using natural ventilation and lighting as much as possible.

4. **Conservation of materials and resources.** Incorporating materials with recycled content, reusing materials, obtaining materials regionally, and using renewable materials reduces the ecological footprint of the project.

5. **Indoor environmental quality.** Linking the outdoors through views and natural light, as well as increasing building ventilation rates that reduce carbon dioxide levels.

A sustainable building strategy has short and long term social, environmental, and economic benefits. Developing an environmentally friendly patient-centered practice can contribute to your community's efforts to improve the environment for all citizens.

Find resources at:

➤ The United States Green Building Council at www.usgbc.org; and

➤ The Green Guide for Health Care at www.gghc.org.

Source: Jeffrey K Griffin, AIA, Principal, Medical Design International and Leadership in Energy and Environmental Design (LEED)-accredited architect

CASE STUDY

A "flowmaster" cuts patient cycle time nearly in half

"I don't have to wait in the waiting room, really? This system is slick. Yep, very slick." That's a typical reaction to the new patient-centered design of practice operations at McKee Family Health Center in San Bernardino, Calif.

With the assistance of the redesign consulting firm Coleman Associates (www.patientvisitredesign.com), McKee Family Health Center dropped its average patient cycle time from 86 minutes to 44 minutes. At the same time, the practice, in which more than 80 percent of patients receive public assistance, managed to increase its providers' daily productivity from 20 patients to more than 40 patients.

In contrast to the traditional model of the front desk, patients walking into McKee are now greeted by a "flowmaster" who welcomes them and verifies their appointment time and demographics. This staff member alerts the practice's patient-care team using a walkie-talkie radio equipped with a headset. When alerted, a team member walks to the front desk and escorts the patient to an exam room where registration is completed and the intake process – including vitals – is performed.

With the patient now fully prepped, a provider with a portable computer enters the exam room and sees the patient. Patients can be discharged directly from the exam room, or if additional services are required, the provider can radio a team assistant or nurse to administer medications, schedule future appointments, tests, or procedures, as well as obtain specimens. By centering its operations on the patient, the health center decreased the number of stops a patient must make in the cycle from eight to three.

McKee accomplished the redesign by removing unnecessary layers of staff hierarchy and making the workplace an exciting place to work. Now, teamwork is the norm and every staff member can work to his or her full potential.

In addition to pleasing patients and providers alike, McKee's efforts have drawn national honors. The health center was awarded a 2006 National Association of Counties Achievement Award for its efforts to improve service and increase access for county residents in need of primary care.

CASE STUDY

One physician's determination to innovate for better patient care

Faced with declining revenue, seemingly endless patient demand, and little time for his family, 25-year veteran Peter Anderson, MD, of Yorktown, Va., decided to forge a new direction for his family medicine practice by implementing what he dubs the "team care" concept.

With his dedication in extensively training clinical personnel and writing guidelines for them to use in taking medical histories, Dr. Anderson knew exactly where to start. He trained an experienced nurse to perform some of the functions that he had previously and exclusively provided, including taking a complete patient history for the visit. He emphasizes that because taking a history involves no medical decision-making, a physician does not have to perform it. He begins each patient visit by having the nurse present this history to him in front of the patient, and then he proceeds to the next phase of the visit – the analysis of data and the pertinent physical exam. He performs the decision making and development of the plan, and then has the nurse execute the plan and provide patient education.

In addition to the nurses' involvement in the patients' care, Dr. Anderson meets with his team once a week to answer questions, improve communication, streamline the process, improve the care given, and foster the relationship among team members. By utilizing such a comprehensive care team, Dr. Anderson is also helping the patient bond to the practice through his staff, not just himself.

Dr. Anderson now employs four clinical assistants, three of whom work part-time. This, he reveals, is helpful because the pace at his practice is hectic.

Patient phone calls have plummeted as a result of the nurse's role in the exam. Because Dr. Anderson can accommodate more patient visits, acute care is handled in the office, not over the phones.

Dr. Anderson's success speaks for itself. Patient satisfaction scores rose almost immediately under the new model as did clinical quality indicators. Financially, gross charges rose 11 percent after adding one assistant and 42 percent after adding two.

The result was $200,000 in additional revenue after one full year of the additional assistance. With the equivalent of one full time assistant, the practice's gross charges increased 25 percent and with the equivalent of two full time assistants gross charges increased by 54 percent as compared with Dr. Anderson handling the delegated functions.

Despite his financial success, says Anderson, "Even if I didn't make a nickel more, I'd never go back because I'm giving better patient care."

Passionate about his team care model, Anderson recorded the details in his book, *Liberating the Family Physician*. For more information, see www.familyteamcare.org.

 CASE STUDY

A clinic reveals its success secret

Embracing the patient-centered practice of the future, Moore Clinic (www.mooreclinic.com) is breaking new ground in patient service and physician productivity. The secret to the Columbia, S.C.-based clinic's success is deceptively simple — improved physician satisfaction.

The numbers show that the clinic's 10 fellowship-trained orthopedic surgeons see patients at the 75th percentile of national
productivity standards. What's not so simple to see on paper is
how much physician satisfaction has improved and how their
improved job satisfaction led to the higher production levels.

Physician satisfaction wasn't always at a high level at Moore
Clinic. In fact, administrator Sean McNally recalls that after
numerous conversations with Moore surgeons it became clear
that the physicians were, in a word, miserable. McNally says he
was challenged to create an environment that sustained the
physicians' productivity levels yet allowed them to achieve
higher levels of customer service. As those early conversations
revealed, the solution started by figuring out how to improve
physicians' work lives at the practice.

McNally says physicians reported especially high levels of frustration when working clinic. Despite having, on paper, seven
staff assigned to each physician, it was common for a surgeon to
step out of an exam room to ask for help only to find no one
around to lend a hand. After McNally heard about the "practice
of the future" concept, he focused on addressing physician dissatisfaction while improving patient service and patient flow.
Here's what Moore Clinic accomplished in less than two years.

Care teams

A key to improving patient and physician satisfaction was developing care teams. The road to building the care teams starting
with a technology shift: installation of a document management solution and a PACS. The new technology created a chart-
less clinic which, in turn, laid the groundwork for staffing
changes. McNally decided to build care teams around each surgeon. In the past, each surgeon had one medical assistant and
shared a large, centralized front desk that performed check-in
and check-out activities. McNally added one medical assistant to
each surgeon's team and reassigned the check-in/check-out staff

to separate teams dedicated to each surgeon. McNally made the shift without adding more staff.

The care teams were augmented by reassigning other staff, too. Previously, each surgeon had a dedicated medical secretary stationed on the third floor of the clinic's five-story building while clinical activities took place on the second floor. Because these secretaries were on a different floor than the clinical activities, they could not be of much assistance to the surgeons during clinic. Also stationed on the third floor were nearly a dozen medical transcriptionists. As the new care team concept was implemented, the secretaries and transcriptionists were asked to apply for jobs in the clinic and make a commitment to train as receptionists or medical assistants.

Today, the clinic's transcription tasks are outsourced and team members continue to perform the former secretary's duties of surgery scheduling, authorizations, etc. What's different is that the cross-trained staff assigned to each physician is just a few steps away from a surgeon who may need help. Patients also love the "solo practice" feel of the new operation. Just as important as the patient reaction has been the favorable reaction of the surgeons.

With the surgeons excited about the new model and the staff clamoring to be part of a "care team," McNally is moving forward to make additional changes, including:

➤ Renaming the centralized appointment staff as the "customer care team";

➤ Initiating cross-training for medical assistants to serve as X-ray and cast technicians, thus collapsing the remaining clinical staff into the cross-trained model; and

➤ Assigning medical assistants to conduct the check out process while the patient is still in the exam room. This process will be aided by locating a credit card swipe machine in each exam room to facilitate point-of-service collections.

Strong supporters of the process include the joint replacement subspecialist physicians who want to avoid making their patients stand in line at a check out counter.

Next steps

What's next for Moore Clinic is an entirely new building, designed by the Columbia-based architectural firm G M K Associates Inc (www.gmka.com). The new structure will be designed to complement the new "solo practice" staffing model. The building will house six surgeons in three "pods" or units – each of which will house the practices of two surgeons. Patients coming into the practice will feel like they've walked into a small office, not a giant clinic. Each practice – called a pod – will have a very small reception area, six exam rooms, and shared imaging and cast rooms accessible from the back of each pod's dedicated hallway. When things get extra busy, the new facility will handle the overflow of waiting patients in a gourmet coffee and Internet café located in a shared space adjacent to the entrances to the pods.

Even though productivity levels and revenue per surgeon are already the highest in the practice's history, McNally is more excited about meeting his original goal of helping the physicians regain the satisfaction of practicing medicine. When one of his spine surgeons pulled him aside and told him to "never go back" to the old model, McNally knew he had hit the mark for success.

• •

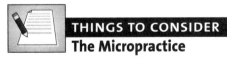

THINGS TO CONSIDER
The Micropractice

Frustrated by high overhead, staff squabbles, and the bureaucracy that often comes with large practices, more physicians are considering downsizing. The model of the new, successful solo practice is different than in years past – today's solo physicians are often looking for ways to reduce staff or even eliminate them altogether. They are making these staffing cuts yet protecting their practice's number one asset: their own time with patients. How? These creative and entrepreneurial physicians harness technology to streamline their workflow, outsource some functions, and do more of the work themselves. Often referred to as a "micropractice", these solo practices can be a realistic vision, but only for physicians with realistic expectations.

Consider the following issues before starting a micropractice:

Staff. Physicians certainly can get along with few or even no staff. They can check in patients, room them, and listen for the phone to ring. After clinic or between patients, they can submit claims and call insurance companies with any questions. That said, be aware of the demands of filling out forms, answering telephones, negotiating insurance contracts, submitting claims, following up on claims denials, inventorying supplies and so on. It's critical to have trusted advisers or an excellent grasp on key financial and other performance indicators to make sure your practice is staying on the right track. It can be exhausting – and complex. To make sure your new micropractice isn't ruining the quality of life that you quit the large practice to obtain, consider hiring at least one assistant. Running with no staff may be unrealistic, depending on your volume; try a fully cross-trained medical assistant to assist.

Revenue. With fewer staff, a solo physician can lower revenue expectations without a drop in income. Spending $100,000 less in staff, for example, can reduce revenue by $100,000 without decreasing income. Simply put, the physician doesn't have to see as many patients to make the practice work. Although having few or no staff greatly reduces overhead, there are many other expenses to running a medical practice –

malpractice liability insurance and other coverage, supplies, equipment, office space, taxes, marketing and so on. Don't forget that a micropractice doesn't mean eliminating the entire overhead of a practice.

Patient demand. Although physicians can see fewer patients, sometimes this can backfire. Since physicians are notoriously bad at saying "no," controlling demand can be a difficult task. If you hear yourself saying, "Oh, I'll just squeeze in a few more patients..." everyday, you may soon find yourself overwhelmed with the demands of seeing patients – and taking care of all of the administrative issues that result. Consider limiting your patient panel by negotiating participation agreements with only certain insurance companies – or better yet, none at all in a cash-only practice – to help control demand.

Technology. Invest in technology – early. Start off your practice with an EHR, a Web portal and automate as much of your workflow as possible. It's much easier to start with a "paperless" office than it is to transition into one.

Career satisfaction. Shedding staff can relieve an incredible emotional burden on physicians who simply don't like to handle conflict or manage people. Some physicians enjoy the reduced complexity and lower overhead of the solo operation. They are comfortable spending part of the day doing nonmedical tasks. And, when faced with repetitive clerical tasks, they try not to say, "I didn't go to medical school to do *this*." Instead, they like the diversity – and the simplicity of it all.

· ·

CHAPTER 15

Summing Up

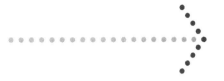

By identifying each stage of the patient encounter – from the moment a new patient calls your practice to his or her exit after the visit is concluded – you can positively affect change. By considering the many processes and tasks your practice performs from the patient's perspective, not just the viewpoint of the unit or department, you are on the road to mastering patient flow.

The initial four steps you must make on this road are to:

1. Embrace the concept of viewing your physician's time as the practice's greatest asset;

2. Create an environment in which each patient encounter provides value for the patient;

3. Root out waste and inefficiency while looking for new ways to do things; and

4. Make an intentional effort to redesign the core process of your practice so they work more seamlessly to bring value to patients.

Let's review the primary lessons that I hope you learned from the book:

➤ Recognize your most precious asset: Your provider's time. Your patients and referring physicians want your providers' time. Based on the current per-unit reimbursement system in our country, this mantra holds true for optimizing earnings. Make providers – and the systems surrounding them – more efficient for delivering care and you create a better bottom line.

➤ Pull in the work. Real-time work processing is more efficient than batching work. Look at the processes in which you are batching work (dictation, scheduling, charge entry, etc.) and convert them to real-time work.

➤ Deploy technology. Technology is often under-utilized in the patient encounter. Seek technology that can work for providers and patients.

➤ Improve your operations by focusing on what your patients and referring physicians want and need from you. Eliminating non-value-added processes can enhance customer service and lead to practice efficiency. Review processes to reduce the components that don't add value to your customers. If you focus on your patients and referring physicians, eliminating non-value-added processes will also benefit your practice.

➤ Create a patient-centered practice. Many medical practices have built systems that work well for their owners but, often, not for their patients. Explore ways to make your practice's patient flow process more patient-friendly.

➤ Don't continue to do things the way you've always done them. Just because you've operated your practice one way doesn't mean that's how it has to be in the future. There is no "right way" to run a medical practice. Stay focused on the patient to create a patient-friendly environment in which your patients are loyal. This effort will pay for itself over and over again.

➤ Use the principles of lean management: Map processes and look at the many steps of each process to determine where value is added and where it is not. Where value from your customer's perspective is not present, eliminate unnecessary steps or even entire processes.

Mastering patient flow is indeed achievable, but for those practices that do reach that goal, the next challenge will be complacency. In many ways, complacency is the greatest challenge of all.

Don't wait for external changes, like a new computer system or a new building, to begin changing work flow and eliminating waste.

Use the techniques of lean management described in the first chapter and throughout this volume to make design decisions and constant refinement part of your practice's value stream.

Once your practice believes the "ideal" has been achieved, it's time to start experimenting to make it better.

With new concepts of resource allocation and new technology on the horizon, the field of medical practice operations continues to be dynamic. Operating a practice will never be an easy task, but working toward the ideal patient flow process can bring a host of opportunities and rewards.

APPENDICES

· · · · · · · · · · · · · ·

APPENDIX A: **Benchmarks for staff performance expectations**

Practice operations task	Workload range
Pre- or site registration with insurance verification	60-80 patients per day
Check-in with registration verification only	100-130 patients per day
Site check-in with registration verification and cashiering only	75-100 patients per day
Appointment scheduling with no registration	75-125 calls per day
Appointment scheduling with full registration	50-75 calls per day
Surgery scheduling	25-30 surgeries per day
Telephones with messaging	300-500 calls per day
Telephones with routing (electronic system) only	1,000-1,200 calls per day
Telephone triage	65-85 calls per day

The workload range depends on patient population, information system, level of automation, and work processes used at the practice. The more information you gather and/or deliver during each function (thus, the higher the transaction time), the lower the productivity you should expect.

Given the multitude of variables, measure the time it takes your staff to handle each telephone call and apply that transaction time to reach your practice's ideal workload range.

APPENDIX B: **Action plan**

Area	Task area	Need? Y/N	Person assigned	Priority* H/M/L	Cost $	Target date	Done Y/N	Reason not done/delayed
The lean-thinking revolution (Chapter 1)								
	Articulate value of work process(es) to patients (and other stakeholders)							
	Identify and measure steps in workflow							
	Establish goals and steps to change/improve/eliminate							
	Implement changes							
	Analyze results							
The physician's time (Chapter 2)								
	Observe and measure physicians' non-clinical tasks							
	Assess facility's impact on provider productivity							
	Target and carry out productivity improvement steps							
	Measure average patient value							
	Implement time management steps							
Telephones (Chapter 3)								
	Track incoming and outgoing call volumes							
	Do "mystery caller" survey and review results							
	Observe and gather telephone system data							
	Ask staff to note topics of incoming calls							
	Analyze outbound calls for patterns (topics)							
	Analyze telephone system's capacities and capabilities							
	Implement steps to: avoid calls, handle issues in live encounters, and/or migrate them to practice Web portal.							

* Priority: H (high impact): critical to practice near-term goals, mission or finances and may require a significant expense or time; M (moderate impact): a desired goal but could be delayed for a short time; L (low impact): a "wish list" item that may not produce immediate, needed practice improvement.

Area	Task area	Need? Y/N	Person assigned	Priority* H/M/L	Cost $	Target date	Done Y/N	Reason not done/delayed
	Assess usage/change voice mail policy							
	Assess/change auto attendant use							
	Evaluate staffing based on per-function benchmarks							
Scheduling (Chapter 4)								
	Evaluate current scheduling process							
	Evaluate (implement) alternative scheduling approaches (group visits, advanced access, etc.)							
	Evaluate use of Web site or portal for scheduling and/or online visits							
	Conduct facility capacity analysis							
	Measure scheduling fluctuations							
	Measure volume, cost and impact on practice from no-shows, cancellations and physician "bumps"							
	Take steps to reduce no-shows, cancellations and physician "bumps"							
	List steps to improve appointment recall and reminder processes							
	Evaluate staffing based on per-function benchmarks							
Patient access (Chapter 5)								
	Begin using Access Performance Dashboard							
	Identify present barriers to meeting patient access demands							
	Examine impact of payer contracting on reimbursement and volume							

* Priority: H (high impact): critical to practice near-term goals, mission or finances and may require a significant expense or time; M (moderate impact): a desired goal but could be delayed for a short time; L (low impact): a "wish list" item that may not produce immediate, needed practice improvement.

Area	Task area	Need? Y/N	Person assigned	Priority* H/M/L	Cost $	Target date	Done Y/N	Reason not done/delayed
	[Specialty practice] List steps of and consider changes to the pre-appointment screening process							
	Appoint team to examine value of using the medical home concept							
	Chart patient access and productivity per provider							
	Establish a new physician integration plan							
Reception services (Chapter 6)	Take steps to improve office environment							
	Consider different ways to pre-register patients							
	Examine insurance verification process							
	Review registration steps for new and established patients							
	Review check-in process steps and identify changes							
	Find alternatives to sign-in lists							
	Review customer service quality at check in							
	Review internal communications systems							
	Evaluate staffing based on per-function benchmarks							
Waiting (Chapter 7)	Analyze patient waiting times							
	Evaluate patient cycle (throughput) time							
	Identify steps to improve quality of waiting							
	Identify options to reduce waiting times							
	Assess communications between staff and patients							

* Priority: H (high impact): critical to practice near-term goals, mission or finances and may require a significant expense or time; M (moderate impact): a desired goal but could be delayed for a short time; L (low impact): a "wish list" item that may not produce immediate, needed practice improvement.

Area	Task area	Need? Y/N	Person assigned	Priority* H/M/L	Cost $	Target date	Done Y/N	Reason not done/delayed
	Calculate impact of process time and staffing levels on wait times							
The patient encounter (Chapter 8)								
	Calculate cost of physician's time							
	Examine ways to reduce "batching" of work							
	Assess staff functions for cross-training opportunities							
	Implement the "virtual patient" concept							
	Adopt steps for more efficient pre-visit planning (chart preview, room stocking, pre-clinic huddles)							
	Create flow sheets and preference cards							
	Examine and revise roles of clinical assistants. Set expectations and establish accountability for rooming and patient preparation.							
	Measure exam room turnover							
	Teach physicians efficient visit and communications techniques							
	Assess opportunity to dictate during exams							
Prescriptions (Chapter 9)								
	Assess process changes to reduce prescription-related paperwork, telephone calls, and errors							
	Implement process changes to reduce staff time spent on prescription renewals and refills							
	Evaluate and improve drug sample management and disbursement practices							

* Priority: H (high impact): critical to practice near-term goals, mission or finances and may require a significant expense or time; M (moderate impact): a desired goal but could be delayed for a short time; L (low impact): a "wish list" item that may not produce immediate, needed practice improvement.

Area / Task area	Need? Y/N	Person assigned	Priority* H/M/L	Cost $	Target date	Done Y/N	Reason not done/delayed
Managing test results (Chapter 10)							
Evaluate current test results management processes, including communications							
Analyze test ordering process							
Evaluate management of inbound results for physician review							
Identify methods to improve patient notification							
Select and integrate technology solutions to improve test results management							
Practice services (Chapter 11)							
Evaluate all checkout processes							
Teach staff and physicians more efficient and accurate charge entry ethods							
Implement more efficient patient follow-up scheduling							
Identify issues in referrals and appointments for ancillary and specialty services							
Improve cash collection performance							
Teach providers more efficient documentation techniques							
Evaluate staffing based on per-function benchmarks							
Technology (Chapter 12)							
Evaluate practice management system							
Use Internet to improve patient flow							

* Priority: H (high impact): critical to practice near-term goals, mission or finances and may require a significant expense or time; M (moderate impact): a desired goal but could be delayed for a short time; L (low impact): a "wish list" item that may not produce immediate, needed practice improvement.

Area	Task area	Need? Y/N	Person assigned	Priority* H/M/L	Cost $	Target date	Done Y/N	Reason not done/delayed
	Develop a Web portal to improve operations and/or patient education							
	Gauge use of document management, PDAs and other technologies							
	Deploy e-prescribing							
	Implement an electronic health record							
	Assess various information technology solutions throughout the practice							
Fundamental financials (Chapter 13)								
	Learn the key financial concepts used in medical practice management							
	Understand fixed vs. variable costs							
	Calculate overhead rates accurately							
	Analyze the practice's breakeven point							
	Select, implement and monitor strategies to cut costs							
The Patient-Centered Practice of the Future (Chapter 14)								
	Reinvent the patient flow process							
	Cross train staff							
	Increase space dedicated to the encounter							
	Center workflow around the patient							
	Consider the care-team approach							

* Priority: H (high impact): critical to practice near-term goals, mission or finances and may require a significant expense or time; M (moderate impact): a desired goal but could be delayed for a short time; L (low impact): a "wish list" item that may not produce immediate, needed practice improvement.

INDEX

· · · · · · ·